Behavioural Medicine

Behavioural Medicine

Psychological Treatment of Somatic Disorders

Edited by

A. A. Kaptein
Leiden University, The Netherlands

H. M. van der Ploeg
Leiden University, The Netherlands

B. Garssen
University of Amsterdam, The Netherlands

P. J. G. Schreurs
Utrecht University, The Netherlands

and

R. Beunderman
University of Amsterdam, The Netherlands

JOHN WILEY & SONS
Chichester · New York · Brisbane · Toronto · Singapore

Other Wiley Editorial Offices

John Wiley & Sons, Inc., 605 Third Avenue,
New York, NY 10158-0012, USA

Jacaranda Wiley Ltd, G.P.O. Box 859, Brisbane,
Queensland 4001, Australia

John Wiley & Sons (Canada) Ltd, 22 Worcester Road,
Rexdale, Ontario M9W 1L1, Canada

John Wiley & Sons (SEA) Pte Ltd, 37 Jalan Pemimpin # 05-04,
Block B, Union Industrial Building, Singapore 2057

Library of Congress Cataloging-in-Publication Data:
Behavioral medicine : psychological treatment of somatic disorders/
    edited by A. A. Kaptein . . . [et al.].
        p.   cm.
    Expanded and updated translation from Dutch.
    Includes bibliographical references.
    ISBN 0-471-92410-5
    1. Medicine and psychology.   2. Sick–Psychology.   I. Kaptein, A. A. (Adrian A.)
    [DNLM: 1. Behavior Therapy–methods.   2. Behavioral Medicine.
3.   Psychophysiologic Disorders–diagnosis.   4. Psychophysiologic Disorders–therapy.
WM 90 B4196]
R726.5.B429   1990
616′.0019–dc20
DNLM/DLC
for Library of Congress   89-16747
                                                                                                CIP

British Library Cataloguing in Publication Data:
Behavioural medicine : psychological treatment of somatic
    disorder.
    1. Man. Psychosomatic diseases
    I. Kaptein, A. A. (Adrian, A.)
    616.08
    ISBN 0-471-92410-5

Typeset by Acorn Bookwork, Salisbury, Wiltshire
Printed and bound in Great Britain by Courier International Ltd, Tiptree, Essex

Contents

Contributors

R. Beunderman	University of Amsterdam, Amsterdam
A. L. Couzijn	Utrecht University, Utrecht
D. J. Duyvis	University of Amsterdam, Amsterdam
H. van Eek	Rehabilitation Center Hoensbroek, Hoensbroek
A. M. C. van der Elst	Utrecht University, Utrecht
R. A. M. Erdman	Erasmus University, Rotterdam
W. Everaerd	University of Amsterdam, Amsterdam
B. Garssen	University of Amsterdam, Amsterdam
G. Godaert	Utrecht University, Utrecht
N. H. Groenman	Limburg University, Maastricht
H. van der Helm-Hylkema	Free University, Amsterdam
M. Johnston	Royal Free Hospital, London
A. A. Kaptein	Leiden University, Leiden
S. Maes	Tilburg University, Tilburg
T. M. Marteau	Royal Free Hospital, London
L. J. M. Pennings-van der Eerden	Utrecht University, Utrecht
H. M. van der Ploeg	Leiden University, Leiden
M. C. Rientsma	Regional Institute for Outpatient Mental Health Care, Hilversum
E. van Rooijen	Utrecht University, Utrecht
H. Rijken	Utrecht University, Utrecht
W. J. G. Ros	Utrecht University, Utrecht
P. J. G. Schreurs	Utrecht University, Utrecht
J. A. Schuerman	Limburg University, Maastricht
M. J. M. van Son	Utrecht University, Utrecht
W. Vandereycken	University Psychiatric Center St Jozef, Kortenberg
M. van Veldhoven	Tilburg University, Tilburg
A. Ph. Visser	Limburg University, Maastricht

J. W. S. Vlaeyen	Limburg University, Maastricht
I. S. Y. Vromans	Institute of Public Health, Utrecht
W. L. Weeda-Mannak	Free University, Amsterdam
J. Weinman	Guy's Hospital, London
J. A. M. Winnubst	Utrecht University, Utrecht
F. M. Zwart	Utrecht University, Utrecht

Introduction

In the development and course of many physical illnesses, behavioural factors play a substantial role. Research on risk factors for the leading causes of mortality and morbidity in western countries (cardiovascular diseases, cancer, respiratory disorders) demonstrates that behavioural factors such as tobacco smoking, unhealthy eating habits, alcohol overconsumption, lack of physical exercise and certain coping behaviours contribute to the development of these disorders. Not only in the development, however, but also during the course of many physical illnesses, the role of behavioural factors (e.g. coping, illness behaviour) is considerable. Adequate coping improves the medical outcome, can make an illness and its consequences bearable, or can reduce the degree to which symptoms interfere with daily activities. Inadequate coping may give rise to increased or prolonged morbidity and even to mortality—for example the man with a myocardial infarction who continues to smoke cigarettes, or the girl with asthma who resists taking measures which help prevent periods of shortness of breath.

The contribution of psychologists to the prevention of somatic disorders, and to the diagnosis (or assessment), treatment and rehabilitation of patients with somatic illness, has grown very rapidly in the past decade. 'Behavioural medicine' is the encompassing term applied to interdisciplinary research and patient care in this field. In this book, the application of behavioural medicine is illustrated with regard to 15 somatic disorders. The disorders have been selected on the basis of their high prevalence and their relevance for health professionals. In each chapter, epidemiological aspects, the clinical picture, behavioural assessment and treatment methods with regard to the somatic illnesses or disorders are presented. Three chapters about theoretical aspects of behavioural medicine precede these chapters.

The book is written for several categories of health professionals. The Editors believe that psychologists working in hospitals will find the book especially useful in patient care and research. Also, psychologists working in university departments (medical psychology, health psychology) and students aspiring to a career in these fields, will, we believe, find inspiring material in this text. Consultation-liaison psychiatrists, health educators involved in self-management programmes, social workers and nurses may benefit from reading about how behavioural methods contribute to prevention, treatment or rehabilitation with regard to medical disorders. Physicians, both general practitioners and medical specialists, similarly will find useful material in this work on the application of behavioural techniques in the care they provide for their patients. Behavioural medicine stresses interdisciplinary cooperation with regard to both treatment and research—the Editors hope this book will help to stimulate interdisciplinary activities concerning the disorders which are dealt with there.

The present book is an expanded and updated version of *Behavioural Medicine* which was published in Dutch in 1986. It is a pleasure to acknowledge the stimulating and supportive work of Wendy Hudlass and her staff at Wiley's in producing this text. We hope the book will contribute to the cause of behavioural medicine and the benefit of health professionals and patients.

ADRIAN A. KAPTEIN
HENK M. VAN DER PLOEG
BERT GARSSEN
PAUL J. G. SCHREURS
RUUD BEUNDERMAN

Leiden, Amsterdam, Utrecht
September 1989

Part 1

Behavioural Medicine in Perspective

CHAPTER 1

Behavioural Medicine—Some Introductory Remarks

A. A. Kaptein[1]

Leiden University, Leiden

and

E. van Rooijen

Utrecht University, Utrecht

ABSTRACT

In this first chapter, the concept of behavioural medicine is introduced and its key characteristics are described:

- It has an interdisciplinary nature.
- Research on the effectiveness of psychological treatment of somatic complaints and disorders are prominent.
- Aetiology and pathogenesis are considered less important than interventions in behavioural factors which lead to health maintenance or the alleviation of negative consequences of illness.
- Research and treatment are not limited to a few specific 'psychosomatic' disorders.

Behavioural medicine, health psychology and consultation-liaison psychiatry are described, and it is stressed that cooperation between these fields is beneficial to patients and health care providers. The classic psychosomatic theories are compared with the theoretical views which guide behavioural medicine.

Behavioural Medicine
Edited by A. A. Kaptein, H. M. van der Ploeg, B. Garssen, P. J. G. Schreurs and R. Beunderman
© 1990 John Wiley & Sons Ltd.

Four applications are described: primary prevention of cardiovascular diseases, secondary prevention in children with asthma and in adults with cancer, and tertiary prevention in patients with chronic obstructive pulmonary disease.

Finally, some recommendations are given regarding research and intervention issues:

- The continuous need for sound research, embedded in elaborate theories.
- Increased emphasis on research and treatment in patients with 'unspectacular' disorders.
- Increased attention to cost-effectiveness.
- The inclusion of health care providers and the health care delivery system as objects of research and intervention.

INTRODUCTION

Behaviour, health, illness and psychological interventions in persons with somatic complaints and diseases—that is the subject of this book. The aim of this first chapter is to introduce the concept 'behavioural medicine' and to illustrate some of the applications of behavioural medicine in an outpatient/hospital setting. We will finish the chapter with some recommendations regarding future research and patient care in behavioural medicine.

BEHAVIOURAL MEDICINE—SOME CONCEPTUAL REMARKS

The term 'behavioural medicine' was not used until 1973. The complementary term for behavioural medicine in children—'behavioural paediatrics'—had already been employed in 1970 in a paper on behavioural factors in the aetiology and course of somatic afflictions in children in a hospital setting (Friedman, 1970; MacMillan, 1985). In 1973, Birk published a book called *Biofeedback: Behavioral Medicine* (Birk, 1973). Some 15 years later, a considerable number of books have appeared that cover theoretical backgrounds and practical applications of behavioural medicine, and congresses, journals and societies are devoted to behavioural medicine (e.g. *Annals of Behavioral Medicine*; Society of Behavioral Medicine (USA); International Society of Behavioural Medicine; European Health Psychology Society; Division of Health Psychology of the American Psychological Association; Bloom, 1988; Miller and Wood, 1980).

Schwartz and Weiss have provided a definition of behavioural medicine which appears to be generally accepted:

> Behavioral Medicine is the interdisciplinary field concerned with the development and integration of behavioral and biomedical science, knowledge and techniques, relevant to health and illness and the application of this knowledge and these techniques to prevention, diagnosis, treatment and rehabilitation. (Schwartz and Weiss, 1978, p. 250)

Some terms and concepts in this definition require elucidation.

Behavioural medicine is an interdisciplinary field—not only psychologists but also physicians, nurses, epidemiologists, health educators and other professionals involved in health care contribute to it. Although this is implicit in the definition, it should be emphasized that research on the effectiveness of interventions has a prominent place in behavioural medicine. Attention is not so much focused on the aetiology and pathogenesis of illness as on the identification of the behavioural factors which, when changed, lead to reductions in the degree or the frequency of illness or complaints. Behavioural medicine is concerned with the whole gamut of somatic diseases—there is hardly a disease or physical complaint which has not been the subject of research or therapeutic endeavour from a behavioural medicine perspective. Behavioural medicine is concerned with 'somatic' health and illness—disorders in the field of 'mental' health (neurosis and psychosis) are generally not the object of research or treatment, unless they contribute to the causation or maintenance of a somatic illness or complaint. Within the definition of behavioural medicine one can see the distinction between primary ('prevention'), secondary ('treatment') and tertiary ('rehabilitation') prevention.

Not unexpectedly, given the recent development of behavioural medicine, much is being written and said about the content of the field, and its relations with associated fields of research and treatment, for example behavioural health (Matarazzo, 1984), medical psychology and health psychology.

A generally accepted definition of health psychology is 'the aggregate of the specific educational, scientific, and professional contributions of the discipline of psychology to the promotion and maintenance of health, the prevention and treatment of illness, and the identification of etiologic and diagnostic correlates of health, illness, and related dysfunction' (Matarazzo, 1980, p. 815). In comparison with the definition of behavioural medicine, two points stand out. First, health psychology is defined as a branch of psychology—the interdisciplinary element is not stressed. Second, health psychology seems to emphasize prevention whereas behavioural medicine is more concerned with treatment and rehabilitation. In real life, we suggest, both terms are not so far apart: most psychologists who work in the field of behaviour, health and illness combine elements from health psychology and behavioural medicine.

Somewhat provocatively, it could be stated that behavioural medicine is the term used by researchers and practitioners who work in medical settings (hospitals, general practices, medical faculties), while health psychology appears to be the term preferred by psychologists who work in research settings in university departments of psychology. We feel that close cooperation between behavioural scientists and professionals with a medical background is a prerequisite for research and patient care in a behavioural medicine perspective. That, we feel, is the real issue—semantic discussions are secondary.

Psychologists engaged in patient care and research in an outpatient/hospital setting will often encounter a medical professional who engages in similar activities—the consultation-liaison psychiatrist. Assessment and treatment of patients with medical disorders which are associated with behavioural and emotional factors that mask or aggravate the medical disorder is a major field of activity of this medical specialist. Power struggles between the hospital psychologist and the consultation-liaison psychiatrist ('you're on my turf') are not really necessary—both professionals should benefit from cooperation. Consultation-liaison psychiatrists recently have emphasized comorbidity in general hospital patients: the combined presence of psychiatric and somatic morbidity in patients with medical complaints and disorders. In recent studies, the prevalence of comorbidity in patients in general practice and hospital settings appears to be 30–40% (Feldman et al., 1987; Lipowski, 1988a). Mayou, Hawton and Feldman (1988) demonstrated that patients with a psychiatric disorder on admission to a general hospital made considerably more use of medical services and showed higher morbidity and mortality than patients without such diseases.

Diagnosing and treating depression in medically ill patients is a major activity in consultation-liaison psychiatry (Rodin and Voshart, 1986). The early detection of organic brain syndromes (Trzepacz, Teague and Lipowski, 1985), the somatic consequences of substance abuse, and somatization (Smith, Monson and Ray, 1986; Lipowski, 1988b) are areas of expertise of the consultation-liaison psychiatrist. In addition, prescribing drugs, where indicated, is an activity performed by the psychiatrist which may help increase the degree to which behavioural treatment by the psychologist is successful. The consultation-liaison psychiatrist, therefore, is an important partner for the psychologist working in a general hospital.

Behavioural medicine is a field of research and treatment which has only recently sprung into full bloom. Psychologists have for a long time been engaged, however, with patients suffering physical illness. In the period from World War II on until about 1975, the activities of many psychologists regarding research and treatment of patients with physical illness were dominated by the so-called 'psychosomatic' theories. Essentially these theories stated that certain personality characteristics, certain interpersonal conflicts and characteristic responses to these conflicts were causative factors in the origin of specific somatic illnesses. An acquired or constitutional vulnerability of a certain organ or organ system would, given the presence of the three factors mentioned before, lead to a specific illness. Asthma, neurodermatitis, ulcus duodeni, ulcerative colitis, rheumatoid arthritis, essential hypertension and diabetes (Alexander's 'holy seven'; Alexander, 1950) were supposed to be psychosomatic illnesses.

Psychosomatic theory has almost completely lost ground in modern theory and practice of behavioural medicine. The theory was based on small numbers of highly selected patients, the methods by which personality characteristics and interpersonal conflicts were assessed must be deemed to have low validity and reliability, and neither research nor treatment in which the theoretical concepts were used resulted in confirmation of the theory or improvement of the medical condition of the patients (see Dorian and Barr Taylor, 1987, for a more extensive coverage of the decline of 'classic' psychosomatic theory).

Since psychosomatic theory was the school of thought that preceded behavioural medicine, the major differences between the two approaches are outlined below:

- In behavioural medicine the medical conditions which are being studied encompass the whole gamut of somatic illnesses and are not limited to the 'classic' psychosomatic illnesses.
- Personality characteristics and/or intrapsychic conflicts in the (supposed) causation of illnesses are in the behavioural medicine approach considered to be not very important. The psychologist who uses behavioural medicine techniques focuses rather on behaviour which maintains or increases physical complaints or illness.
- Empirical studies have led to theories in which the relations between the application of behavioural intervention techniques and the reduction or disappearance of somatic complaints or illnesses are delineated. As illustrated in the various chapters in Part 2 of this book, many patients do benefit from the application of these techniques.

Major shifts in morbidity and mortality patterns in industrialized western societies, growing awareness of the importance of behavioural factors in the development of chronic illness (various forms of cancer, cardiovascular diseases, AIDS, emphysema, diabetes mellitus), the relatively modest contribution of purely medical interventions in patients with chronic illnesses and the rather successful interventions by psychologists in patients with various medical disorders, the efficacy of self-management programmes in patients with chronic illnesses—all these developments have boosted the field of behavioural medicine. In Chapter 3 of this book some of these topics are illustrated in more detail.

BEHAVIOURAL MEDICINE—SOME APPLICATIONS

In this section we will briefly describe four studies which illustrate central issues in behavioural medicine: prevention, treatment and rehabilitation. In selecting the studies we are somewhat guilty of selection bias: the illustrations are 'success stories'. We intend to portray some methods from behavioural medicine applied to various categories of persons or patients and illustrate some of the results in terms of health benefits such as reductions in limitations in daily activities, morbidity and mortality and improvements in psychological outcome measures such as anxiety or depression.

Primary Prevention

The first illustration concerns the primary prevention of coronary heart disease, the major cause of death in western societies. Patel *et al.* (1985) conducted a randomized controlled trial in subjects aged 35–64 who were employed in a large factory near London. Subjects had to satisfy two or more of the following selection criteria: blood pressure higher than 140/90 mmHg, high plasma cholesterol concentration, and smoking 10 cigarettes or more per day.

The participants in the study were allocated to an experimental and a control group. Both groups received written information stressing the importance of stopping smoking, reducing the intake of dietary cholesterol and animal fat, and reducing high blood pressure. The experimental group additionally participated in group sessions of one hour a week for eight weeks to learn breathing exercises, deep muscle relaxation, meditation, and how to cope with stressful situations. Participants were asked to practise relaxation and meditation for 15–20 minutes twice daily and to try to relax during everyday activities, such as while waiting for red traffic lights, before picking up a telephone, and every time they looked at their wristwatches.

After four years the subjects in the two groups were examined again with respect to risk factors for coronary heart disease and cardiovascular morbidity and mortality. The results showed significant reductions in blood pressure and cholesterol levels in the experimental group while cigarette smoking was reduced in both groups. More of the controls had symptoms of angina, ischaemia or possible myocardial infarction, as assessed by electrocardiogram, and more often received long-term treatment for hypertension and its complications. In addition, it was found that those subjects in the treatment group who had applied the relaxation procedures showed greater health gains than those who had not. The authors conclude that 'if the results of this study could be obtained in a larger study the financial and health care implications would be enormous' (p. 1103).

Behavioural Treatment—Reducing the Negative Consequences of Illness

People who become ill or who are ill differ in the way they cope with their illness. Inadequate illness behaviour is associated with, for example, a longer than usual length of hospitalization, more postoperative infections, or an increased rate of rehospitalization (Kaptein, 1988). Behavioural interventions aimed at changing inadequate illness behaviour may lead to a better medical outcome. We will present two illustrations of behavioural treatment in patients with somatic disorders where a behavioural medicine approach leads to reductions in morbidity.

The first study concerns children with asthma. Asthma is a serious health problem: in children asthma is the leading cause of absence from school, the incidence of asthma is rising, and so are the morbidity and mortality of this respiratory illness (Kaptein and Maillé, 1990). Medical management of asthma is aimed at preventing attacks of shortness of breath and alleviating asthma attacks if they occur. Due to the intermittent nature of asthma, the self-care skills of a patient are essential in preventing or stopping asthma attacks. However, research consistently shows that many patients with asthma lack these skills or are unwilling to perform them (Kaptein et al., 1988).

Fireman and colleagues randomized asthmatic children and their mothers in an experimental and a control group (Fireman et al., 1981). The experimental group met five times for a 1½-hour group session in which the children and their mothers were taught about the anatomy and physiology of the lungs, how to prevent asthma attacks, and the correct use of medication. A nurse educator telephoned the participants during the study in order to give additional information and support if necessary. Compared to the children in the control group who received normal care, the children in the experimental group showed a significant decrease in number of visits to a hospital emergency room, days absent from school due to asthma, and number of asthma attacks. The authors give figures which demonstrate that in this study the experimental intervention led to a financial gain of some $50,000. Like Patel *et al.* (1985) in the previous example, the authors state that the cost effectiveness of their intervention is considerable.

Another example of the application of techniques from behavioural medicine to patients with a somatic illness is given by Burish *et al.* (1987). These authors applied progressive muscle relaxation training and guided relaxation imagery in patients with cancer who had to undergo chemotherapeutic treatment and who had developed conditioned nausea and vomiting. In an experimental design, patients in the treatment group received the two techniques on an outpatient basis. In comparison with a control group, ratings by patients and nurses of nausea, anxiety, and frequency of vomiting were all significantly reduced, suggesting that 'behavioral changes may be effective in preventing, or at least retarding the development of, conditioned responses in cancer chemotherapy patients . . . many patients are able to successfully induce self-relaxation after several therapist-directed sessions, thereby increasing the likelihood of relaxation's continued protective effects and its overall cost effectiveness' (p. 48).

Rehabilitation

A chronic illness, almost by definition, cannot be cured—therefore patients who suffer from, for example, rheumatoid arthritis, spinal cord injury, diabetes or emphysema will have to 'learn to live' or cope with the chronic condition. Increasingly, physicians and psychologists have turned their attention to therapeutic approaches which help patients in living or coping with their illness. Emphysema is a typical example of an illness where increased attention to self-management by providers of health care appears to result in positive health outcomes (Kaptein and Dekker, 1987).

In emphysema, irreversible structural damage in lung tissue leads to continuous shortness of breath, serious limitation of daily activities and, often, premature death (Petty, 1985). Medical management consists of medication and physical therapy. Only recently have psychologists 'discovered' the patient with chronic respiratory illness. Therapeutic pessimism regarding these patients, in physicians and psychologists, seems to disappear (Agle and Baum, 1977). Pulmonary rehabilitation programmes traditionally consisted of breathing exercises, physical therapy, trying to restore daily activities as much as possible, and graded exercise training. In 1984, Atkins *et al.* published a paper where cognitive behavioural therapy was applied to a group of emphysema patients. Self-statements by the patients such as 'I cannot walk this far, so why would I try' were replaced by more positive cognitions, such as 'this walking is quite hard, but I'll manage. In a while I'll be able to walk further than now'. In addition, physical exercise and group discussions on coping with emphysema were part of the rehabilitation programme. It was found that in comparison with various control groups, patients in the cognitive behavioural therapy condition improved significantly on a measure of well-being and in the distance they were able to walk.

In these examples we have tried to illustrate how the application of various techniques from the behavioural medicine repertoire may lead to the prevention of illness and to reductions in morbidity (both physically and psychologically). More examples could be given, for example concerning preoperative preparation for surgery (Anderson, 1987), therapeutic suggestions during general anaesthesia (Evans and Richardson, 1988), or psychoeducational interventions (Mullen *et al.*, 1987). The chapters in Part 2 of this book contain many more illustrations of behavioural medicine. Behavioural medicine provides healthy persons and patients with behavioural skills which may help to prevent illness or help in experiencing less illness and disability. In all the examples physicians and psychologists cooperated. 'Underlying' personality characteristics are irrelevant, and in all the examples the methodology with which the effects of the intervention were studied was sound.

BEHAVIOURAL MEDICINE—SOME CLOSING NOTES

In this section we present a few observations which in our opinion may be relevant for a further growth in the practice and theory of behavioural medicine.

- Many authors emphasize and we concur with them, the importance of research on the effectiveness of different intervention methods for various disorders and illnesses. As early as 1973 Birk warned against the danger that *furor therapeuticus* would dominate the field, instead of careful research which is necessary to establish a sound theoretical basis for behavioural medicine. In this book, Maes and van Veldhoven (Chapter 3) make an equally strong statement in this respect. Evans, discussing the role of psychologists in health promotion and prevention of illness, stated '. . . the perhaps too enthusiastic promotion of certain health practices in our culture may not be entirely warranted on the basis of sufficient evidence for such practices . . . Science, not ideology, should drive health promotion' (1988, p. 204).
  Second, various authors (e.g. Edwards and Cooper, 1988; Rosenstock, Strecher and Becker, 1988) encourage researchers in behavioural medicine to incorporate concepts from the literature on coping, stress, cognitive psychology, social learning theory, self-efficacy and health belief model into elaborate theories on health, illness, illness behaviour and behavioural interventions. Research and treatment which is guided by sound theoretical underpinnings will help behavioural medicine to flourish.
- Psychologists who work in a hospital setting sometimes tend to be attracted to patients in the more 'spectacular' and prestigious departments (e.g. cardiac

surgery or intensive care). In our opinion, it would be worthwhile for practitioners of behavioural medicine to explore other patient categories as well, for example patients with arthritis or patients on geriatric wards.

- In this chapter, the focus of research and treatment up to now has been the patient. This emphasis may carry with it the danger of 'blaming the victim' (Kronenfeld, 1979): the patient is blamed for a complicated course of the medical treatment or is being suspected of 'sabotaging' the therapy. Research, however, has shown that providers of medical care (e.g. physicians, nurses) may induce non-compliance themselves (Meichenbaum and Turk, 1987). In Chapter 2 of this book, Johnston, Weinman and Marteau elaborate on these issues. We hope that psychologists in hospitals keep an eye open for the possibility that the physician and/or the medical staff can also be the object of intervention.
- Finally, the substantial costs of the health care system offer practitioners of behavioural medicine excellent opportunities. Increasingly, research on the cost effectiveness of behavioural treatment of patients with medical disorders demonstrates that length of hospitalization, number of hospital admissions, and number of diagnostic and therapeutic interventions can be reduced by applying principles from the field of behavioural medicine (Evans, 1988; Holtzman *et al.*, 1987; Jacobs, 1987). Explaining the cost effectiveness of behavioural medicine to governments and third-party payers should be beneficial for patients and for researchers and practitioners involved with behavioural medicine.

Behavioural medicine as a concept was introduced in the Index Medicus—a prestigious medical literature retrieval system—only in 1983. In that year only 12 papers on behavioural medicine were indexed. In 1988, some 80 papers were included under that heading. In 1985, Basmajian published a provocative paper called 'The next clinical revolution—behavioural medicine'. In this paper the author analyses developments that have had dramatic impact on medicine as an art and a science. The first revolution, according to the author, concerned the development of modern surgery at around the turn of the century. Some 50 years later, breakthroughs in biochemistry and the associated increase in the application of therapeutic drugs accounted for the second revolution. The third revolution, in his opinion, is the rise of behavioural medicine: behavioural factors play a considerable role in the initiation and course of physical illness, and interventions in these behavioural factors will lead to reductions in morbidity and mortality.

Interdisciplinary cooperation in research and patient care, adequate theoretical models which guide research and treatment, and attention to the cost effectiveness of behavioural treatment of patients with medical disorders—behavioural medicine seems to have a bright future if its practitioners take these three issues into account. Psychologists, consultation-liaison psychiatrists, nurses, medical specialists and members of other disciplines involved in medical care can, through cooperative efforts, help reduce morbidity and mortality and improve the quality of life of patients.

NOTES

[1]Addresses for correspondence: A. A. Kaptein, Department of General Practice, Leiden University, PO Box 2088, 2301 CB Leiden, The Netherlands; E. van Rooijen, Department of Psychiatry, Utrecht University, PO Box 85500, 3508 GA Utrecht, The Netherlands.

REFERENCES

Agle, D. P. and Baum, G. L. (1977). Psychological aspects of chronic obstructive pulmonary disease. *Medical Clinics of North America*, **61**, 749–758.

Alexander, F. (1950). *Psychosomatic Medicine: Its Principles and Applications*. London: Allen & Unwin.

Anderson, E. A. (1987). Preoperative preparation for cardiac surgery facilitates recovery, reduces psychological distress, and reduces the incidence of acute postoperative hypertension. *Journal of Consulting and Clinical Psychology*, **55**, 513–520.

Atkins, C. J., Kaplan, R. M., Timms, R. M., Reinsch, S. and Lofback, K. (1984). Behavioral exercise programs in the management of chronic obstructive pulmonary disease. *Journal of Consulting and Clinical Psychology*, **52**, 591–603.

Basmajian, J. V. (1985). The next clinical revolution—behavioral medicine. *Journal of the American Osteopathic Association*, **85**, 592–594.

Birk, L. (1973). *Biofeedback: Behavioral Medicine*. New York: Grune & Stratton.

Bloom, B. L. (1988). Topical review: Primary prevention and the partnership of clinical, community, and health psychology. *Journal of Primary Prevention*, **8**, 149–163.

Burish, T. G., Carey, M. P., Krozely, M. G. and Greco, F. A. (1987). Conditioned side effects induced by cancer chemotherapy: Prevention through behavioral treatment. *Journal of Consulting and Clinical Psychology*, **55**, 42–48.

Dorian, B. J. and Barr Taylor, C. (1987). Psychosomatic medicine. In: Morrison, R. L. and Bellack, A. S. (Eds) *Medical Factors and Psychological Disorders*. New York: Plenum Press, pp. 267–286.

Edwards, J. R. and Cooper, C. L. (1988). Research in stress, coping, and health: Theoretical and methodological issues. *Psychological Medicine*, **18**, 15–20.

Evans, R. I. (1988). Health promotion—science or ideology? *Health Psychology*, **7**, 203–219.

Evans, C. and Richardson, P. H. (1988). Improved recovery and reduced postoperative stay after therapeutic suggestions during general anaesthesia. *Lancet*, August 27, 491–493.

Feldman, E., Mayou, R., Hawton, K., Ardern, M. and Smith, E. B. O. (1987). Psychiatric disorder in medical inpatients. *Quarterly Journal of Medicine*, **63**, 405–412.

Fireman, P., Friday, G. A., Gira, C., Vierthaler, W. A. and Michaels, L. (1981). Teaching self-management skills to asthmatic children and their parents in an ambulatory care setting. *Pediatrics*, **68**, 341–348.

Friedman, S. B. (1970). The challenge in behavioral pediatrics. *Journal of Pediatrics*, **77**, 172–173.

Holtzman, W. H., Evans, R. I., Kennedy, S. and Iscoe, I. (1987). Psychology and health: Contributions of psychology to the improvement of health and health care. *Bulletin of the World Health Organisation*, **65**, 913–935.

Jacobs, D. F. (1987). Cost-effectiveness of specialized psychological programs for reducing hospital stays and outpatients visits. *Journal of Clinical Psychology*, **43**, 729–735.

Kaptein, A. A. (1988). Psychological determinants of length of hospitalization in patients with acute severe asthma. In: Spielberger, C. D., Sarason, I. G. and Defares, P. B. (Eds) *Stress and Anxiety*, Vol. 11. Washington: Hemisphere, pp. 197–205.

Kaptein, A. A. and Dekker, F. W. (1987). CARA—een uitdaging voor de gezondheids-psycholoog (Respiratory illness—a challenge for the health psychologist). *Gedrag & Gezondheid*, **15**, 49–57.

Kaptein, A. A., Dekker, F. W., van der Waart, M. A. C. and Gill, K. (1988). Health psychology and asthma: Current status and future directions. In: Maes, S., Spielberger, C. D., Defares, P. B. and Sarason, I. G. (Eds) *Topics in Health Psychology*. Chichester: Wiley, pp. 157–170.

Kaptein, A. A. and Maillé, R. (1990). Self-management in children with asthma. *The American Journal of Asthma & Allergy for Pediatricians*, in press.

Kronenfeld, J. J. (1979). Self-care as a panacea for the ills of the health care system: An assessment. *Social Science & Medicine*, **13**, 263–267.

Lipowski, Z. J. (1988a). Linking mental and medical health care: An unfinished task. *Psychosomatics*, **29**, 249–253.

Lipowski, Z. J. (1988b). Somatization: The concept and its clinical application. *American Journal of Psychiatry*, **145**, 1358–1368.

MacMillan, H. (1985). Behavioral pediatrics: What has it achieved and where is it going? A resident's perspective. *Developments in Behavioral Pediatrics*, **6**, 100–103.

Matarazzo, J. D. (1980). Behavioral health and behavioral medicine—frontiers for a new health psychology. *American Psychologist*, **35**, 807–817.

Matarazzo, J. D. (1984). Behavioral health: A 1990 challenge for the health sciences professions. In: Matarazzo, J. D., Weiss, S. M., Herd, J. A., Miller, N. E. and Weiss, S. M. (Eds) *Behavioral Health, A Handbook of Health Enhancement and Disease Prevention*. New York: Wiley, pp. 3–40.

Mayou, R., Hawton, K. and Feldman, E. (1988). What happens to medical patients with psychiatric disorder? *Journal of Psychosomatic Research*, **32**, 541–549.

Meichenbaum, D. and Turk, D. C. (1987). *Facilitating Treatment Adherence*. New York: Plenum.

Miller, R. W. and Wood, M. S. (1980). Journals in behavioral medicine. *Behavioral & Social Sciences Librarian*, **1**, 303–319.

Mullen, P. D., Laville, E. A., Biddle, A. K. and Lorig, K. (1987). Efficacy of psychoeducational interventions on pain, depression, and disability in people with arthritis: A meta-analysis. *Journal of Rheumatology*, **14**, 33–39.

Patel, C., Marmot, M. G., Terry, D. J., Carruthers, M., Hunt, B. and Patel, M. (1985). Trial of relaxation in reducing coronary risk: Four year follow up. *British Medical Journal*, **290**, 1103–1106.

Petty, T. L. (Ed.) (1985) *Chronic Obstructive Pulmonary Disease*, 2nd edn. New York: Marcel Dekker.

Rodin, G. and Voshart, K. (1986). Depression in the medically ill: An overview. *American Journal of Psychiatry*, **143**, 696–705.

Rosenstock, I. M., Strecher, V. J. and Becker, M. H. (1988). Social learning theory and the health belief model. *Health Education Quarterly*, **15**, 175–183.

Schwartz, G. E. and Weiss, S. M. (1978). Behavioral medicine revisited: An amended definition. *Journal of Behavioural Medicine*, **1**, 249–251.

Smith, G. R., Monson, R. A. and Ray, D. C. (1986). Psychiatric consultation in somatization disorder. *New England Journal of Medicine*, **314**, 1407–1413.

Trzepacz, P. T., Teague, G. B. and Lipowski, Z. J. (1985). Delirium and other organic mental disorders in a general hospital. *General Hospital Psychiatry*, **7**, 101–106.

CHAPTER 2

Health Psychology in Hospital Settings

M. Johnston[1]

Royal Free Hospital School of Medicine, London

J. Weinman

Guy's Hospital, London

and

T. M. Marteau

Royal Free Hospital School of Medicine, London

ABSTRACT

Hospitals are organized on the basis of disease subsystems and medical specialization. However, some psychological aspects of care are relevant in all clinical
departments. This chapter deals with:

- Perceptions of health and illness.
- Communication between patient and staff.
- Uptake of treatment and compliance with medical advice.
- Stressfulness of medical procedures.
- Coping with chronic illness.

First, health professionals' and patients' perceptions of health, illness, diagnosis
and treatment, and differences in outcome expectations of medical interventions
are illustrated. Secondly, communication between patients and staff are discussed. Several areas where improvements can be achieved are identified. The
value for both patients and health care providers of providing information about

Behavioural Medicine
Edited by A. A. Kaptein, H. M. van der Ploeg, B. Garssen, P. J. G. Schreurs and R. Beunderman
© 1990 John Wiley & Sons Ltd.

the illness, its diagnosis, investigation, treatment and prognosis is demonstrated. Thirdly, the acceptance of medical treatment and compliance with medical advice is discussed. Fourthly, the stressfulness of medical procedures and possible ways to reduce this, are dealt with. By applying psychological techniques, patients and physicians experience less stress and more satisfaction. Finally, the contribution of psychologists to coping with chronic illness is outlined.

INTRODUCTION

Hospitals are organized on the basis of disease subsystems and medical specializations. As outpatients attending hospital, individuals will be seen by specialists in their particular presenting disease or complaint and as a consequence the problems are likely to be investigated and defined primarily in terms of that area of specialization. Similarly, the hospital inpatient will be diagnosed or treated by specialists either in the presenting disease or in a particular treatment procedure.

Psychological contributions have also been framed in this way, tailoring investigations, treatments and clinical approaches to specific diseases such as coronary heart disease (see Chapter 9) and cancer (see Chapter 16) or matching the work to a particular medical speciality (see Broome, 1989). However, some aspects of care, including some behavioural aspects, transcend these subdivisions and permeate all clinical departments.

This chapter deals with cognitive, emotional, behavioural and interpersonal issues which affect all inpatients and outpatients. We have chosen to deal with five psychological issues which go beyond the specific diseases or treatments and which identify aspects of human behaviour common to many areas of hospital inpatient or outpatient life. In each case, it is widely recognized that behaviours can be the source of problems in the conventional delivery of health care and that these problems are not readily solved using available medical and biomechanical wisdom. Clarification and resolution have come instead from the behavioural sciences and especially from the relatively new field of health psychology.

The issues chosen illustrate the diversity of approaches, with contributions from disparate theoretical perspectives including cognitive-behavioural, social/attributional and psychophysiological. Theoretical models have suggested analyses of behaviour in the health setting that have wide applicability. For example, what has been learned about coping with stress has been applied to facilitate both coping with disease and coping with medical procedures. In return, these theories have been advanced by their application and testing in medical environments. Attempts at solutions reflect the rich variety of techniques available and the value of having different techniques for different behaviourally defined problems.

The level or target of the intervention may vary too, providing alternatives to changing the behaviour of the individual patient. Thus some studies direct their efforts at groups of patients, some at health care professionals and still others at the health care delivery system. The first issue to be addressed is the perception of health and illness, an issue that has salience for all clinical settings as well as for health decisions and behaviours outside the clinical situation. Following this there are separate considerations of communication, adherence to advice and/or treatment, coping with stressful medical procedures and coping with chronic illness. In each of these areas there is a very brief overview of some of the key issues and findings from research studies as well as some indication of the contributions which psychologists can make. Finally, there is discussion of the challenges which a health psychology perspective poses for traditionally organized hospital settings and of the obstacles to implementing psychological approaches.

PERCEPTIONS OF HEALTH AND ILLNESS

How people perceive their health and factors influencing it will influence the health care behaviours they engage in. Similarly, people's perception of a symptom or an illness will determine whether they seek help and what kind of help they seek. Perceptions of the diagnosis and any treatment offered will in turn determine response to the illness and what advice they follow. For example, in a study of patients with hypertension, whether or not patients took antihypertensive medication depended upon how they interpreted their condition (Meyer, Leventhal and Gutmann, 1985). Patients who thought hypertension was an acute condition with a limited time course were more likely to stop taking medication and subsequently had higher blood pressure than those who thought the condition was chronic and persisted in taking the drugs.

How doctors and other health professionals perceive an illness, its treatment as well as the patient's state of health, will also influence their response to the illness and the patient. Variations in perceptions of staff can result in different approaches to the same illness and patient. Johnston and coworkers (Johnston *et al.*, 1989) compared assessments of disability made on the same patient by occupational therapists and physiotherapists with those made by nurses. While there was some agreement between therapists and nurses, they only agreed on one patient of the 84 studied. Disagreements were not randomly distributed: therapists consistently rated patients as less disabled than nurses and therefore were likely to have higher expectations of what the patients could achieve. Physicians also vary in their assessment and diagnostic practices. For example, some physicians are more likely to make the diagnosis of asthma in a wheezy child than others (Anderson, Freeling and Patel, 1983). These differences are in turn reflected in different approaches to treatment. In a study examining the variation in admission rate to neonatal care units, variation in doctors' attitudes towards need for admission was one factor accounting for some of the variance (Campbell, 1984).

Patients and health professionals do not always share the same view of an illness, its course or treatment and these differences in perspective may lead to communication difficulties and an ineffective therapeutic alliance. In a study comparing parents' and physicians' perceptions of facial plastic surgery in children with Down's syndrome, the vast majority of parents felt that their child was well accepted and that facial plastic surgery was not indicated: only 13% thought that they might want to have plastic surgery for their child. By contrast, almost half of the physicians were in favour of the operative procedure in children with Down's syndrome (Pueschel, Monteiro and Erickson, 1986).

Health professionals and patients are also likely to differ in their explanations for the outcome of treatment. Gamsu and Bradley (1987) compared staff and patient explanations for positive and negative outcomes of diabetes. Negative outcomes included having high blood sugar levels for a few days and becoming unacceptably overweight; positive outcomes included being well controlled for a period of several weeks and avoiding the complications of diabetes. Different patterns of explanations were apparent for the two groups: medical and nursing staff considered positive outcomes were due more to medical control than negative ones, whereas patients felt that they had more personal control over positive outcomes than the staff attributed to them.

In part stemming from their different perspectives on an illness and factors influencing its course, patients and health professionals are liable to hold different goals of treatment. For example, significant differences were evident in the goals of treatment held by parents of children with diabetes and those held by physicians (Marteau et al., 1987). Parents' goals of treatment were governed more by avoidance of the short-term threat of diabetes (hypoglycaemia); doctors' goals more by the long-term threat of diabetes (diabetic complications). The outcome of treatment (diabetic control) was more closely related to parents' than doctors' goals of treatment.

While it is unlikely that patients and staff will always share the same perceptions of health, illness and treatment, if staff are able to elicit the patient's perspective the patient is likely to be more actively involved in treatment with beneficial results. For example, Inui, Yourtree and Williamson (1976) gave doctors treating patients with hypertension a single tutorial about the nature and importance of patients' beliefs. These doctors subsequently spent more time discussing the patients' ideas, and these patients were then found to adhere more rigidly to their recommended drug regimen and compared with a control group had better control of their blood pressure.

Where perceptions of health and illness are not shared between health care staff and patients, there are likely to be difficulties in communication. Communication problems have frequently been noted.

COMMUNICATION BETWEEN PATIENTS AND STAFF

In surveys of patients' reactions to health care, probably the most consistent complaints are those concerned with aspects of communication. These complaints have been levelled at all departments—medical, surgical, paediatric, oncology, and at both inpatient and outpatient care. Many studies have revealed that patients complain that they are given insufficient information about their condition and their treatment. Also, communication between health care staff and patients has often been shown to be poor because of the health professional's use of jargon and other terms which are misunderstood or because of their failure to take account of the concerns and emotional needs of the patient (e.g. Korsch and Negrete, 1972; Stiles *et al.*, 1979).

As regards information provision, there appear to be a number of areas where improvements can be made. First, there are specific situations, such as prior to a medical investigation, where patients benefit from the provision of information either about the procedure that they will undergo or about the sensations they will experience while in the situation. Moreover, this is often associated with an improved outcome in terms of recovery or reduced pain (Weinman and Johnston, 1988). In the outpatient setting, patients may often present for special tests or investigations. Here it is especially important to provide good information about the nature of the investigations and about any painful or stressful aspects of it. If this is not provided, the patient may arrive for special tests without making the necessary dietary or medicinal preparations, or may even fail to arrive. This can result in apparent failure to comply with medical advice or accept medical investigations (see next section).

It is also necessary to ensure that the results of investigations are clearly communicated back to the patient and that there are adequate opportunities for clarification and further discussion which takes account of the patients' perceptions of and attitudes towards their conditions. Here the timing and content of communication can be crucial and late or incomplete feedback can result in unnecessary distress to patients. For example, in studies of women undergoing prenatal investigations, significant elevations in anxiety have been found to be generated by either delayed or insufficient feedback of the results (Robinson, Hibbard and Laurence, 1984; Field *et al.*, 1985). The provision of information about the illness, its diagnosis, investigations, treatments and prognosis is valuable in a number of ways. Information may reduce anxiety, either by reducing uncertainty about the severity of the condition, the painfulness of the procedures or the long-term outcomes, or by giving patients the opportunity to muster their coping resources and to engender the participation of their social supports. Patients' needs here vary since information provision should relate to the coping style and attitude of the individual patient. For example, individuals with high external locus of control showed better adjustment following the provision of general information whereas more 'internal' individuals adapted better with more specific information (Auerbach *et al.*, 1976). Moreover, the informational needs of the same individual may change as his/her coping style changes as part of the development of the disease or the adjustment to it.

Health care staff have been cautious about information-giving which might result in patients' distress. The provision of difficult or emotionally laden information, particularly 'bad news', is another area where there are major communication problems. Here there is need for health care staff to become much more aware of patients' needs for open communication and for the opportunity to discuss areas of uncertainty and particular fears.

In a review of work in this area, Maguire (1984) maintains that many of the problems or worries experienced by patients are not attended to or dealt with by health care staff. For example, a study of mothers and children attending a paediatric outpatient department revealed that only a quarter of the mothers had been given the opportunity to discuss their main concerns about their child (Korsch and Negrete, 1972). Similarly, Maguire (1976) observed that surgeons made relatively little attempt to identify the worries experienced by women with breast cancer. As a result, their endeavours at reassurance were ineffective since they did not take account of the women's concerns.

One consistent finding to emerge from work in this area is that patients not only want the opportunity to discuss their anxieties but they also would like to be given more information about their condition. This is not only for 'routine' consultations but also for patients with serious and life-threatening illnesses. For example, Reynolds et al. (1981) found that over 90% of cancer patients wanted to know about their diagnosis and their treatment. The evidence from studies in this field indicates that medical staff are not only rather poor at detecting emotional concerns in patients but also both unskilled and unwilling to communicate effectively in response to these.

In addition to identifying the nature of patients' communication needs in hospital settings, psychologists also have a major contribution to make in the training of students or staff in these areas. Many psychologists have helped to develop communication skills teaching for medical and other health professional students. These have ranged from packages designed to teach basic information-gathering skills (Rutter and Maguire, 1976) to those concerned with very specific problems and patient groups (e.g. talking to dying patients; giving 'bad news' to parents; talking to children). In order to ensure that these packages are successful, it may be necessary to provide very structured learning experiences where the students are able to see, at first hand, the importance of good communication skills.

Weinman and Armstrong (1986) provide a good example of this approach to communication skills teaching. Their training takes place in small groups in a primary care setting and uses patient volunteers who have recently consulted the general practitioner. Students are required to interview these patients with two or three other students and a tutor observing; the interviewer's task is to find out why the patient recently sought medical help. Each patient is interviewed by two separate students and, following this, the patient, tutor and students all compare and discuss the two interviews and identify other areas which were not covered. All the students have the opportunity to carry out an interview and to observe others doing so. The important features of this type of training are based on the comparison of the interviews, the feedback to students from patients, tutors and peers and the detailed discussion of the patient's reasons for seeking medical help. Formal evaluation of this teaching has shown that it not only provides basic training in interviewing skills but, more important, it also gives rise to important insights that patients' problems exist in psychological and social dimensions as well as organic and that these three are strongly linked. These insights also prove to be important in motivating students not only to participate in more structured communication skills training but also to increase their understanding of health and illness behaviour.

UPTAKE OF MEDICAL TREATMENT AND COMPLIANCE WITH MEDICAL ADVICE

A limiting factor on the effectiveness of almost any form of disease prevention, investigation or treatment is that recommendations from health professionals are not always followed. When treatments or investigations are available, eligible patients frequently fail to receive them. When diseases are avoidable by changing behaviours, the risky behaviours often persist. When a cure is available, patients have been shown to undermine its effectiveness by failure to comply with the treatment required. There are numerous studies of patient non-adherence in many different areas of health care, including non-adherence to medication required, to advice about preventive health behaviours and to advice about attending screening check-ups. These have been reviewed recently by Becker and Rosenstock (1984) and Meichenbaum and Turk (1987).

The extent of patient non-adherence varies enormously and depends on many factors including the nature of the proposed treatment or advice, the perceived severity of the disease, the perceived advantages and disadvantages associated with the recommended behaviours, the patient's social and physical environment and the quality of the relationship between the patient and the health care professional. Typically it has been found that about 50% of patients fail to follow advice or treatment in a significant way (Ley, 1977). Lower rates of adherence tend to be found with prophylactic medication or advice, particularly in patients with chronic diseases. Perhaps this is understandable since no immediate adverse consequences are experienced, but significant levels of non-adherence are also seen in groups of patients such as those with glaucoma (Vincent, 1971) or diabetes (Cerkoney and Hart, 1980), where the effects can be more immediate and severe.

The contribution of psychologists to this area has been significant and can be discussed under two broad headings. First, psychological studies have provided important insights into the nature and extent of non-adherence, as well as into the types of factors which can affect it. Second, psychologists have developed teaching packages and other interventions for work with health care staff and with patients. Examples of work in both these areas are now discussed.

In attempting to understand the causes of non-adherence, psychological research has tended to concentrate on two different types of psychological explanation, namely, patients' beliefs and the quality of patient–health professional communication. Much of the original work on the health belief model was concerned with using various patient health beliefs to explain the failure to take up preventive measures or to adhere to treatment. While the original model has been justly criticized, there are many studies which have demonstrated a relationship between particular patient beliefs and non-adherence (Janz and Becker, 1984).

Other patient cognitions, such as perception of control, have also been found to have explanatory value, particularly if the measures have been specifically adapted to focus on a particular disease, treatment or patient group. Wallston and colleagues (e.g. Wallston *et al.*, 1987) have recently reviewed the various ways in which different aspects of perceived control can have health outcomes. They maintain that perceptions of control can reflect the extent to which individuals believe their health is influenced by their own behaviour (internal locus of control), by powerful others (e.g. health professionals) or by 'chance' factors. From their work, they conclude that beliefs in internal or chance factors are useful in predicting whether an individual engages in preventive behaviour, whereas beliefs in 'powerful others' will predict adherence to treatment, particularly in those with chronic conditions. However, others (e.g. Bradley *et al.*, 1984) have shown that general beliefs in these three different aspects of control are not necessarily predictive of specific behaviour and that it may be necessary to focus on more specific perceptions of control (e.g. about a specific treatment or a specific disease) in order to see a clear relation between individuals' cognitions and their health-related behaviour.

Research on the relationship between communication and compliance has tended to focus either on the quality of the relationship between patient and health care professional or on the way in which information is transmitted to the patient. As was indicated in the previous section, higher rates of patient satisfaction and adherence are found when communication is more open and shared, particularly when patients are provided with sufficient opportunities to discuss their own concerns and ideas. In addition, the work of Ley (1977) has demonstrated that the information presented to patients is often not sufficiently clear or organized with the result that it is easily forgotten or misunderstood.

Ley's work has shown that patients are often given information which is not comprehensible (e.g. medical jargon) and therefore has relatively little meaning. In addition, the amount of information given often exceeds what can be reasonably retained in memory, particularly when patients are anxious, which is very often the case in medical consultations. Apart from ensuring that information is clear and comprehensible, Ley and colleagues also recommend that it should be categorized into content areas (e.g. 'the symptoms you are experiencing are due to . . .'; 'the treatment will consist of . . .'; 'you need to make the following dietary changes . . .', etc., etc.), and that particularly noteworthy information or advice should be stressed and given at the beginning and/or end of the consultation. These relatively straightforward communication skills can go a long way to ensuring that patients understand and retain the information presented by health care professionals.

Research on the nature of non-adherence has given rise to some very specific guidelines for work with staff and patients. At the simplest level, there is considerable scope for teaching the value of providing clear, organized and jargon-free information for patients. Also, the value of good written information has been described by Ley and Morris (1984) and others. A more difficult objective for teaching health care staff and students is the development of appropriate attitudes and a commitment to a more open and explanatory style of communication, including attention to the patient's own concerns and beliefs. Some attempts to develop teaching approaches in these areas were mentioned in the previous section.

In addition to these general strategies for changing staff behaviour and communication, there are an increasing number of specific psychological techniques which can be used for facilitating adherence (see Meichenbaum and Turk (1987) for a comprehensive recent review). These techniques can either be used directly by psychologists involved in health care teams or be taught to health care professionals. They include behavioural approaches such as the use of goal-setting contracts and various reinforcement strategies in planning and overseeing treatment. In addition, Meichenbaum and Turk outline a range of other approaches including those based on problem-solving skills and attribution-retraining, which is designed to increase patients' belief in the treatment and their sense of mastery and self-confidence in adhering to it over a sustained period.

Finally, it is also important to mention that psychologists can play a role in working with individual patients who are having problems in undergoing investigations or in adhering to medical advice or treatment. This can be particularly important if patients reject treatment or investigations because they are frightened of the procedures.

For example, many patients do not present for dental check-ups or treatment because of their fears of pain or of a specific procedure such as an injection or drilling (Lindsay, 1984). A range of behavioural and cognitive-behavioural techniques are now available for helping patients with these sort of specific fears (Kent, 1984). Psychology departments frequently assist in the care of patients who are frightened of injections. We have been asked to treat a patient who left the surgical ward after receiving premedication for surgery as he was too frightened of anaesthesia to remain on the ward. He responded well to simple cognitive-behavioural approaches, including training in relaxation and desensitization to the frightening thoughts. A colleague recently described an intervention with a patient who was excessively fearful about being in an enclosed space and who needed a neurological examination using nuclear magnetic resonance techniques. The patient absolutely refused to lie down in the enclosed chamber, but, following four fairly brief behavioural sessions involving modelling and desensitization, the investigation was carried out successfully.

Thus the general principles of behavioural and cognitive-behavioural treatments can be successfully used for helping patients come to terms with specific fears about investigative or treatment procedures in various hospital settings.

STRESSFULNESS OF MEDICAL PROCEDURES

Many medical procedures are stressful both for staff and for patients, taxing the resources of the individual to cope with the procedures and resulting in the experience of distress, disruptions in behaviour and physiological changes (Johnston and Wallace, 1990). The stressfulness of the procedure for the individual may detract from its success. As illustrated above, patients may be so frightened that they avoid participating in stressful procedures. Tense patients may make the procedure more difficult, for example in passing a gastric endoscope or in dressing severe burns; anxious surgical patients will require more anaesthetic to achieve adequate levels of sedation; and anxiety in any department will make communication more difficult and misunderstandings more common. Patients who are anxious prior to a surgical procedure are likely to have a slower recovery than those who are less anxious (Johnston, 1986). Various studies have shown that the anxious patients are more distressed postoperatively and they may have increased pain, drug use and total length of hospital stay. Procedures may be stressful for many different reasons. Some are painful, some involve unconsciousness and lack of control, whereas others are life-threatening or may involve techniques which are unfamiliar to the patient. In addition to the stresses inherent in the procedure, the outcome of the procedure may also add to the stressfulness of the experience. Thus minor surgical procedures undertaken to diagnose an unexplained condition may be more stressful than a major but routine therapeutic surgical procedure. Clinical interviews may be just as stressful as major surgery if they determine the patients' acceptance for *in vitro* fertilization (IVF) treatment for infertility (Johnston, Shaw and Bird, 1987) or communicate the results of amniocentesis investigations (Robinson, Hibbard and Laurence, 1984). In these studies IVF patients attending a clinic interview were as anxious as those undergoing surgery, and those anticipating the results of amniocentesis reported considerably higher anxiety levels.

Procedures may also be stressful because they disrupt the individual's normal routine, involving travel to the hospital, time off work, arrangements for child care and for inpatient procedures, preparation for being away from home. In the midst of their worries about the procedures and their outcome, patients frequently cite home matters as a main worry (Johnston, 1987).

The experience of distress is accompanied by physiological changes, and while some changes such as palmar sweating and pupil dilation may have little apparent significance for the patient's treatment, others such as changes in heart rate and respiration rate or increases in catecholamine and corticosteroid output may not only make the patient more vulnerable during the procedure but also more likely to experience later complications and slower to recover.

It is not surprising then that interventions have been devised which attempt to moderate the effects of the stress of the procedures. Well-controlled clinical trials of interventions to prepare patients for diagnostic investigations, medical and surgical procedures have been conducted on children and on adults. These have demonstrated significant benefits in terms of a range of outcomes including the patient's emotional state, behaviour during the procedure, recovery from the procedure, use of medication especially analgesic medication and need for extended medical care (Mathews and Ridgeway, 1984; Weinman and Johnston, 1988). The value of information about the procedure has already been mentioned, but information about the sensory experience associated with the procedure has proved even more effective. It would appear that such information allows patients to evaluate the threats of the procedure realistically so that they are not then overwhelmed by unexplained and therefore potentially dangerous sensory signals. Sensory information appears to be particularly valuable in circumscribed routine procedures where sensations follow a reliable pattern. In more complex or unpredictable procedures, cognitive approaches which teach the patients techniques for dealing with unpleasant or frightening thoughts have been more successful, perhaps because they elaborate the individual's capacity to deal with any form of threatening signal.

Work with surgical patients has been particularly intensive and is well reviewed elsewhere (e.g. Mathews and Ridgeway, 1984). For example, these authors include in their review their own research on patients undergoing gynaecological surgery. In a well-controlled study with random allocation to experimental and control conditions, they demonstrate the effectiveness of training patients to recognize their negative interpretations of events and to reinterpret the same events in a more positive light.

Patients facing medical procedures adopt a variety of coping strategies which have been described along two main dimensions: approach–avoidance and control. Approach–avoidance has been labelled monitoring–blunting, sensitization–repression, vigilance–avoidance, etc., but in each case, the approach/monitoring/sensitizing or vigilant patient is the one who is highly attentive to threat cues and actively seeks information, while those at the other extreme avert attention from threat, distract themselves and limit their information. The control dimension indicates the extent to which patients perceive the situation to be under their own control. At the other extreme, patients may see control as resting with powerful others or they may see no evidence of control and believe that outcomes will be due to chance (Wallston *et al.*, 1987). No single strategy is clearly more effective than others although avoidance strategies appear to be more successful for surgical patients (Cohen and Lazarus, 1973; Wilson, 1981).

In each case, the patients who sought more information and attended to threats showed poorer adjustment in the postoperative period. Avoidance might prove a less successful strategy where participation is involved, and where, for example, it might prevent recognition of symptoms and attendance for treatment. It has frequently been observed that patients may delay in coming for treatment for conditions where early detection is important and in these cases avoidance may prove a dangerous strategy. The effectiveness of various control strategies has been explored but with inconsistent results; success may depend on the opportunities for control in the situation.

This is particularly obvious if procedures carried out with conscious patients are contrasted with procedures under anaesthetic. Patients having surgery under general anaesthetic cannot control what happens in the operating theatre and even their control over postoperative care may be limited. On the other hand, patients having gastroendoscopy may be able to exert control over muscle tension and gagging and thereby reduce both the discomfort and the duration of the procedure.

Interventions can conflict or be compatible with patients' style, and as mentioned earlier, patients with high levels of perceived personal control, i.e.

internal control, have been shown to benefit more from specific than general information while the opposite is true for those with 'external' control. For patients with avoidance styles, providing additional information may disrupt their coping, and other forms of preparation which facilitate their own coping style may be more useful.

Stress for Staff

Medical and surgical procedures may be stressful not only for patients but also for staff. They may be stressful because they demand a high level of technological and interpersonal skill in carrying out the procedure and in discussing it with patients, relatives and other staff and also because they may elicit emotions which are difficult to cope with in professional settings. Some of this stress will come in communicating with patients, especially if the staff are providing undesirable results of investigations or if they are dealing with patients who are anxious about the procedures. In addition, clinicians must make difficult treatment decisions, such as the choice between radical mastectomy and lumpectomy in the treatment of breast cancer, and about executing more complex procedures. These stresses may be exacerbated by the organization of medical and nursing care, which may prove punitive and judgemental for junior staff and isolating and unsupporting for senior staff. Increases in patient throughput, associated with the pressure to increase efficiency of services, can result in a higher rate of procedures being undertaken without the reassurance of continuing care of recovering patients, who are now being discharged from inpatient care at an earlier stage. Staff stress may also be increased by the growing burden of caring for chronically ill patients and the lack of effective therapy or even strategies of care (see next section). While there are many reports of hospital staff stress (e.g. see review by Moos and Schaefer, 1987), there has been much less work on stress-reducing interventions than with patients.

Hospital and clinic settings may create an environment which is in itself stressful, sometimes because many stressful procedures are being conducted and sometimes because the procedure may require an adapted environment. For example, evidence of stress in special care baby units has been described in both paediatricians and nurses by Astbury and Yu (1982).

COPING WITH CHRONIC ILLNESS

In the hospital inpatient and outpatient setting, a very large proportion of patients have diseases which may be lifelong. Many will show inevitable deterioration and some are clearly life-threatening. For patients with these chronic, degenerative or terminal illnesses the ability to cope with the limitations and demands of their illness is a central issue, regardless of the underlying condition. The contribution of psychologists here has been threefold. First, in defining the nature of coping and the various ways in which coping manifests itself and affects illness or treatment outcome. Second, psychologists have also been instrumental in developing teaching packages and skills training for staff involved in the care of the chronically ill. Finally, psychologists have developed various treatment approaches for helping patients cope better not only with aspects of their disease and its consequences but also with external factors which may directly or indirectly affect the disease (e.g. stress management, smoking cessation). Each of these contributions is now briefly reviewed.

Coping is recognized as an important factor influencing the outcome of an illness, as well as in relation to more specific stresses in the hospital, as was discussed in the previous section. The term 'coping' is used to refer to behaviours engaged by individuals to manage environmental or internal demands which exceed their immediate psychological resources. The demands can be in the form of immediate threats or may reflect forthcoming or anticipated threats. Coping behaviours may either be direct attempts to change a threatening or unpleasant situation (problem-focused) or may serve to manage the emotional distress accompanying the threats (emotion-focused). Although apparently a straightforward concept, there is still disagreement about the nature and measurement of coping (Cohen and Lazarus, 1983; Cohen, 1987). Even so, it has provided an important perspective in understanding the effects of chronic illness and the associated treatments and treatment settings.

A particularly important insight from psychological studies of chronic illness has been that an individual's mode of coping and responding arises not from the disease itself but from the individual's perception of the threats and demands associated with it. Moreover, as the perceived threats and demands will often change over time, so the patterns of coping will also change in response to these. For example, Mages and Mendlesohn (1979) have illustrated the changing perceptions and adaptations of patients with cancer. Leventhal, Nerenz and Steele (1984) have suggested that patients' model of the illness incorporates a time component and that perceptions of an illness as acute, cyclic or chronic can significantly modify their response to changes in their condition or to their unchanging condition. Clearly an acute model may result in disappointment and resistance to treatment in patients whose condition proves to be chronic. Long-term coping with disability, essential hypertension or multiple sclerosis demands a different kind of adaptation to acute conditions such as appendicitis or mumps.

Psychological studies have also shown that individuals do not just use one mode of coping but are most likely to draw upon problem- and emotion-focused modes in many situations (Folkman and Lazarus, 1980). Also, there may well be different ways of coping with different aspects of the same illness. For example, different modes of coping have been found to be used for dealing with the pain of a disease and with the threats to self-esteem posed by it (Cohen et al., 1986).

Staff working with the chronically sick or terminally ill may often have limited views about the nature of patients' responses to the illness. For example, they may believe that because individuals react in a certain way, then they will always react in that way. Also, they may believe that one particular way of coping is intrinsically better or more adaptive or, correspondingly, that some modes of coping are unhelpful or bizarre. As Cohen (1987) points out, health practitioners want to know which mode of coping is most adaptive. She demonstrates the impossibility of providing a firm answer to this question by providing examples where particular modes of coping have different outcomes, depending on the situation. Thus the use of an avoidant coping style has been found to be associated with a better initial outcome in patients in a coronary care unit but with decreased compliance with medical treatment after one year. Similarly, the expression of emotion may worsen the symptoms of patients with some diseases but may be helpful for others.

There are also more specific psychological approaches for helping patients cope with terminal illness. Weisman, Worden and Sobel (1980) and Sobel (1981) have developed specific psychological and behavioural packages for work with dying patients. Specific psychological techniques used in other areas can be adapted for use with dying patients where goals are similar. Recently, we were asked to help a dying patient who was extremely depressed, having withdrawn from treatment with the expectation of dying immediately. The support team responsible for her care felt helpless in caring for her and concerned that work they might do at a later stage in minimizing pain and discomfort might become impossible. The patient was asked to keep a diary of her mood, thoughts and activities and to increase activities associated with more positive moods. This simple cognitive-behavioural intervention was followed by clear mood improvements which were sustained for two weeks before the patient became too ill to maintain the diary and died two weeks later (Jones, Johnston and Speck, 1989).

There are a growing number of psychological approaches to treatment which are particularly suitable for many chronically ill patients. Various approaches for pain management have been developed by psychologists (Linton, 1982) and, while these have not been adequately evaluated, they do appear to be helpful in reducing complaints of pain or in facilitating coping with chronic pain. It has been pointed out that the success of these treatments may depend as much on the increased feelings of self-efficacy or control which they engender in the individual patient. Thus they may also serve to facilitate coping in this way and may actually improve rehabilitation and recovery as a result (Partridge and Johnston, 1989).

For other chronic diseases behaviour change may be particularly important to prevent recurrence or exacerbation. Stress-management approaches have proved useful since they are designed to help the individual cope better with actual or potential stressors and, hopefully, avoid the physiological consequence of poor or maladaptive attempts at coping (e.g. Frasure-Smith and Prince, 1987). There are also an increasing number of studies demonstrating the value of self-management packages for the control of symptoms of many chronic diseases (see Holroyd and Creer, 1986 for a comprehensive account).

IMPLEMENTING THE PSYCHOLOGICAL PERSPECTIVE

The five areas described above illustrate the application of psychological approaches for clarifying problems and improving the clinical care of patients. Each has a widespread relevance, as there is no clinical specialty where an understanding of the perceptions of illness, communication between staff and patients, the uptake of medical procedures and compliance with medical advice, the stressfulness of medical procedures and coping with chronic illness would not contribute to better patient care. There have been perceptible increases in the contribution of psychologists in each of these areas of health care. Yet the majority of health care settings have no specific psychology input. There are several possible explanations.

First, as discussed in the opening section, many of the critical behaviours in health care are not specific to any particular medical specialty and therefore tend not to be fostered by that specialty. In presenting information about coping with chronic illness, one needs to present data on coronary heart disease to cardiologists, bronchitis to thoracic physicians, diabetes to endocrinologists and arthritis to rheumatologists. This has been the approach of psychologists working within a behavioural medicine framework, as illustrated elsewhere in this book, but even that approach has had limited impact.

Second, the basic models used by psychologists and the majority of health professionals differ. While psychological models can incorporate the biomechanical perspective, the reverse may not be true. Lack of training in measurement and research in the behavioural domain may leave the health professional unable to evaluate evidence about psychological phenomena and therefore as likely to be swayed by opinion as by evidence.

Third, there are relatively few psychologists working in the health field compared with the numbers of medical, nursing and paramedical staff. There may be too few to even create awareness of what they might do if available.

In planning to integrate psychology and health care further, at least two tasks need to be considered: first, the creation of a recognized need for psychology in medicine; and second, the strengthening of psychology to accomplish this task.

In creating a recognized need for psychology, the lead has to come from psychologists, as medicine is currently in a strong position, unaware of what it may gain, but aware of what it may lose (resources, power and status, to name a few). Persuasion needs to be aimed at doctors and other health professionals, health service managers as well as patients. Attitudes of doctors are perhaps best changed by their working alongside psychologists within a research or a clinical context.

Beliefs and attitudes will also be changed by making behavioural sciences more integrated into medical education. The beliefs and attitudes of health service managers are perhaps also best changed by exposure to the skill of psychologists in achieving objectives they value. this can be effected by inviting them to seminars and departmental meetings. For patients, the main source of information about medicine is from the media. While reporting about medicine is often mixed, medicine and its practitioners are presented as high-technology life-savers. Coverage of psychology, and its success in promoting health and making medical care more effective, is poor.

Currently, dissatisfaction is being expressed by patients as well as health service managers about the way health care is provided in western culture. The focus on technological acute medicine can be in conflict with goals of quality of life and the objectives of coping with more enduring morbidity. This provides an opening for psychology. However, in order for psychologists to take advantage of this opportunity, it is necessary that they act as a united force and that they are able to demonstrate to health professionals, politicians, the public and health service managers alike that they have something of value to offer.

NOTES

[1] Addresses for correspondence: M. Johnston and T. M. Marteau, Royal Free Hospital School of Medicine, University of London, Royal Free Hospital, Pond St, London NW3 2QG, UK; J. Weinman, Department of Psychology as Applied to Medicine, Guy's Hospital, University of London, London Bridge, London SE1 9RT, UK.

REFERENCES

Anderson, H. R., Freeling, P. and Patel, S. P. (1983). Decision-making in acute asthma. *Journal of the Royal college of General Practitioners*, **33**, 105–108.

Astbury, J. and Yu, V. Y. H. (1982). Determinants of stress for staff in a neonatal intensive care unit. *Archives of Diseases in Childhood*, **57**, 108–111.

Auerbach, S. M., Kendall, P. C., Cuttler, H. F. and Levitt, N. R. (1976). Anxiety, locus of control, type of preparatory information and adjustment to dental surgery. *Journal of Consulting and Clinical Psychology*, **44**, 809–818.

Becker, M. H. and Maiman, L. A. (1975). Sociobehavioural determinants of compliance with health and medical care recommendations. *Medical Care*, **13**, 10–25.

Becker, M. H. and Rosenstock, I. M. (1984). Compliance with medical advice. In: Steptoe, A. and Mathews, A. (Eds) *Health Care and Human Behaviour*. New York: Academic Press.

Bradley, C., Brewin, C. R., Bamsu, D. and Moses, J. L. (1984). Development of scales to measure perceived control of diabetes mellitus and diabetes-related health beliefs. *Diabetic Medicine*, **1**, 213–218.

Broome, A. (1989). *Health Psychology*. London: Croom Helm.

Campbell, D. H. (1984). Why do physicians in neonatal care units differ in their admission threshold? *Social Science & Medicine*, **18**, 365–374.

Cerkoney, A. B. and Hart, K. (1980). The relationship between the health belief model and compliance of persons with diabetes mellitus. *Diabetes Care*, **3**, 594–598.

Cohen, F. (1987). Measurement of coping. In: Kasl, S. V. and Cooper, C. L. (Eds) *Stress and Health: Issues in Research Methodology*. New York: Wiley.

Cohen, F. and Lazarus, R. S. (1973). Active coping processes, coping dispositions, and recovery from surgery. *Psychosomatic Medicine*, **35**, 375–389.

Cohen, F. and Lazarus, R. S. (1983). Coping and adaptation in health and illness. In: Mechanic, D. (Ed.) *Handbook of Health, Health Care and the Health Professions*. New York: Free Press.

Cohen, F., Reese, L. B., Kaplan, G. A. and Riggio, R. E. (1986). Coping with the stresses of arthritis. In: Moscowitz, R. W. and Haig, M. R. (Eds) *Handbook of Health, Health Care and the Health Professions*. New York: Springer.

Field, T., Sandberg, D., Quetel, T. A., Garcia, R. and Rosario, M. (1985). Effects of ultrasound feedback on pregnancy anxiety, fetal activity and neonatal outcome. *Obstetrics and Gynaecology*, **66**, 525–528.

Folkman, S. and Lazarus, R. S. (1980). An analysis of coping in a middle-aged community sample. *Journal of Health and Social Behaviour*, **21**, 219–239.

Frasure-Smith, N. and Prince, R. (1987). The ischaemic heart disease life stress monitoring program: Possible therapeutic mechanisms. *Psychology and Health*, **1**, 273–286.

Gamsu, D. S. and Bradley, C. (1987). Clinical staff's attributions about diabetes: Scale development and staff vs patient comparisons. *Current Psychological Research and Reviews*, **6**, 69–78.

Holroyd, K. A. and Creer, T. L. (1986). *Self-Management of Chronic Disease*. New York: Academic Press.

Inui, T. S., Yourtree, E. L. and Williamson, J. W. (1976). Improved outcomes in hypertension after physician tutorials: A controlled trial. *Annals of Internal Medicine*, **84**, 646–651.

Janz, N. K. and Becker, M. H. (1984). The health belief model: A decade later. *Health Education Quarterly*, **11**, 1–147.

Johnston, M. (1986). Pre-operative emotional states and post-operative recovery. *Advances in Psychosomatic Medicine*, **15**, 1–22.

Johnston, M. (1987). Emotional and cognitive aspects of anxiety in surgical patients. *Communication & Cognition*, **20**, 245–260.

Johnston, M., Bromley, I., Boothroyd-Brooks, M., Dobbs, W., Ilson, A. and Ridout, K. (1989). Behavioural assessments of physically disabled patients: Agreement between rehabilitation therapists and nurses. *International Journal of Research in Rehabilitation*, **10** (Suppl. 5), 205–213.

Johnston, M., Shaw, R. and Bird, D. (1987). Test-tube baby procedures: Stress and judgements under uncertainty. *Psychology and Health*, **1**, 25–38.

Johnston, M. and Wallace, L. M. (1990). *Stress and Medical Procedures*. Oxford: Oxford University Press.

Jones, K., Johnston, M. and Speck, P. (1989). Despair felt by the patient and the professional carer: A case study of the use of cognitive behavioural methods. *Journal of Palliative Care*, **3**, 39–46.

Kent, G. G. (1984). *The Psychology of Dental Care*. Bristol: John Wright.

Korsch, B. M. and Negrete, V. F. (1972). Doctor–patient communication. *Scientific American*, **227**, 67–74.

Leventhal, H., Nerenz, D. R. and Steele, D. (1984). Disease representations and coping with health threats. In: Baum, A., Taylor, J. and Taylor, S. (Eds) *Handbook of Psychology and Health*, Vol. IV. Hillsdale NJ: Erlbaum.

Ley, P. (1977). Psychological studies of doctor–patient communication. In: Rachman, S. (Ed.) *Contributions to Medical Psychology*, Vol. 1. Oxford: Pergamon.

Ley, P. and Morris, L. A. (1984). Psychological aspects of written information for patients. In: Rachman, S. (Ed.) *Contributions to Medical Psychology*, Vol. III. Oxford: Pergamon.

Lindsay, S. J. (1984). The fear of dental treatment: A critical and theoretical analysis. In: Rachman, S. (Ed.) *Contributions to Medical Psychology*, Vol. III. Oxford: Pergamon.

Linton, S. J. (1982). A critical review of behavioural treatments for chronic benign pain other than headache. *British Journal of Clinical Psychology*, **21**, 321–337.

Mages, N. L. and Mendelsohn, G. A. (1979). Effects of cancer on patients' lives; A personological approach. In: Stone, G. C., Cohen, F. and Adler, N. (Eds) *Health Psychology—A Handbook*. San Francisco: Jossey-Bass.

Maguire, P. (1976). The psychological and social sequelae of mastectomy. In: Howells, J. S. (Ed.) *Modern Perspectives on Psychiatric Aspects of Surgery*. New York: Bruner Mazel.

Maguire, P. (1984). Communication skills and patient care. In: Steptoe, A. and Mathews, A. (Eds) *Health Care and Human Behaviour*. London: Academic Press.

Marteau, T. M., Johnston, M., Baum, J. D. and Bloch, S. (1987). Goals of treatment in diabetes: A comparison of doctors and parents of children with diabetes. *Journal of Behavioural Medicine*, **10**, 33–48.

Mathews, A. and Ridgeway, V. (1984). Psychological preparation for surgery. In: Steptoe, A. and Mathews, A. (Eds) *Health Care and Human Behaviour*. London: Academic Press, pp. 231–259.

Meichenbaum, D. and Turk, D. C. (1987). *Facilitating Treatment Adherence: A Practitioner's Guidebook*. New York: Plenum.

Meyer, D., Leventhal, H. and Gutmann, M. (1985). Common-sense models of illness: The example of hypertension. *Health Psychology*, **4**, 115–135.

Moos, R. H. and Billings, A. G. (1982). Conceptualising and measuring coping resources and processes. In: Goldberger, L. and Breznitz, S. (Eds) *Handbook of Stress: Theoretical and Clinical Aspects*. New York: Free Press.

Moos, R. H. and Schaefer, J. A. (1987). Evaluating health care work settings: A holistic conceptual framework. *Psychology and Health*, **1**, 97–122.

Partridge, C. and Johnston, M. (1989). Perceived control of recovery from physical disability: Measurement and prediction. *British Journal of Clinical Psychology*, **28**, 53–59.

Pueschel, S. M., Monteiro, L. A. and Erickson, M. (1986). Parents' and physicians' perceptions of facial plastic surgery in children with Down's Syndrome. *Journal of Psychosomatic Research*, **28**, 163–169.

Reynolds, P. M., Sanson-Fisher, R., Poole, A. and Harker, J. (1981). Cancer and communication: Information giving in an oncology clinic. *British Medical Journal*, **282**, 1449–1451.

Robinson, J. O., Hibbard, B. M. and Laurence, K. M. (1984). Anxiety during a crisis: Emotional effects of screening for neural tube defects. *Journal of Psychsomatic Research*, **28**, 163–169.

Rutter, D. R. and Maguire, G. P. (1976). History taking for medical students: II— Evaluation of a training programme. *Lancet*, **ii**, 558.

Sobel, H. (1981). *Behavioural Therapy in Terminal Care: A Humanistic Approach*. Cambridge, Mass: Balinger.

Stiles, W. B., Putnam, S. M., Wolf, M. H. and James, S. A. (1979). Interaction exchange structure and patients' satisfaction with medical interviews. *Medical Care*, **17**, 667–669.

Vincent, P. (1971). Factors influencing patient non-compliance: A theoretical approach. *Nursing Research*, **20**, 509–516.

Wallston, K. A., Wallston, B. S., Smith, S. and Dobbins, C. J. (1987). Perceived control and health. *Current Psychological Research and Reviews*, **6**, 5–25.

Weinman, J. and Armstrong, D. (1986). Using interview training as a preparation for behavioural science teaching. In: Aldridge-Smith, J., Butler, A., Dent, H. and Mindham, R. H. S. (Eds) *Proceedings of First Conference of Behavioural Sciences in Medical Undergraduate Education*. Leeds: Leeds University Press, pp. 20–29.

Weinman, J. and Johnston, M. (1988). Stressful medical procedures: An analysis of the effects of psychological interventions and of the stressfulness of the procedures. In: Maes, S., Spielberger, C., Defares, P. B., and Sarason, I. G. (Eds) *Topics in Health Psychology*, pp. 205–217. Chichester: Wiley.

Weisman, A. D., Worden, J. W. and Sobel, H. J. (1980). Psychosocial screening and intervention with cancer patients: Research report. Cambridge, Mass: Shea.

Wilson, J. F. (1981). Behavioural preparation for surgery: Benefit or harm? *Journal of Behavioural Medicine*, **4**, 79–102.

CHAPTER 3

From Health Behaviour to Health Behaviour Change

S. Maes[1] and M. van Veldhoven

Tilburg University, Tilburg

ABSTRACT

Health psychology is defined, and conceptualized as an important discipline contributing to behavioural medicine. The reasons for the fast growth of health psychology are described. Three major objects of study are identified:

- Behaviour which may have direct physiological effects that affect health.
- Certain life-styles and daily habits.
- Perceptions of and coping with illness.

A distinction is made between 'basic' and 'applied' health psychology research. The authors critically describe relevant research examples and suggest ways to improve the quality and relevance of the two types of health psychology research. It is stressed that health psychology benefits from linking basic and applied research. The authors conclude that health psychology has great potential for contributing to primary and secondary prevention of disease. The importance of continuous critical reflection on the quality of the methodology used in health psychology research is also stressed.

WHAT IS HEALTH PSYCHOLOGY?

In a way, health psychology does not, as many people think, originate from North America but from ancient Greece. According to the legend, Zeus, the chief Olympian god, brought the healer Asclepius into the heavens because of

Behavioural Medicine
Edited by A. A. Kaptein, H. M. van der Ploeg, B. Garssen, P. J. G. Schreurs and R. Beunderman
© 1990 John Wiley & Sons Ltd.

his healing skills. Asclepius had two daughters, Hygeia and Panacea. Hygeia, known as the goddess of health and prevention, taught the Greeks they could be healthy if they were moderate in all forms of behaviour. Panacea, the other daughter, was known as the goddess of medicine and represented the continuous search for treatment of all illnesses (Lyons and Petrucelli, 1978). As health psychology studies the role of behaviour in health and illness, we can think of Hygeia as being the goddess of health psychology.

The definition of Matarazzo (1980, p. 815) describes health psychology elaborately: 'Health psychology is the aggregate of the specific educational, scientific and professional contributions of the discipline of psychology to the promotion and maintenance of health, the prevention and treatment of illness, and the identification of etiologic and diagnostic correlates of health and illness, and related dysfunctions'. It states that as health psychology focuses more on prevention than on treatment of illness, health behaviour as well as illness behaviour is the object of study. In addition, the present state of the art (Stone, Cohen and Adler, 1979; Millon, 1982; Matarazzo et al., 1984; Feuerstein, Labbé and Kuczmierczyk, 1986; Taylor, 1986) demonstrates that health psychologists tend to apply their knowledge more to physical than mental health. As such, they are more interested in 'normal', everyday life behaviours which lead to or are the consequence of somatic pathology or dysfunction, and less interested in psychopathology or abnormal behaviour. Salutogenesis, rather than psychopathology, forms the base for health psychology. Health psychology may be differentiated from other related fields of knowledge as follows: traditional clinical psychology is more interested in psychopathology, mental health and treatment; medical psychology can be defined as psychology in medicine rather than as a subdiscipline of psychology and focuses on illness behaviour and treatment rather than on health behaviour and prevention (Schmidt, 1984); behavioural medicine is considered the interdisciplinary field and concerns itself with behaviour and medicine. Health psychology is only one of the contributing disciplines together with, for example, biology and physiology (Matarazzo et al., 1984).

THE GROWTH OF THE DISCIPLINE

Health psychology is a recent and very fast growing subdiscipline of psychology. Since the American Psychological Association (APA) founded the first health psychology division in 1979, many European and international health psychology groups have been formed; among these are the European Health Psychology Society and the Health Psychology Division of the International Association of Applied Psychology. National health psychology groups have also been established in several European countries.

There are at least three good reasons for the fast growth of the discipline, the *first* being the dramatic change in the causes of mortality in western Europe. At the beginning of the twentieth century, communicable diseases such as influenza, pneumonia, diphtheria, tuberculosis and gastrointestinal infections were the main causes of death. However, mortality caused by these diseases has dropped to a very low level in the western world during the last few decades, this being due to improved sanitation, the development of effective vaccines, mass immunization and pharmacological treatment. Today cardiovascular diseases and cancer are responsible for more than two-thirds of the mortality in western countries (Matarazzo *et al.*, 1984).

The principal risk factors for these diseases and for accidents (which are the next major cause of death in western countries) are strongly linked to behavioural factors such as smoking, nutritional habits, alcohol abuse and lack of physical exercise. A group of American experts have suggested that perhaps as much as half of the present mortality is due to unhealthy behaviour: 20% to environmental factors, 20% to human biological factors, and 10% to inadequacies in health care (Shirrefs, 1982). As psychology may be defined as the science of behaviour, there can be no doubt that psychologists may contribute to community health by studying the onset and development of unhealthy behaviours.

The *second* reason for the fast growth of the discipline is that in the 1970s it became apparent that national health care expenditures in western countries were rapidly growing out of control. As a consequence, apart from direct measures such as cuts in the health care budget, there is now an ever-growing interest in disease prevention. As health education may be considered the most powerful preventive strategy in the present health context, there is an interest on government level for behavioural scientists in the prevention of disease. As psychology can be considered the basic discipline as far as information processing and inducing behavioural changes are concerned, several health psychologists have made significant contributions in the field of health promotion and disease prevention (Matarazzo *et al.*, 1984).

Finally, the *third* reason for the growth of the discipline is closely linked to the development of psychology itself. The successful application of psychological principles and techniques in the field of compliance with some medical regimens and to various disorders and health problems such as pain, coronary heart disease and diabetes has increased the belief that psychologists have the tools to influence health conditions. In addition, modern psychology is characterized by an expertise in research methodology, which puts psychologists in a position to carry out research in health care settings.

THE OBJECT OF STUDY

As already pointed out, the object of study is the relationship between behaviour and (physical) health. Krantz, Grunberg and Baum (1985) distinguished three possible relationships between behaviour and health: (a) behaviour may have direct physiological effects affecting health; (b) lifestyles and daily habits may endanger or enhance health; and (c) the way in which people perceive and cope with illness may affect their health. An example of each of these relationships is given below.

Psychophysiology and Health

Psychophysiological effects imply physiological reactions to psychosocial stimuli. Research has demonstrated direct physiological effects of stress. Stress can be defined as the subjective experience of tension, which occurs when there is a perceived discrepancy between certain environmental demands and individuals' capacities to cope with them (Chalmers, 1981). Good examples of short-term physiological effects of stress are increased heart rate and blood pressure. Long-term effects of stress may lead, for example, to chronic disorders of the cardiovascular or the gastrointestinal system (Baum, Grunberg and Singer, 1982).

Recent research in the field of psychoneuroimmunology provides a good example of this type of relationship. Experimental research with animals and humans has demonstrated that specific stressors may have a reducing effect on the number of lymphocytes (blood cells which play an important role in the immune process) as well as on the level of interferon (a substance influencing the spread of cancer cells in the body) (Ader, 1981). Although the mechanism is not very well understood, it is generally accepted that 'stress hormones' such as adrenaline, noradrenaline and cortisol play an important role in this process. An example of this line of research is the study carried out by Kiecolt-Glaser et al. (1984). They measured the activity (vigour of attack) of the natural killer cells (which play a crucial role in the defence against infectious agents) in both a non-stressful (mid-term) and a stressful condition (end of term before exams) in a student population. It was found that the activity of natural killer cells was reduced significantly in the stressful condition. In addition, the students were asked, both at mid-term and before the exams, whether they had recently experienced stressful events. It was found that the activity of the natural killer cells in students who had experienced the most stressful events was significantly lower at both measuring points than that of students who reported having experienced less stressful events. Consequently, it may be argued that stress may increase susceptibility to various infectious diseases.

Several authors have argued that stress may also play an important role in the onset and development of coronary heart disease and cancer, in which physiological processes would play a mediating role (Fox, 1982; Maes et al., 1987b). Although there is evidence supporting the relationship between stress and the onset and course of infectious diseases, there is no sound research demonstrating a direct link between stress and the onset of coronary heart disease or cancer (Maes, Vingerhoets and Van Heck, 1987). It has been shown, however, that psychological factors may play an important role in the course of established breast cancer, and that feelings of vital exhaustion and depression are precursors of myocardial infarction (Appels, 1988).

Lifestyles and Health

Unhealthy lifestyles and daily habits are strongly related to the onset of disease. By means of a nine-year follow-up study, Belloc and Breslow (1972) and

Breslow and Enstrom (1980) investigated the relationship between health behaviour and life expectancy in a population of nearly 7000 adults from Alameda County, California, USA. It was shown that daily habits such as sleeping seven to eight hours a night, eating breakfast regularly, avoiding snacks, maintaining desirable weight for height, moderate or no use of alcohol, regular physical exercise, and not smoking proved to increase health status and average life expectancy. It was calculated that a 45-year-old man who engaged in six to seven of these behaviours had a life expectancy of 78 years of age, whereas the life expectancy of a 45-year-old man who engaged in none to three of these behaviours was only 67 years of age. This means that these simple daily behaviours can account for a difference of 11 years in the average life expectancy. A remarkable fact is that there is a smaller life expectancy difference (seven years) for comparable 45-year-old women. Among other explanations, women seem to be hormonally protected against the effects of unhealthy habits.

In addition, psychosocial factors seem to mediate or influence the relationship between lifestyles, health status and mortality. Berkman and Syme (1979) showed, from the already cited Alameda County follow-up study, that (after being matched for initial health, health status and social class) men as well as women with strong social support networks were on the whole in better health and lived longer than comparable men and women reported to have poor or no social support. The results of this epidemiological study show, for example, a difference of 21.2% in mortality after nine years between men with the strongest and men with the weakest social support in the age group 50–59. A comparable difference of 19.7% in mortality was found for women in the age group 60–69. Perceived social support as well as many other personality variables (e.g. self-efficacy or hardiness) should be taken into account as possible social/behavioural modulators of behaviour–illness relationships (Feuerstein, Labbé and Kuczmierczyk, 1986).

However convincing the results of the Alameda County study may be, there is still a long way to go. Not only must similar studies be undertaken in other populations and societies, but sound knowledge must be gained with respect to factors which influence the onset and the development of healthy (or unhealthy) behaviour, as this lack of knowledge is turning most interventions in health behaviour into processes of trial and error. In the case of the 'Alameda 7', which is what the seven health habits described above are called, we only have relevant data for a US population, as the US National Health Interview Survey (NHIS) has included questions on these habits since 1977. The most recent survey shows, for example, that only 12% of men and 11% of women have six or seven good health habits. This type of survey may allow one to identify target groups for each of the habits in terms of intervention (Schoenborn, 1986).

As a consequence of studies which demonstrated the relationship between lifestyles and health, primary prevention programmes have been developed to promote health and to alter risk behaviour prior to illness. Here one can differentiate between two possible strategies, the first of which attempts to prevent healthy people from developing bad habits and/or promote good habits, and the second, which focuses on risk groups, to alter existing bad habits. These strategies imply health education and health promotion on a general-population level (mass media campaigns, health promotion in industrial, school or leisure settings) or for specific risk groups in the population (e.g. people who are overweight, people who smoke, people with a high alcohol consumption and people doing little or no physical exercise). We should keep in mind that health psychologists are not only able, but also expected, to make major contributions in the field of disease prevention and health promotion by contributing to larger-scale programmes. A good example of the possible effectiveness of such programmes is presented by recent evaluation studies of health promotion programmes in work settings which prove to be effective in improving the average health status of the participants and in reducing their use of medical resources and absence from work (Cataldo and Coates, 1986). Other successful examples can be found in the field of prevention of coronary heart disease on a population level. These include programmes focusing on high-risk individuals and on the community at large. In some cases, for example the North Karelia Project in Finland (Puska, 1984) and the Controlled Multifactorial Preventive Trial in Belgium (Kittel, 1986), these large-scale interventions succeeded in altering risk behaviour related to cardiovascular diseases and in the reduction of subsequent mortality. For further information, the interested reader is referred to an excellent overview chapter by Kornitzer (1987).

Coping with Illness

Whereas the first two paths focus on the role of behaviour in the development of disease, the third concerns behavioural consequences of disease and illness. In other words, this third pathway is concerned with illness behaviour and sick role behaviour in the various stages of disease: diagnosis, treatment and psychosocial reintegration. Although there is a vast amount of literature on a wide variety of illness and sick role behaviours, it would appear that a lot of these behaviours can be described along an approach–avoidance dimension (Roth and Cohen, 1986). At one end of this dimension we have patients who tend to exaggerate or aggravate their symptoms and health conditions, and at the other patients who seem to minimize or deny them. It is quite clear that both types of behaviour may lead to a variety of consequences in terms of health, the use of medical resources, and psychological and social functioning.

The magnitude of non-compliance is perhaps the best example of the avoidance side of the continuum, at least if patients are well informed about their medical condition and treatment. It is a well-known fact that in many cases about half the patients do not comply with medication prescriptions, and that about the same amount do not comply with medical advice concerning physical exercise or diets (Di Matteo and Di Nicola, 1982; Ley, 1979, 1982; Martin and Dubbert, 1982; Sackett and Snow, 1979). Compliance with medical advice to stop smoking is even worse: on average, eight to nine out of every 10 patients who smoke prove to be non-compliant one year after medical advice (Lichtenstein and Brown, 1981; Burling et al., 1984). Dropout from rehabilitation programmes and not keeping hospital appointments are just two other examples of the problem at hand. Although there are many reasons for non-compliance, a considerable part of it can be explained by avoidant behaviour with regard to disease, diagnosis, treatment or the sick role. Where the medical profession can be blamed for giving poor information which leads to non-compliance, we cannot blame physicians for the more voluntary forms of non-compliance, which are often caused by the fact that personal beliefs, goals and expectancies of patients and/or their social environments interfere with the advice given. There are, however, many psychological techniques such as stimulus control, self-control, self-monitoring and reinforcement as well as other cognitive and social psychological strategies which have proved to be successful in increasing compliance with different types of medical advice (Di Matteo and Di Nicola, 1982; Feuerstein, Labbé and Kuczmierczyk, 1986). Although some people agree with Seneca that some treatments are worse than the disease itself, there is a proven need for psychologists in medical settings to alter patients' perceptions and attitudes in order to improve compliance.

Other behavioural consequences of illness lie in the opposite direction, and can be characterized by the approach end of the dimension. Overemphasizing symptoms or health conditions may have even more severe consequences than avoidant behaviour in terms of overuse of medical resources and inadequate social functioning. In a recent study it was demonstrated that apart from disease variables, a considerable part of the variance in hospital admission and absence from work in asthmatic patients could be explained by psychological variables such as focusing on asthma in daily life and reacting emotionally in attack situations (Maes and Schlösser, 1987). Other studies have demonstrated that an overpreoccupation with personal health may lead to chest pain and use of various medical resources despite insignificant or no coronary artery disease (Wieglosz et al., 1984). In order to reduce the overuse of medical resources, health psychologists can design intervention programmes based on social learning theory, stress management techniques and cognitive behaviour modification (Feuerstein, Labbé and Kuczmierczyk, 1986).

RESEARCH IN HEALTH PSYCHOLOGY: SOME CRITICAL REMARKS

If the first part of this chapter attempts to demonstrate the potential contributions of health psychology, the second aims to formulate critical remarks on the present research in health psychology. These critical remarks are by no means an attempt to discount the value of current research. They should be seen as reflections, mainly stemming from our own research. As such, for many of the questions raised in this part there are no definite answers.

In the following paragraphs, we differentiate between basic and applied health psychology research. *Basic* health psychology research aims at discovering the relationship between specific behaviours and the development or maintenance of health or development of illness. *Applied* health psychology research implies interventions aiming at the enhancement of health behaviour or the modification of illness behaviour.

Some Remarks on Basic Health Psychology Research

According to Kaplan (1984), basic health psychology research should provide answers to the following relevant questions:

1. Which behaviours increase the risk of damage to health?
2. Can changes in specific behaviours reduce the probability of risk of disease?
3. Can these behaviours be changed?

The first question seems to be a simple one. Agreement on relevant health criteria is, however, already a problematic issue. It has recently been suggested that mortality is too crude to use as a criterion and that a combination of mortality and morbidity (including various quality of life aspects) is more suitable (Kaplan, 1984). However, many health psychologists develop interventions directed at the reduction of risk factors for mortality, as in the case of coronary heart disease. Although this is a defendable strategy, in order to make relevant contributions to health and health care on a population level there is a need for additional research which includes quality of life aspects. For example, what do we know about the relationship of various health behaviours with absence from work in patients with chronic obstructive pulmonary disease (a group of diseases responsible, according to the Dutch Asthma Fund, for about 20% of the total absence from work)? As the state of the art may show, this type of research is only in its initial stages (Kaplan, 1985).

When we turn to the other aspect of the first question (the identification of risk behaviours), it is quite clear that these so-called risk behaviours depend largely upon the health criteria used. A behavioural factor which proves to influence return to work does not necessarily relate to mortality. As such, the validity of risk factors for relevant health criteria is the main issue. In this respect we would like to plead for solid proof which, in the case of some psychological risk factors, is absent. As an example we wish to stress that the causal relationship between type A behaviour pattern and coronary heart disease, which seemed firmly established in the Western Collaborative Group Study (Rosenman et al., 1975), has recently been challenged. At present many researchers are of the opinion that the coronary risk factor could be the hostility component of the behaviour pattern and not the behaviour pattern as a whole (Maes, Van Elderen and Haarbosch, 1986). In other words, apart from many other criteria, the validity of risk factors should not only be proved in one prospective longitudinal study establishing risk over time, but be replicated in different populations and cultures before a specific behaviour (or behaviour pattern) is proclaimed as a recognized risk factor. With this information in mind, one can ask serious questions about efforts at altering type A behaviour on a population level even if there is evidence that this may be a defendable strategy for a patient population (Thoresen, Telch and Eagleston, 1981).

Another problem is associated with the assessment of relevant health behaviours (e.g. physical exercise, smoking or dietary intake). In many cases health behaviours are assessed by means of weak criterion variables, such as medical diagnosis, clinical ratings or self-reports. The overuse of self-reports contains a danger (Prokop and Bradley, 1981). It should be standard procedure that various forms of assessment of risk behaviours are used, including self-reports and more objective and observational measures. Apart from this, reliable and comparable instruments should be used in studies within one area of research. The main problem here seems to be that we are more interested in establishing possible relationships between behavioural factors and disease than we are in developing adequate measures for the assessment of these factors. Part of the conflicting evidence concerning the coronary risk of the type A behaviour pattern may be due to the fact that different measures are used in different studies for the assessment of type A.

The second question: 'Can changes in these behaviours reduce the probability of risk for these diseases?' is an even more critical one. Although the evidence showing the relationship between the restriction of alcohol consumption and automobile accidents or the beneficial effects of smoking cessation is plentiful, there is, for example, less evidence on beneficial effects of physical exercise programmes for cardiac patients or specific diets for cancer patients (WHO Report, 1982). In other words, interventions should be founded on basic studies which assess the effects of alterations in unhealthy behaviours on various outcome criteria.

The third question implies research on: (a) factors influencing the onset and the development of various health behaviours, and (b) the development of effective methods for change.

First, it is difficult to produce effective changes in relevant health behaviours without knowledge of factors that influence the onset and the course of these behaviours. As Taylor (1986) pointed out, the exact point where one should intervene to offset a developing bad habit may differ from habit to habit (e.g. smoking, lack of physical exercise, alcohol abuse, poor diet), but remains basically unknown. Must we present interventions to enhance physical exercise when a child is offered regular physical exercise at school, or much later when sluggishness may set in? If the latter is the case, when should we approach these young people? When is the best time to offer a child a smoking prevention programme: before smoking the first cigarette or, as Leventhal and Cleary (1980) suggest, after smoking the first cigarette?

An example of the possible consequences of this type of knowledge is derived from a study by Leventhal, Fleming and Glynn (1988). It was found that, apart from peer pressure, tolerance by parents is a strong predictor for the onset of smoking. Hence, almost all existing attempts in the area of smoking prevention focus mainly on children and young adolescents, and not on their parents. The same applies for prevention programmes concerning overweight and alcohol abuse in adolescent populations (Taylor, 1986). These are only a few examples. We do not even know whether different healthy or unhealthy habits and behaviours are linked, or to what degree they may influence each other (Leventhal, Prohaska and Hirschman, 1985). Answers to this type of question can, without any doubt, enhance the effectiveness of interventions. Thus it is important that health psychologists engage in this type of research.

Another aspect of the question whether relevant health behaviours can be changed is related to the existence of effective methods for behavioural change. There is much research demonstrating the effectiveness of principles and methods from operant conditioning and associative learning theories, cognitive behavioural, self-management and social learning theories (Lee and Owen, 1985). There are also, however, many criticisms that can be made in this respect, the main one being lack of basic knowledge of the process of behavioural change involved. Everyone will agree that behavioural change is a process rather than an event and that it occurs through at least three basic stages: (a) the decision to change; (b) active changing; and (c) maintenance of the new behaviour (Di Clemente and Prochaska, 1982). All existing models of behavioural change place considerable emphasis on the last phase. The reason for this is that relapse rates following behavioural change tend to be 50% or more within one year (Lee and Owen, 1985). In contrast, most interventions concentrate on the first two stages. This is because there is a lack of knowledge concerning factors and methods which may enhance the maintenance of new behaviours. In brief, one of the main targets of basic health psychology research may be to determine which methods are most effective for which stage.

We also lack knowledge on mediating factors such as cognitions and coping. Although many models (e.g. Lazarus' stress model) suggest that cognitive processes mediate behavioural change, the nature of this process remains unknown. This lack of knowledge has far-reaching consequences, of which Karoly (1985) gives a good example: 'Physicians, psychologists, nurses and other health professionals are seeking to teach their intractable or high-risk patients to think different thoughts about themselves, their bodies, their illness, their relationship with the medical system and the like. The essence of the plan is the substitution of new ideas for old ones. Although this scheme seems reasonable, it has one major drawback—it usually does not work' (p. 22).

In conclusion, what we do not know is sometimes more impressive than what we do know. The following questions, which, until now, have only poor answers may summarize the problem at hand and can be considered guidelines for future research: 'What are relevant criteria for health?' 'How can we measure quality of life?' 'On what conditions can health behaviours be considered risk behaviours for disease?' 'How can we assess relevant health behaviours in a valid and reliable way?' 'Which changes in which risk behaviours can reduce the probability of risk?' 'Which factors influence the onset and the development of relevant health behaviours?' 'Which methods for behavioural change are effective at which stage in the process?' 'What is the nature of the process of change?' and 'How can we maintain behavioural effects?'

Some Remarks on Applied Health Psychology Research

Applied health psychology research can be defined as research on the effectiveness and/or efficiency of interventions in health or illness behaviours. In terms of interventions, one can differentiate between primary prevention (directed at healthy people on a general population level or at specific risk groups in the population) and secondary prevention. Secondary prevention is usually directed towards identified groups of patients in a rehabilitation and/or community setting. If not offered to individual patients, secondary preventive interventions are usually designed for smaller groups. Stop smoking programmes for patients with CHD or COPD are a good example.

There seems to be a strange controversy throughout these preventive approaches. As can be seen from the present state of research, interventions tend to be more effective when targets become more specific and allow for interpersonal communication between the influencer and the target group (Lee and Owen, 1985). As such, many secondary preventive approaches seem to be the most effective. Nevertheless, we should remember that they contribute less to health on a population level as they are mostly designed for small groups.

Many other observations can be made with respect to existing intervention research. An important one is that published studies do not seem to meet expectancies in terms of research methodology. During the process of writing a review article on studies on psychological interventions in patients with CHD, we identified from approximately 100 studies only 17 that had made use of a control group. Studies without control groups teach us very little in terms of effects of the intervention. Most of these 17 studies made use of non-treatment control groups, or were not randomized trials, meaning that the reported effects might be due to an attention placebo effect or sampling error (Maes, Van Elderen and Bruggemans, 1987). The same applies to evaluation studies carried out without specific intervention objectives defined prior to the intervention: if there are no objectives, there is nothing to evaluate. Of the few experimental studies meeting these criteria, most only assess short-term intervention effects. The researcher may, however, make two mistakes in omitting long-term measuring points: underestimation or overestimation of the results. The former may be illustrated by a recent effect study on a health education programme for patients with coronary heart disease, where significant long-term effects were found in terms of enhancement of physical exercise and compliance with prescribed diets, but almost no short-term effects (Maes and Van Elderen, 1988). The latter may be illustrated by the fact that encouraging short-term effects were found (e.g. on medication consumption) in a comparable health education programme for asthmatic patients. These effects were, however, no longer seen after one year (Maes and Schlösser, 1988a).

Another critical observation may be that we seem to overestimate the importance of statistical significance. Statistical significance is not necessarily clinical significance, may be due to chance (the effect must be replicated) and is mostly used as an 'overall' measure of effect. This last observation deserves more comment. It seems as if we are currently asking the wrong question. The right question is most probably not 'Do people profit from an intervention?', but 'Which people profit from which type of intervention?' Thus the conclusion of effect studies should perhaps not be whether all patients profit in the same way from a specific intervention, but which patients profit (most) in which respect from which intervention. This type of research would make possible a relevant selection of patients prior to the intervention, thus enhancing the efficiency of existing interventions.

In conclusion, future applied research should: (a) pay as much attention to the efficiency as to the effectiveness of interventions; (b) learn from previous intervention studies and from basic health psychology research before developing interventions; (c) use strict methodological criteria for the design of applied studies; (d) assess short- and long-term effects; and (e) assess differential effects of different types of interventions for various subgroups in order to develop screening measures.

A POSSIBLE STRATEGY FOR THE FUTURE: LINKING BASIC AND APPLIED RESEARCH

Ideally, research in health psychology should be characterized by a strong interplay between the two branches, basic research giving answers about the components that should be influenced by intervention programmes and applied research posing questions as to the fundamental knowledge required for the designing of programmes.

One way to guarantee such interplay is to integrate basic and applied research into a single, although often multiphasic, research programme. Behind this model of working lies the idea that it is not enough to investigate health behaviour in one setting and evaluate a programme in another. Health psychology may profit from such research in a single specific setting or population.

Examples of such an approach are given in the way Leventhal, Fleming and Glynn (1988), starting from basic research concerning factors which influence the onset of smoking, developed a smoking prevention programme for children and young adolescents. Adopting a similar approach, Rosemeier and Saupe (1985) conducted basic studies on attitudes to menstruation prior to developing intervention programmes. Likewise, prior to the development of an intervention aimed at altering cognitions and coping in order to affect relevant outcomes such as the use of medication, frequency and duration of hospital stay and absence from work because of asthma, Maes and Schlösser (1988b) set up a study to identify the role of cognition and coping factors in health behaviour outcomes of asthmatic patients.

In both basic and applied health psychology research, we should also pay more attention to the broader context in which health and illness behaviour is situated. As Winett (1985) pointed out, health psychology seems to focus on individual behaviours, thus neglecting social, economic and political factors which influence these behaviours. We should never forget that many health behaviours are largely influenced by the environment, for example most forms of physical exercise require access to place, availability of time, money and social acceptance. These environmental conditions are more widespread among the upper and middle classes than among the lower social classes. Health psychology should, in other words, adopt an ecobehavioural approach in order to escape, for example, the danger of promoting survival of the fittest among the richest.

CONCLUSION

Considering what has been presented in this chapter, the reader may have got a distorted impression. The first part is indeed written from a positive point of view. It shows the relevance of health psychology research in the domain of psychophysiology or lifestyles and health, and coping with physical illness, and may demonstrate that health psychology has great potential for contributions to primary and secondary prevention of disease. The second part is written from a more critical point of view, and tries to point out some shortcomings in basic and applied health psychology research. Although many of these shortcomings may apply more to our own research than to the chapters included in this book, we considered that they might be of broader use. In any case, they may demonstrate that health psychology is in full process of development rather than being a well-established discipline with a long research tradition.

NOTES

[1]Address for correspondence: S. Maes and M. van Veldhoven, Health Psychology, Tilburg University, PO Box 90153, 5000 LE Tilburg, The Netherlands.

REFERENCES

Ader, R. (Ed.) (1981). *Psychoneuroimmunology*. New York: Academic Press.

Appels, A. (1988). Vital exhaustion as a precursor of myocardial infarction. In: Maes, S., Spielberger, C. D., Defares, P. B. and Sarason, I. G. (Eds) *Topics in Health Psychology*, pp. 31–35. Chichester: Wiley.

Baum, A., Grunberg, N. E. and Singer, J. E. (1982). The use of psychological and neuroendocrinological measurements in the study of stress. *Health Psychology*, **1**, 217–236.

Belloc, N. B. and Breslow, L. (1972). Relationship of physical health status and health practices. *Preventive Medicine*, **1**, 409–421.

Berkman, L. F. and Syme, S. L. (1979). Social networks, host resistance, and mortality: A nine year follow-up study of Alameda county residents. *American Journal of Epidemiology*, **109**, 186–204.

Breslow, L. and Enstrom, J. E. (1980). Persistence of health habits and their relationship to mortality. *Preventive Medicine*, **9**, 469–483.

Burling, T. A., Singleton, E. G., Bigelow, G. E., Baile, W. F. and Gottlieb, S. H. (1984). Smoking following myocardial infarction: A critical review of the literature. *Health Psychology*, **3**, 83–96.

Cataldo, M. F. and Coates, T. J. (1986). *Health and Industry: A Behavioral Medicine Perspective*. New York: Wiley.

Chalmers, B. E. (1981). A selective review of stress: Some cognitive approaches taken a step further. *Current Psychological Review*, **1**, 325–344.

Di Clemente, C. C. and Prochaska, J. O. (1982). Self-change and therapy change of smoking behaviour: A comparison of processes of change in cessation and maintenance. *Addictive Behaviors*, **7**, 133–142.

Di Matteo, M. R. and Di Nicola, D. D. (1982). *Achieving Patient Compliance*. New York: Pergamon.

Feuerstein, M., Labbé, E. E. and Kuczmierczyk, A. R. (1986). *Health Psychology: A Psychobiological Perspective*. New York: Plenum.

Fox, B. H. (1982). Endogenous psychosocial factors in cross-national cancer incidence. In: Eiser, J. R. (Ed.) *Social Psychology and Behavioural Medicine*. Chichester: Wiley, pp. 104–141.

Kaplan, R. M. (1984). The connection between clinical health promotion and health status. *American Psychologist*, **39**, 755–765.

Kaplan, R. M. (1985). Quality-of-life measurement. In: Karoly, P. (Ed.) *Measurement Strategies in Health Psychology*. New York: Wiley.

Karoly, P. (1985). The logic and character of assessment in health psychology: Perspectives and possibilities. In: Karoly, P. (Ed.) *Measurement Strategies in Health Psychology*. New York: Wiley, pp. 3–45.

Kiecolt-Glaser, J. K., Garner, W., Speicher, C., Penn, G. M., Holiday, J. and Glaser, R. (1984). Psychosocial modifiers of immunocompetence in medical students. *Psychosomatic Medicine*, **46**, 7–14.

Kittel, F. (1986). Type A and other psychosocial factors in relation to coronary heart disease. In: Schmidt, T. H., Dembroski, T. M. and Blümchen, G. (Eds) *Biological and Psychological Factors in Cardiovascular Disease*. Heidelberg: Springer Verlag, pp. 63–84.

Kornitzer, M. (1987). Controlled trials in cardiovascular diseases: Some lessons for chronic non-communicable disease control. In: Leparski, E. (Ed.) *The Prevention of Non-Communicable Diseases: Experiences and Prospects*. Copenhagen: WHO, pp. 123–149.

Krantz, D. S., Grunberg, N. E. and Baum, A. (1985). Health psychology. *Annual Review of Psychology*, **36**, 349–383.

Lee, C. and Owen, N. (1985). Behaviourally-based principles as guidelines for health promotion. *Community Health Studies*, **9**, 131–138.

Leventhal, H. and Cleary, P. D. (1980). The smoking problem: A review of the research and theory in behavioural risk modification. *Psychological Bulletin*, **88**, 370–405.

Leventhal, H., Fleming, R. and Glynn, K. (1988). A cognitive-developmental approach to smoking intervention. In Maes, S., Spielberger, C. D., Defares, P. B. and Sarason, I. G. (Eds) *Topics in Health Psychology*, pp. 79–105. Chichester: Wiley.

Leventhal, H., Prohaska, T. R. and Hirschman, R. S. (1985). Preventive health behavior across the life span. In: Rosen, J. and Solomon, L. (Eds) *Prevention in Health Psychology*. New York: University Press of New England.

Ley, Ph. (1979). Giving information to patients. In: Eiser, J. R. (Ed.) *Social Psychology and Behavioral Medicine*. New York: Wiley, pp. 339–373.

Ley, Ph. (1982). Satisfaction, compliance and communication. *British Journal of Clinical Psychology*, **21**, 241–254.

Lichtenstein, E. and Brown, R. A. (1981). Smoking cessation methods: Review and recommendations. In: Miller, W. R. (Ed.) *The Addictive Behaviors*. New York: Pergamon.

Lyons, A. S. and Petrucelli, R. J. (1978). *Medicine, an Illustrated History*, New York: Abrams.

Maes, S. and Schlösser, M. (1987). The role of cognition and coping in health behavior outcomes of asthmatic patients. *Current Psychological Research and Reviews*, **6**, 79–90.

Maes, S. and Schlösser, M. (1988a). Changing health behaviour outcomes in asthmatic patients: A pilot intervention study. *Social Science & Medicine*, **26**, 359–364.

Maes, S. and Schlösser, M. (1988b). The cognitive management of health behaviour outcomes in asthmatic patients. In Maes, S., Spielberger, C., Defares, P. and Sarason, I. G. (Eds) *Topics in Health Psychology*, pp. 171–189. Chichester: Wiley.

Maes, S. and Van Elderen, T. (1988). Effects of psycho-educational programmes in cardiac rehabilitation. *Dutch Journal of Cardiology*, **1**, 30.

Maes, S., Van Elderen, T. and Bruggemans, E. (1987). Effecten van voorlichting aan coronaire hartpatiënten, een literatuuroverzicht. *Gezondheid en Samenleving*, **8**, 60–76.

Maes, S., Van Elderen, T. and Haarbosch, J. (1986). De invloed van rationeel-emotieve groepstherapie op woede en Type-A gedrag. *Gedrag & Gezondheid*, **14**, 27–35.

Maes, S., Vingerhoets, A. and Van Heck, G. (1987). The study of stress and disease: Some developments and requirements. *Social Science and Medicine*, **25**, 567–578.

Martin, J. E. and Dubbert, P. M. (1982). Exercise applications and promotion in behavioural medicine: Current status and future directions. *Journal of Consulting and Clinical Psychology*, **6**, 1004–1017.

Matarazzo, J. D. (1980). Behavioral health and behavioral medicine, frontiers of a new health psychology. *American Psychologist*, **35**, 807–817.

Matarazzo, J. D., Weiss, S. M., Herd, J. A., Miller, N. E. and Weiss, S. M. (1984). *Behavioral Health; A Handbook of Health Enhancement and Disease Prevention*. New York: Wiley.

Millon, T. (1982). On the nature of clinical health psychology. In: Millon, T., Green, D. and Meagher, R. (Eds) *Handbook of Clinical Health Psychology*. New York: Plenum, pp. 1–27.

Prokop, C. K. and Bradley, L. A. (1981). *Medical Psychology: Contributions to Behavioural Medicine*. New York: Academic Press.

Puska, P. (1984). Community-based prevention of cardiovascular disease: The North Karelia Project. In: Matarazzo, J. D., Weiss, S. M., Herd, J . A., Miller, N. E. and Weiss, S. M. (Eds) *Behavioural Health: A Handbook of Health Enhancement and Disease Prevention*. New York: Wiley, pp. 1140–1147.

Rosemeier, H. P. and Saupe, R. (1985). The Berlin study on female attitudes towards menstruation. In: Sanchez-Sosa, S. S. (Ed.) *Health and Clinical Psychology*. Amsterdam; North-Holland.

Rosenman, R. H., Jenkins, C. D., Brand, R. J., Friedman, M., Straus, R. and Wurm, M. (1975). Coronary heart disease in the Western Collaborative Group Study: Final follow-up experience of 8.5 years. *JAMA*, **233**, 872–877.

Roth, S. and Cohen, L. S. (1986). Approach–avoidance and coping with stress. *American Psychologist*, **41**, 813–819.

Sackett, D. L. and Snow, J. C. (1979). The magnitude of compliance and non-compliance. In: Haynes, R. B., Taylor, D. W. and Sackett, D. L. (Eds) *Compliance in Health Care*. Baltimore: Johns Hopkins Press.

Schmidt, L. (1984). *Psychologie in der Medizin*. Stuttgart: Thieme.

Schoenborn, C. A. (1986). Health habits of US adults, 1985; The 'Alameda 7' revisited. *Public Health Reports*, **101**, 571–580.

Shirrefs, J. H. (1982). *Community Health: Contemporary Perspectives*. Englewood Cliffs: Prentice-Hall.

Stone, G. C., Cohen, F. and Adler, N. E. (1979). *Health Psychology—A Handbook*. San Francisco: Jossey Bass.

Taylor, S. E. (1986). *Health Psychology*. New York: Random House.

Thoresen, C. E., Telch, M. J. and Eagleston, J. R. (1981). Approaches to altering the type A behaviour pattern. *The Journal of the Academy of Psychosomatic Medicine*, **22**, 472–479.

WHO Report (1982). *Prevention of Coronary Heart Disease*. Geneva: World Health Organization.

Wieglosz, A. T., Fletcher, R. H., McCants, C. B., McKinnis, R. A., Haney, T. L. and Williams, R. B. (1984). Unimproved chest pain in patients with minimal or no coronary disease: A behavioral phenomenon. *American Heart Journal*, **108**, 67–72.

Winett, R. A. (1985). Ecobehavioural assessment in health life-styles: Concepts and methods. In: Karoly, P. (Ed.) *Measurement Strategies in Health Psychology*. New York: Wiley, pp. 147–181.

Part 2

Behavioural Medicine—Applications

CHAPTER 4

Chronic Pain

N. H. Groenman[1]

Limburg University, Maastricht; Academic Hospital Maastricht, Maastricht

J. W. S. Vlaeyen

Limburg University, Maastricht; Institute for Rehabilitation Research, Hoensbroek

H. van Eek

Rehabilitation Center Hoensbroek, Hoensbroek

and

J. A. Schuerman

Limburg University, Maastricht; Lucas Foundation for Rehabilitation, Hoensbroek; Rehabilitation Center Hoensbroek, Hoensbroek

ABSTRACT

Chronic pain is conceptualized on the basis of a theoretical model in which nociception, the sensation of pain, suffering, and pain behaviour form four elements. Acute pain, experimental pain and clinical pain are distinguished, and epidemiological data on the incidence and prevalence of chronic pain are presented. The stimulus—organism—response—consequence scheme is applied to a case study in which the assessment phase is elaborated upon. The treatment of a patient with chronic low back pain illustrates the value of a behavioural medicine approach. Also, respondent techniques and cognitive approaches to chronic pain are described. In a review of evaluation studies on behavioural treatment of pain, the authors conclude that pain behaviour modification programmes, conducted on an inpatient or outpatient basis, are an effective extension of the therapeutic arsenal of behavioural medicine.

Behavioural Medicine
Edited by A. A. Kaptein, H. M. van der Ploeg, B. Garssen, P. J. G. Schreurs and R. Beunderman
© 1990 John Wiley & Sons Ltd.

INTRODUCTION

The International Association for the Study of Pain (IASP) defines pain as 'an unpleasant sensory and emotional experience associated with actual and potential tissue damage, or described in terms of such damage' (1979, p. 250). Pain, according to this definition, has both a sensory (physiological) and an emotional side to it. Both are important. The distinction that was once made between organic (real) and psychogenic (imaginary) pain is no longer considered relevant. Only in cases where pain symptoms are deliberately simulated can one speak of imaginary pain. Such cases are, however, quite rare.

Fordyce (1987) uses the following psychophysiological phenomenon to illustrate the irrelevance of distinguishing between the two types of pain referred to above. 'Imagine that you have not eaten for a long time. Someone happens to start talking about one of your favourite meals. What happens? Your mouth begins to water. Yet, there is no food. Is the saliva real or imaginary? Naturally, it is real. A physiological process—in this case, salivation—can be set off just by thinking about food. With pain, the same phenomenon can occur.' Fordyce thus describes the classical conditioning paradigm, which is based on the experimental work of Pavlov.

Not every pain scientist agrees with the IASP definition. Booy (1984) for one makes a distinction between real pain and psychogenic pain, the latter consisting of various forms of misery which the patient experiences as pain and then labels as such. According to Booy, a somatic cause can always be found for real pain; the ultimate criterion for determining whether or not there is pain is the presence of a somatic cause and not pain behaviour.

These authors agree with the IASP definition. Loeser and Fordyce's definition (1983) fits our conceptual framework even better. Because this definition is

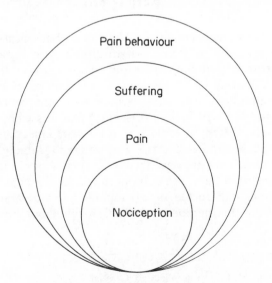

Figure 4.1. Loeser's concept of pain

included in that of the IASP, there can be no objections to it. Loeser's model is graphically represented by four concentric circles (see Figure 4.1). The smallest circle represents *nociception* and indicates that aspect of pain for which a physiological explanation is possible. The second circle represents (*the sensation of*) *pain*, that is, the registering of the nociception by the central nervous system. In order for a pain stimulus to be experienced, the boundary between nociception and perception must be crossed. A person does not remain emotionally aloof when experiencing pain; pain leads to *suffering*, represented by Loeser's third circle. If a person who is experiencing pain does not communicate this in some way to others, then he and he alone will be aware that a pain problem exists. In other words, pain needs to be communicated in order for others to become aware of its existence. This pain communication is what Loeser calls '*pain behaviour*' (his fourth and largest circle). According to his definition, pain behaviour includes grimacing, moaning, sweating, crying, taking sick leave from work and staying in bed. In other words, any and all behaviour that suggests the existence of pain is called pain behaviour. The dimensions and components of observed pain behaviour have been recently examined by Vlaeyen *et al.* (1987). As pain is described as a form of behaviour, it is only logical then that one would try to apply what is known about the onset, development and continuation of behaviour in general to the phenomenon of pain in particular.

EXPERIMENTAL PAIN AND CLINICAL PAIN

A distinction needs to be made between experimental pain and clinical pain. Experimental pain refers to pain reported by subjects undergoing laboratory experiments. What is experienced as pain in the laboratory cannot necessarily be generalized to the pain which occurs in clinical situations. A clinical situation can be an inpatient or an outpatient facility. Clinical pain can be broken down into three categories: acute pain, chronic benign pain and chronic malignant pain.

Acute pain is caused by tissue damage (as in the case of infection, inflammation, surgery or burns) and is characterized by a relatively isomorphic relationship between the nociceptive stimulus and the pain behaviour. The most important aspect of acute pain is that which arises in an emergency situation, with the concomitant psychophysiological changes (increases in blood pressure, heart and respiratory frequency, pupil dilatation) which are similar to those of anxiety attacks. The pain experience in the acute phase is dominated by anxiety, not only because of the pain itself, but also because of the attribution the individual assigns to the pain felt. Beecher (1959) reported that wounded soldiers at the Anzio Front (Italy) requested fewer analgesics than a comparable group of civilians with surgical wounds in a civilian hospital. For the soldiers pain meant evacuation from an extremely dangerous front, thus relief from suffering, something positive. The civilians could only attach a negative meaning to the pain. Anxiety-reducing techniques, such as relaxation, reassurance and feedback on what is happening, often result in patients reporting less pain.

When dealing with acute pain, somatic-oriented treatments tend to produce good results. A fast, effective treatment for acute pain is the best strategy against the development of chronic pain.

Chronic pain is different from long-standing acute pain (Aronoff, 1985). A rule of thumb is that any pain which lasts for more than six months can be considered chronic. Some researchers, however, such as Schmidt (1986) do not agree; to them any pain which lasts longer than the expected healing time can be called chronic. With chronic pain, the role of nociception is seldom demonstrable. Moreover, not only do neural mechanisms appear to be far more complex in this situation than in acute pain, but the psychological and social variables involved also show a more complex pattern of interactions. This in itself is not surprising. The long duration of the complaint makes it possible to repeat certain learning processes, something which, in the long run, develops into a negative spiral. Clinical experience shows that the duration of the complaint is inversely proportional to the chance of a successful treatment. How these learning processes can be responsible for the maintenance of pain behaviour will be discussed later. In the case of chronic pain, the pattern of suffering is characterized by a depressive mood. Chronic pain patients are almost always depressed although they do not always complain about it. The depression is sometimes masked by preoccupation with somatic symptoms. Whereas a relationship between chronic pain and depression has often been observed, the source, strength, and nature of the linkage between these two conditions remains not very well understood (Romano and Turner, 1985).

Chronic malignant pain contains elements of both acute and chronic pain. There seem to be not unimportant differences between chronic malignant pain, chronic benign pain and acute pain. Despite the paucity of studies on this subject, the following comments seem to be warranted. In the case of cancer pain—in contrast with chronic benign pain and acute pain—personality factors do play an inconsistent role in the modulation of pain, there is only a weak association between social network and pain intensity, and between affective state and pain only a minimal relationship exists (Dalton and Feuerstein, 1988; Cohen *et al.*, 1985; Foley, 1985).

SOME EPIDEMIOLOGICAL DATA ON CHRONIC PAIN

Haanen (1984) carried out an epidemiological study on chronic low back pain in The Netherlands. On the basis of a literature survey, he concludes that the annual incidence of chronic low back pain is around 20%. Furthermore, he concludes that between 50 and 60% of the population at large at some time suffer from low back pain. In 90% of the cases complaints disappear spontaneously after three weeks. Haanen's data concern the Dutch situation. In the USA according to Deyo (1983), almost 80% of all adults suffer from low back pain some time during their lives. On the basis of his study Haanen concludes that at the time of his interview, 25% actually did have such complaints. One-third of the group which had had low back pain at some time in the past were unable to continue with their work and 10% had to leave their jobs for more than six months.

Bonica (1985) estimates that in the USA more than 86 million people suffer from some type of chronic pain. According to Clark, Gosnell and Shapiro (1977), more than eight million Americans were disabled by chronic low back pain in 1977. Seres (1985) estimated that $11 billion in income is lost annually in the USA because of work disability, a significant amount of which is caused by chronic pain. Turk, Meichenbaum and Genest find that in excess of $900 million is spent each year on over-the-counter medications for pain (Turk, Meichenbaum and Genest, 1983). Anderson, Hegstrum and Charboneau (1985) conclude that pain is one of the most complex and most expensive problems of modern medicine.

CHRONIC PAIN AS LEARNED BEHAVIOUR

Pain behaviour can be maintained even after the original tissue damage has healed. How is this to be explained? One way to represent the relationship between environment and behaviour is by constructing a stimulus, organism, response, and consequence (SORC) scheme (see Figure 4.2). When the SORC scheme is applied to pain, the latter is seen as a response following diverse stimuli (e.g. a physical trauma) to a specific organism (e.g. a depressed patient), leading to certain consequences (e.g. increased attention from the spouse).

Fordyce (1976) assumes that pain behaviour which in the acute phase is determined largely by nociceptive stimuli can eventually come to be controlled by the consequences in the chronic phase. He claims that this is operant pain

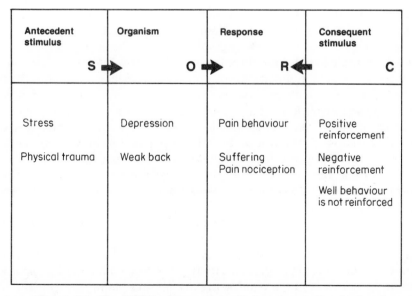

Figure 4.2. The SORC scheme as applied to chronic low back pain

and describes three ways in which pain can become operant:

1. First, pain behaviour can be positively reinforced. Examples of positive reinforcers include resting in bed, taking medication, receiving attention from one's physician and family members and, in certain cases, receiving financial benefits. The prescription of pain medication on a pain-contingent basis (i.e. 'take when necessary') means creating a situation in which the patient has to display pain behaviour in order to receive the medication, which is often positively experienced. Medication thus becomes contingent upon pain behaviour, which then becomes positively reinforced. Advising the patient to 'rest when it hurts' promotes chronicity in the same way.
2. Pain behaviour can also be negatively reinforced. Negative reinforcement occurs when the consequences of pain behaviour are such that unpleasant situations are avoided. All activities associated with immediate pain decrease are negative reinforcers. By resting or staying in bed, conflicts at work, feared personal confrontations or the need to assume responsibilities can be avoided. Cosyns and Vlaeyen (1984) present a case study in which pain behaviour was maintained so that a marital conflict between the patient and her spouse could be avoided. In elderly people, pain behaviour can serve as a way of avoiding situations which become difficult to handle due to cognitive deficiencies.
3. A third possibility is that 'well behaviour' is not reinforced any more. When a patient wants to undertake some activity, his social environment can hamper him by stressing his unhealthy condition. Activities and responsibilities are taken over by well-meaning family members. The patient is encouraged to take his medicine, to rest in bed, to consult his doctor and in no way to overexert himself. The resumption of activities by the patient sometimes becomes inconvenient for family members, who, for whatever reason, are not willing to assume their previous family roles.

It is worth noting that with chronic pain, as opposed to acute pain, stimuli other than the original traumatic ones can elicit pain behaviour. Such situations resemble those in which positive or negative reinforcement has frequently occurred. As an illustration, let us consider a patient with chronic low back pain whose pain had followed a rather erratic course. Pain peaks occurred most often in the evenings and during the weekend. It appeared to be very unlikely that nociception was responsible for this course. Behaviour analysis revealed that the spouse, who had become very supportive after the onset of the pain, was a significant positive reinforcer for the patient behaviour. The spouse's presence in the evenings and during weekends became a stimulus which systematically elicited pain behaviour (Vlaeyen, Groenman and Legrelle, 1987). Clinicians need to be aware of this phenomenon, for their presence can elicit pain behaviour through pain-reinforcing interventions such as repeated diagnostic procedures, prescriptions for other types of medication, referrals to other medical specialists and even the advice 'call me when you have a lot of pain'.

The factors mentioned in the SORC scheme influence each other. Inactivity leads to muscle disuse and a deterioration of one's overall condition. Activities which were once performed with relative ease become more difficult and lead to new nociception, giving yet another reason to avoid activity.

Pain behaviour also has long-term consequences. The increasing inactivity and pain give rise to a feeling of powerlessness. Patients see their future as bleak and they become depressed. A decreased level of activity deprives patients of daily reinforcers (social contact, leisure activities, work, etc.) and this may lead to depression (Lewinsohn, 1974). In short, the interaction of various factors causes the pain problem to grow worse. As in a spiral movement, the existing components are reinforced. Inactivity increases. The patient feels his condition deteriorating. The label 'serious illness' is used. Anticipation anxiety increases. Still more activities are avoided. Increasing pain behaviour is further reinforced by the environment and a depressive mood takes hold of the patient. He finds himself caught in the deadlock of the chronic pain syndrome.

ASSESSMENT

Chronic pain is difficult to treat (Bonica, 1985). In most cases, somatic and traditional approaches have met with little, if any, success. Chronic pain behaviour is often accompanied by other significant behaviour problems. Not only do depression and anxiety occur regularly with chronic pain, but also unresolved mourning, obsessive compulsiveness, phobias and lack of assertiveness (Turk, Meichenbaum and Genest, 1983). What is clear is that the assessment phase is of crucial importance. Not only does it reveal essential information about the complexity of the individual chronic pain problem, but it also provides the necessary clues to a coherent tailor-made treatment programme (Turk and Rudy, 1987; Bradley, 1988).

The assessment phase in the case of chronic pain consists of three components:

- The history-taking,
- The behavioural analysis, and, if necessary,
- Psychological tests (Fordyce, 1979; Karoly, 1985).

Each of these components reveals information that brings one closer to answering the key question: 'Which factors maintain pain behaviour?'

The phase of history-taking is primarily concerned with the nature of the complaint, how it has been treated in the past, the patient's thoughts and feelings about both his pain complaint and past treatment, as well as the life history of the patient, his social circumstances and vocational background. The purpose of this part of the assessment is to gain some insight into the background of the patient and this is achieved by approaching the patient in an open, empathic way using a non-directive interview. Special attention is focused on the following:

- The patient's family (illness) history, in order to find out whether the complaints may be considered a type of learned behaviour. That is to say, is the patient simply imitating his parents' way of coping with psychosocial stressors by means of bodily complaints?
- The history of the complaint, in order to discover whether the illness behaviour has been reinforced and whether its frequency has gradually increased; and
- Any traumatic life events which coincide with the onset of the complaints.

The behavioural analysis (Fordyce, 1976) consists of a number of directed, closed questions to which the patient must react with a short answer. In this behavioural analysis the psychologist is directed towards the complaint pattern in daily life through such questions as: 'How does your wife know when you are in pain?', 'What does she do then?', 'Does your wife notice that you are awake at night?', 'How do you know that?'. This way of analysing behaviour is, in fact, a systematic way of looking for relationships between behavioural stimuli and pain. The same analysis is repeated with the spouse. This repetition is important, because the spouse often sees different behavioural connections from the patient himself.

Another source of information is the so-called 'activity diary'. This diary, originally developed by Fordyce (1976), is kept by the patient for a period of three to seven days. By this means the patient is monitoring his activities on an hourly basis.

The psychodiagnostic assessment leads to a psychological report. A number of sentences have been taken from one such report and are presented here as an illustration:

> The patient is a 36-year-old married plumber who complains of sharp chronic low back pain, radiating into his left leg. Walking is quite difficult and as a consequence, he has had to use crutches for quite a long time. The patient is completely disabled. It is no longer possible for him to do his job. He depends on social security disability income. A somatic cause for his pain has not been found, in spite of intensive neurological and orthopaedic examinations. Several treatments, including pharmacotherapy, physiotherapy, massage, epidural blocks and rest, have had no lasting effects. Painkillers have not helped either. At the age of 18, the patient had back pain problems for the first time. Between his nineteenth and twenty-fifth years the pain abated. During the last four years, his complaints have become more severe. The patient had been planning to take over the family plumbing business. Yet, in the end, he decided against it. It would simply have been too much for him to take on. The patient is intellectually gifted (IQ = 131). His personality is that of a depressive, tense, highly achievement-oriented, rigid and shy person. He severely lacks interpersonal skills. He is very dependent on other people. He avoids expression of his feelings.

The data on this patient fit into the SORC scheme as follows:

S: (Avoided) situations are those which call for social contact or in which assertiveness and autonomy are to be expressed. Some examples of these situations are contact with his family, the presence of his spouse, sexuality, financial management, taking the initiative and giving guidance.

O: The various tests and interviews portray a person who is strongly achievement-oriented and who pursues his goal in a rather rigid way. In connection with this, there have in the past been a number of failures, something which was not, or could not be, verbalized. This resulted in a lack of assertiveness, depression and an increasing level of tension. In the course of time, the patient found that having and exhibiting back problems could mean a temporary escape from the various situations described above.

R: Partly as a result of the learning experience referred to above (i.e. that pain can mean a temporary escape from stress), a chronic immobilization has developed which takes various forms: walking with crutches, lying down frequently for long periods of time, feeling that the left leg is completely paralysed. An appeal is made to the social environment verbally and regularly to acknowledge this immobilization.

C: The immediate consequence of both the verbal and non-verbal pain behaviour is the avoidance of all tension-producing stimuli. The negative long-term consequence, however, is the continuation of what has already become a rather established personality structure, characterized by depression, lack of social skills and a gradually increasing social isolation.

The conclusion is drawn that over a number of years this man has learned that pain behaviour makes it possible for him to avoid situations in which assertiveness is required. His pain can be considered as largely operant in character.

One possible treatment that can be administered by a clinician (physician or clinical psychologist) includes:

1. Antidepressive medication, in combination with counselling focused on the depression;
2. Training in assertiveness and social skills; and
3. The prescription of time-contingent medication and the gradual reduction of analgesics.

Although these treatment aims are justified, one important problem still remains: the pain behaviour itself. It is unrealistic to expect a person who has been using crutches for more than five years to develop a normal pattern of walking on his own. This well behaviour will have to be relearned by way of a behaviour modification programme. Although some clinicians claim that such a programme can be done on an outpatient basis (Roberts, 1986), it seems that the best results are achieved in a clinical inpatient setting.

THE OPERANT TREATMENT OF CHRONIC PAIN—CHRONIC LOW BACK PAIN AS AN EXAMPLE

For the sake of clarity and brevity, the discussion of the treatment of chronic pain is confined to a description of the operant treatment of chronic low back pain. This type of treatment is well documented in literature (Linton, 1986; Fordyce, Roberts and Sternbach, 1985; Fordyce, 1988). Critical treatment outcome studies on this subject will be dealt with in a section to follow.

The treatment programme for the case study described above consists of the following components:

- Extinction of the verbal and non-verbal pain behaviour
- Increase in the activity level
- Exploration of new leisure activities
- Supportive contacts with the spouse
- Involvement of the general practitioner

One hopes that by treating the overt pain behaviour, changes will occur that will cause pain cognitions, muscular tension, depression and lack of social skills to become reduced. If such changes are not demonstrated by continuous measurements, further treatment for these problems is indicated. In order to evaluate the treatment effect on pain behaviour as well as on other problems, various measurements are taken before, during and after the treatment.

Extinction of the Verbal and Non-verbal Pain Behaviour

The approach used here with this intelligent, non-assertive man has appeared to work well. He has been told that he may talk about his pain complaints if he feels the need to, but that the staff will not pay any attention to it. After three days this problem behaviour is no longer observed.

Increase in the Activity Level

The irregular pattern of walking is chosen as the most direct relevant pain behaviour of the patient. By means of a 'shaping' procedure (i.e. the step-by-step relearning of behaviour which no longer belongs to the patient's behaviour repertoire), normal walking (without crutches) is relearned. In the first phase, a baseline walking distance is established. Then, the patient is provided with a wheelchair and asked to use it during treatment except when doing physical therapy. In this way, the old, unhealthy walking pattern cannot be maintained. The gait-retraining programme consists of 17 steps which gradually take the patient out of the wheelchair and to the point where he can again resume a normal gait. This procedure is described in detail by Fordyce (1976). A very important aspect of this approach is that the patient is asked to perform only those activities which he is capable of doing. Throughout this training programme attention is given to the general improvement of the patient's physical condition.

Leisure Time

During the treatment, a programme is designed to provide the patient with a structured and full day. Therapist and patient together plan ways in which the patient, once he has been discharged, will be able to further increase the distance or time he can walk, bicycle, swim, etc.

Supportive Contacts With the Spouse

The ideal situation is one in which the spouse continuously reinforces newly learned well behaviour in the same way as the team of therapists, that is, through the extinction of pain behaviour and the reinforcement of realistic motor achievements. The spouse is given the opportunity to change her behaviour in this direction through regular contacts with the psychologist. Practical considerations, however, such as travel time, child care and vacations often present obstacles to achieving this goal. Consequently, attempts at behaviour modification are often limited to talks, during which information and insight are passed on to the spouse.

Involvement of the General Practitioner

It is still not completely clear just what the role of the general practitioner is in the treatment of chronic pain. However, in our opinion, he assumes a central position after discharge of the patient, at which time he supports the results achieved during the clinical treatment programme. The results of the assessment procedure are discussed with him in order to establish what course of action is to be followed. Patient and practitioner also agree that:

1. Home visits will be planned at fixed intervals, irrespective of pain decreases or increases;
2. Increased activity, in the form of leisure activities, will receive the general practitioner's full attention; and
3. The general practitioner will help and encourage the spouse with regard to her changed attitude towards the patient.

Results

The patient came in on crutches and left the treatment centre on a bicycle. The goal was achieved after an inpatient rehabilitation programme of eight weeks. The treatment period was both preceded and followed by a period of six weeks, during which measurements of all relevant problems and aspects of pain behaviour were taken every two weeks. Six weeks after the treatment period, the following observations were made:

- Even after discharge, activities (walking, swimming, bicycling) continue to increase;
- Verbal and non-verbal pain behaviours have not reoccurred;
- Lack of social skills, depression, preoccupation with physical symptoms and intake of medication have decreased slightly.

RESPONDENT TECHNIQUES

Chronic pain can also be controlled by antecedent factors. Viewed like this, the classic conditioning paradigm comes into play. In the course of time patients with chronic pain may have become entangled in a vicious circle of pain–anxiety–pain. In the acute stage pain is associated with fear and the enhanced arousal that goes with it (increased muscular tension, heart rate, respiration, etc.). When the painful event is repeated a number of times, situations related to the original pain situation will provoke the cluster anxiety, pain perception and pain behaviour, *via* classical conditioning. This leads to a continuous or frequent elevation of the arousal level, even when there is no longer any tissue damage at all. Moreover, increased muscular tension causes renewed nociceptive stimulation, which in turn feeds the pain problem. From this point of view, chronic pain can be treated by breaking through the vicious circle. This can be done by teaching the patient a 'relaxation response' (Benson, 1975) incompatible with an elevated arousal level. During treatment this relaxation response is systematically coupled to diverse pain-provoking stimuli. This procedure is known as systematic desensitization. The relaxation response can be acquired by means of progressive relaxation (Jacobson, 1938) or autogenic training (Schultz and Luthe, 1959).

THE COGNITIVE APPROACH

Adherents of the cognitive approach assume that behaviour is mainly determined by the way in which events are experienced and by the meaning attributed to them. Under the influence of continuously repeated learning processes all sorts of false and unadapted 'cognitions' come about, which eventually maintain all sorts of emotional and behavioural disturbances. There is, however, much confusion about the concept of 'cognition' so that widely divergent definitions like 'attitudes, beliefs and expectancies' (Turner and Chapman, 1982), 'things inside the head, private events' (Jaremko, 1978) or 'appraisal of the environment, expectancies and ideas' (Tan, 1982) are encountered in the literature. The cognitive approach to pain aims at a reevaluation of the pain sensation and strives for a feeling of self-control over the pain. Holzman, Turk and Kerns (1986) go so far as to include in the cognitive treatment all the techniques that help the patient to attain this goal. Thus, for the individual treatment divergent procedures are available, for example relaxation exercises, biofeedback, self-hypnosis, assertiveness training, diversion of attention, and thought stop, besides operant manipulation and family treatment. In general, cognitive treatment is carried out on an outpatient basis, which minimizes the cost, increases the chance of generalization of the results and facilitates quick testing in real life of the things learned. At the moment, the cognitive treatment of chronic pain enjoys great popularity and has been found practicable in clinical practice (Linton, 1986). Because of the confusion of concepts, however, it is difficult to determine which ingredients are effective.

EVALUATION

In this section, the results of recent research on the psychological treatment of chronic pain will be discussed. For the sake of brevity, only four evaluation studies regarding the effectiveness of pain behaviour modification programmes are mentioned. These studies have been chosen because of their high methodological quality, which is lacking in many others. For more extensive reviews, the reader is referred to Aronoff, Evans and Enders (1983) and Fordyce, Roberts and Sternbach (1985).

The study which prompted a series of approximately 30 evaluation studies is that of Fordyce *et al.* (1973). These researchers describe 36 single case studies. After a mean follow-up period of 22 months, all patients appeared to be considerably more active than they were prior to treatment and exhibited fewer movement restrictions. Cairns *et al.* (1976), in a second study, report that 10 months after termination of their modification programme, 74% of their patients no longer sought any contact with the health care system for the relief of pain. A third study, that of Anderson *et al.* (1977), states that after termination of treatment, 74% of the patients treated appeared to be living a 'normal' life. The follow-up period in this case ranged from six months to seven years. Finally, Roberts and Reinhardt (1980) compare 26 chronic pain patients who were treated in a clinical operant pain programme with 20 patients who, for various reasons, were turned down by the staff and 12 patients who were accepted but later decided not to enter the programme. Of the 26 patients who were treated, 77% led a 'normal' life after treatment; by contrast, this was the case in only one of the 32 untreated patients. Follick, Zitter and Ahern (1983), by focusing their attention on treatment failures, attempt to gain insight into the effectiveness of the pain behaviour modification programmes. They come to the conclusion that approximately 30% of all chronic pain patients do not show any improvement with such a programme. As in the above-mentioned studies, Follick *et al.*'s (1983) review concerns patients who, prior to treatment, were seriously disabled, both somatically and socially. They all had an extensive medical history.

The maintenance and generalization of results have been closely examined by most researchers. What happens to the pain behaviour when the patient returns home? Linton (1986) searches the literature for an answer to this question and concludes that patients resort back to pain behaviour only relatively rarely. The attained therapeutic gain is maintained in most of the cases.

From a review of the literature, it is generally accepted that the clinical pain behaviour modification programme, conducted on an inpatient or outpatient basis, is an effective extension of the therapeutic arsenal. Linton (1986) presents a comparable conclusion, stating that the operant variant is effective in increasing activity levels and decreasing the intake of medication. He goes on to say that the operant programme is apparently also effective in improving the patient's mood and in decreasing the reported pain level.

Turk, Meichenbaum and Genest (1983) do not agree with this last statement. According to them, patients learn to tolerate pain—the experienced pain intensity does not change.

Fordyce, Roberts and Sternbach (1985) react to this criticism by stating that pain behaviour modification programmes are aimed at improving the patient's ability to function in daily life; they are not meant to directly modify the pain experience itself. It is our opinion that whether it is the pain itself or its behavioural expressions that need to be treated is a question of semantics rather than one of substance. Pain, whether expressed overtly or covertly, is regarded as a form of behaviour. Thus, pain behaviour modification programmes are behaviour-oriented.

CONCLUSIONS

What has been discussed here are diagnostic procedures and one treatment modality for chronic low back pain. Treatment modalities for chronic pain such as relaxation, cognitive behavioural programmes and so-called 'back schools' are not mentioned or only sketchily. This chapter was not intended, as mentioned in the opening sentences, to function as an overview of all the possible behavioural endowments to the treatment of chronic pain: the example of the operant approach to chronic low back pain is used to illustrate the contribution of the behavioural-oriented clinical psychologist to patients with chronic pain.

NOTES

[1]Addresses for correspondence: N. H. Groenman, J. W. S. Vlaeyen and J. A. Schuerman, Department of Medical Psychology, Limburg University, PO Box 616, 6200 MD Maastricht, The Netherlands; H. van Eek, Rehabilitation Center Hoensbroek, 6432 CC Hoensbroek, The Netherlands.

REFERENCES

Anderson, E. F., Hegstrum, J. A. and Charboneau, G. J. (1985). Multidisciplinary management of patients with chronic low back pain. *Clinical Journal of Pain*, 1, 85–90.
Anderson, T. P., Cole, T. P., Gulickson, G., Hudgens, A. and Roberts, A. H. (1977). Behavior modification of chronic pain: A treatment program by a multidisciplinary team. *Clinical Journal of Orthopedics and Related Research*, 129, 96–100.
Aronoff, G. M. (1985). Editorial. *Clinical Journal of Pain*, 1, 1–13.
Aronoff, G. M., Evans, W. O. and Enders, P. L. (1983). A review of follow-up studies of multidisciplinary pain units. *Pain*, 16, 1–11.
Beecher, H. K. (1959). Relationship as significance of wound to the pain experienced. *Journal of the American Medical Association*, 161, 1609–1613.
Benson, H. (1975). *The Relaxation Response*. New York: Morrow.
Bonica, J. J. (1985). Introduction. In: Aronoff, G. M. (Ed.) *Evaluation and Treatment of Chronic Pain*. Baltimore–München: Urban and Schwarzenberg, pp. xxxi–xliv.
Booy, L. H. D. J. (1984). Organization of a university pain centre in Amsterdam. *Applied Neurophysiology*, 47, 171–175.
Bradley, L. A. (1988). Assessing the psychological profile of the chronic pain patient. In: Dubner, R., Gebhart, G. F. and Bond, M. R. (Eds) *Proceedings of the Vth World Congress on Pain*. Amsterdam: Elsevier, pp. 251–262.

Cairns, D., Thomas, L., Mooney, V. and Pace, J. B. (1976). A comprehensive treatment approach to chronic low back pain. *Pain*, **2**, 301–308.

Clark, M., Gosnell, M. and Shapiro, D. (1977). The new war on pain. *Newsweek*, April 25, 48–50.

Cohen, R. S., Brechner, Th. F., Pavlov, A. and Reading, A. E. (1985). Comparison of cancer pain and chronic benign pain patients on dimensions of pain intensity, affect and approach to treatment. *Clinical Journal of Pain*, **4**, 205–210.

Cosyns, P. and Vlaeyen, J. (1984). La douleur chronique rebelle. In: Fontaine, O., Cottraux, J. and Ladouceur, R. (Eds) *Cliniques de Therapie Comportementale*. Liège: Mardaga, pp. 371–384.

Dalton, J. A. and Feuerstein, M. (1988). Biobehavioral factors in cancer pain. *Pain*, **33**, 137–149.

Deyo, R. A. (1983). Conservative therapy for low back pain. *Journal of the American Medical Association*, **250**, 1057–1062.

Foley, K. M. (1985). The treatment of cancer pain. *New England Journal of Medicine*, **313**, 84–95.

Follick, M. J., Zitter, R. E. and Ahern, D. K. (1983). Failures in the treatment of chronic pain. In: Foa, E. B. and Emmelkamp, P. M. G. (Eds) *Failures in Behavior Therapy*. New York: Wiley, pp. 311–334.

Fordyce, W. E. (1976). *Behavioral Methods for Chronic Pain and Illness*. St Louis: C. V. Mosby.

Fordyce, W. E. (1979). *The Use of the MMPI in the Assessment of Chronic Pain*, Part III. Rochester: Hoffman-LaRoche.

Fordyce, W. E. (1987). Personal communication. Vth World Congress on Pain, Hamburg, 2–7 August.

Fordyce, W. E. (1988). Pain and suffering: A reappraisal. *American Psychologist*, **43**, 276–283.

Fordyce, W. E., Fowler, R. E., Lehmann, J., Delateur, B., Sand, P. and Trieschmann, R. (1973). Operant conditioning in the treatment of chronic clinical pain. *Archives of Physical and Medical Rehabilitation*, **54**, 399–408.

Fordyce, W. E., Roberts, A. H. and Sternbach, R. H. (1985). The behavioral management of chronic pain: A response to critics. *Pain*, **22**, 113–125.

Haanen, H. C. M. (1984). Een epidemiologisch onderzoek naar lage rugpijn. Thesis, Erasmus University of Rotterdam.

Holzman, A. D., Turk, D. C. and Kerns Jr, R. D. (1986). The cognitive-behavioral approach to the management of chronic pain. In: Holzman, A.D. and Turk, D. C. (Eds) *Pain Management, A Handbook of Psychological Treatment Approaches*. New York: Pergamon, pp. 31–50.

International Association for the Study of Pain, Subcommittee on Taxonomy (1979). Pain terms: A list with definitions and notes on usage. *Pain*, **6**, 249–252.

Jacobson, E. (1938). *Progressive Relaxation*. Chicago: University of Chicago Press.

Jaremko, M. E. (1978). Cognitive strategies in the control of pain tolerance. *Journal of Behavior Therapy and Experimental Psychiatry*, **9**, 239–244.

Karoly, P. (1985). The assessment of pain: Concepts and procedures. In: Karoly, P. (Ed.) *Measurement Strategies in Health Psychology*. New York: Wiley, pp. 461–515.

Lewinsohn, P. M. (1974). A behavioral approach to depression. In: Friedman, R. J. and Katz, M. M. (Eds) *The Psychology of Depression: Contemporary Theory and Research*. New York: Wiley, pp. 157–178.

Linton, S. J. (1986). Behavioral remediation of chronic pain: A status report. *Pain*, **24**, 125–141.

Loeser, J. D. and Fordyce, W. E. (1983). Chronic pain. In: Carr, J. E. and Dengerink, H. A. (Eds) *Behavioral Science in the Practice of Medicine*. Amsterdam: Elsevier Biomedical, pp. 331–346.

Roberts, A. H. (1986). The operant approach to the management of pain and excess disability. In: Holzman, A. D. and Turk, D. C. (Eds) *Pain Management, a Handbook of Psychological Treatment Approaches*. New York: Pergamon, pp. 10–30.

Roberts, A. H. and Reinhardt, L. (1980). The behavioral management of chronic pain: Long-term follow-up with comparison groups. *Pain*, **8**, 151–162.

Romano, J. M. and Turner, J. A. (1985). Chronic pain and depression: Does the evidence support a relationship? *Psychological Bulletin*, **97**, 18–34.

Schmidt, A. J. M. (1986). Persistence behavior of chronic low back patients. PhD thesis, University of Limburg, Maastricht.

Schultz, J. H. and Luthe, W. (1959). *Autogenic training*. New York: Grune & Stratton.

Seres, J. (1985). Comments at the Boulder Conference on Pain, Aspen CO, Feb. 1985. As mentioned in: Anderson, E. F., Hegstrum, J. A. and Charboneau, G. J. (1985). Multidisciplinary management of patients with chronic low back pain. *Clinical Journal of Pain*, **1**, 85–90.

Tan, S. Y. (1982). Cognitive and cognitive behavioral methods for pain control: A selective review. *Pain*, **12**, 201–228.

Turk, D. C., Meichenbaum, D. and Genest, M. (1983). *Pain and Behavioral Medicine. A Cognitive-Behavioral Perspective*. New York: Guilford.

Turk, D. C. and Rudy, T. E. (1987). Towards a comprehensive assessment of chronic pain patients. *Behavioral Research and Therapy*, **25**, 237–249.

Turner, J. A. and Chapman, C. R. (1982). Psychological interventions for chronic pain: A critical review. II. Operant conditioning, hypnosis and cognitive behavioral therapy. *Pain*, **12**, 23–46.

Vlaeyen, J. W. S., Groenman, N. H. and Legrelle, T. (1987). Traitement multimodal et interdisciplinaire de la douleure chronique. *Revue de Modification du Comportement*, **176**, 95–113.

Vlaeyen, J. W. S., Van Eek, H., Groenman, N. H. and Schuerman, J. A. (1987). Dimensions and components of observed chronic pain behavior. *Pain*, **31**, 65–76.

CHAPTER 5

Headache

H. van der Helm-Hylkema

Free University, Amsterdam

ABSTRACT

In this chapter, migraine and tension headaches are listed according to the recent classification of headaches provided by the Headache Classification Committee of the International Headache Society. Various forms of migraine and tension headache and their trigger factors and symptomatology are delineated. Some epidemiological data are presented on both these conditions in children and adults. Theories on the pathophysiological mechanisms of migraine and tension headache (as disorders of the vascular, neural, or muscular system) are discussed. The psychological treatment of headache is elaborated upon. In two case studies, behaviour therapy (relaxation training, biofeedback training, assertiveness training, rational emotive training) is illustrated as applied to patients with headache. A review of research on the effectiveness of behaviour therapy and hypnotherapy is given. It is concluded that both behaviour therapy and hypnotherapy can reduce headache in a considerable proportion of patients.

HEADACHE: CLASSIFICATION AND SYMPTOMATOLOGY

The Ad Hoc Committee on the Classification of Headache in 1962 described 15 categories of headache. In 1988 the Headache Classification Committee of the International Headache Society proposed a new classification, giving more accurate descriptions and diagnostic criteria of the various categories of headache. In the classification scheme it is stressed that any form of headache in a particular patient must fit one set of criteria and only one. However, a patient may very well have more than one form of headache. After some years of

Behavioural Medicine
Edited by A. A. Kaptein, H. M. van der Ploeg, B. Garssen, P. J. G. Schreurs and R. Beunderman
© 1990 John Wiley & Sons Ltd.

testing, this classification will be used in the future as the 'International Headache Classification'.

In most categories of the classification scheme headache is considered to be caused by organic factors or to be a side-effect of a somatic disorder. Headache may occur with epilepsy, intracranial tumors, cerebral circulatory disorders, infections, and diseases of eyes, ears, nose, sinuses and teeth. In other words, headache can be a symptom of a more or less serious disease. Often, however, there is no apparent organic cause, though the sensation of pain can be very intense and can be a serious impediment to the individual's ability to function well. Headache categories without apparent organic cause are 'migraine' and 'tension headache', from which over 90% of all headache patients suffer. In this chapter the symptomatology, epidemiology, development of the disorder, theories of pathological mechanisms, psychological treatment and results of psychological treatment of both migraine and tension headache will be described.

Migraine

The mention of migraine dates back to ancient times. An Egyptian papyrus found in the nineteenth century, written in 1550 BC, contains a clear description of migraine. In later times Hippocrates (400 BC) and Boerhaave (AD 1668–1737), among others, paid attention to headache and the treatment of it (Danby, 1977). In the recently proposed Headache Classification System 'migraine' is defined as: an idiopathic (originating independently of other diseases) chronic headache manifesting in attacks lasting 4–72 hours. Typical characteristics of headache are unilateral location, pulsating quality, moderate or severe intensity and association with nausea or photo-phonophobia. The headache attacks are separated by pain-free intervals. This description refers to a form of migraine from which most patients suffer and which is called 'common migraine' or 'migraine without aura'. The other form, which is less frequently seen, involves headache preceded by an aura and is called 'classical migraine' or 'migraine with aura'.

The aura is a neurological symptom due to shunting away of blood from various areas of the cerebral cortex or the brainstem. Disturbances in the blood supply cause visual symptoms such as flashing lights (photopsia) or fortification spectra (teichopsia). They occur in 33% of patients with classical migraine. Others suffer from disturbances of the brainstem such as double vision (diplopia), dizziness (vertigo), disturbance in forming syllables (dysarthries) and a dyscoordination of voluntary muscles movement (ataxie). Other less common observed symptoms are: loss of memory, feeling weak, fainting, hallucination, sensations of numbness, tingling of pins and needles (Lance, 1975). Numerous autonomic symptoms can accompany migraine such as nausea, vomiting, anorexia, pallor, cold extremities, perspiration, diarrhoea and polyuria. When the aura symptoms occur in isolation, without headache, they are called 'migraine equivalents' or 'isolated neurological migraine accompaniments'.

Children suffering from migraine display more abdominal complaints, travel sickness and sleep disorders than control children without headache. Child and adult migraine patients differ in the following respects: in children the attacks are more frequent, of shorter duration, more often accompanied by nausea and vomiting, and less often preceded by prodromal phenomena (Hoelscher and Lichstein, 1984).

Tension Headache

'Tension headache' is characterized by recurrent episodes of headache lasting minutes to days. The pain is typically pressing/tightening in quality, of mild or moderate intensity, bilateral in location and does not worsen with routine physical activity. Nausea is absent, but photophobia or phonophobia may be present. In the literature this kind of headache is known under a lot of different names, such as tension headache, muscle contraction headache, psychomyogenic headache, stress headache, ordinary headache, idiopathic headache, and psychogenic headache.

There are many headache patients (30–40%) suffering from both migraine and tension headache (Kunkel, 1976). There are no research data on the differences in symptoms between children and adults with tension headache.

EPIDEMIOLOGY

The following data sometimes refer to headache in general and sometimes to migraine or tension headache specifically. In comparison with data on tension headache the data on migraine are in the majority. Epidemiological studies show that headache is widespread and related to sex and age. There are more women than men suffering from headache, particularly the more serious kinds of headache. From a survey of five epidemiological studies which were conducted by different researchers between 1974 and 1978, it appears that 9.8–16.7% of men and 20.8–26.6% of women suffer from severe headache (Goldstein and Chen, 1982).

Headache can already be found in the very young. Swedish research has shown that at the age of seven some 4% of children frequently suffer from headache (Bille, 1987). Migraine is observed in 1.4% of these seven-year-olds, who on average suffered their first attacks when they were 4.8 years old. At the age of 10–15 the number of migraine patients has gone up to 5.3%. At first there is no difference between the proportions of boys and girls suffering from migraine, but from the age of 10 onwards there are more female than male migraine patients (Bille, 1987). From the results of another epidemiological study it appears that 12% of boys aged 10–11 and 10% of boys aged 12–18 suffer from headache recurring at least once a week. For girls in the same age groups the figures are 22% and 24% respectively (Passchier and Orlebeke, 1985).

As for the occurrence of migraine in adults, the figures of various epidemiological studies over the past 20 years differ widely. This probably has to do with the lack of clear criteria for the diagnosis of migraine. The figures on men vary from 2.1 to 14.9%, on women from 6.3 to 25.4% (Goldstein and Chen, 1982).

What is clear is that more women than men suffer from this kind of headache.

The epidemiological studies also indicate that the occurrence of migraine increases until the age of 20–25, then remains at the same level until about the age of 40, after which it decreases gradually. For headache in general the same pattern has been observed (Goldstein and Chen, 1982). No connection has been established between headache and various demographic factors like education, intelligence, socioeconomic background or marital status.

Bille carried out a longitudinal study on migraine over a 30-year period (Bille, 1987). About 30 years after the study had begun—by which time the children had grown into adults of 37–40 years old—it appeared that one-third of the subjects had suffered from recurrent migraine without large intervals since childhood. Another 20% had remained migraine patients but had been free from symptoms for some years before the complaint returned. This leads to the conclusion that some 50% of the children suffering from migraine maintain the complaint into adulthood.

Many headache patients find it difficult or impossible to work during attacks of headache. This highlights the fact that, apart from the personal suffering, headache accounts for an enormous loss of working hours. It has been estimated that in the United States those who suffer from migraine with aura (classical migraine) alone are responsible for a social and economic loss of $512 million per year (Bruyn, 1983). There is no consensus about the prevalence of tension headache. This is probably due to a lack of clear diagnostic criteria for this disorder. Some authors report a higher percentage (Bakal, 1976; Philips, 1977), others (Korczyn, Carel and Pereg, 1980) a lower percentage of patients with tension headache in comparison with patients with migraine. Korczyn, Carel and Pereg (1980) found that more men than women suffered from tension headache.

DEVELOPMENT OF HEADACHE; CONTRIBUTING FACTORS

Migraine

There are many factors that can bring about a migraine attack, for example too little or too much sleep, foods and stimulants (cheese, chocolate, alcohol), hormonal changes that accompany menstruation, and meteorological conditions (snow and wind) (Danby, 1977; van den Bergh, Amery and Waelkens, 1987).

Apart from factors of a physiological nature, psychological and/or social factors may also play a role in the development of both migraine and tension headache. In the literature on headache these psychological factors are referred to as 'stress'. There are many definitions of stress. In the current text stress is defined as 'an inability to cope adequately with difficult situations in life, including small irritations'.

Many (85%) migraine patients are aware of factors that bring about an attack, so-called 'trigger factors'. The most important trigger factors mentioned are menstruation (48.0%) or ovulation (8.5%), certain foods (44.7%), alcoholic drinks (51.6%) and stress (48.8%) (van den Bergh, Amery and Waelkens, 1987). Women mention more trigger factors than men, even if menstrual cycle or ovulation are not counted. The same holds true for older patients and patients with a longer duration of headache—they also mention more trigger factors. Women with menstruation-related migraine report more other trigger factors, especially in the field of food and drink, than women who do not experience a correlation between menstruation and migraine (van den Bergh, Amery and Waelkens, 1987).

Tension Headache

Less is known about the trigger factors of tension headache. Tension headache patients appear to experience more day-to-day irritation at work and socially, to judge this more negatively, and to apply more non-effective coping strategies than controls (Holm *et al.*, 1986). During a study on headache (migraine and tension headache) in schoolchildren, out of all the children that could identify some cause for their headache, 60% of preparatory school pupils and 85% of secondary school pupils mentioned stress (in the above-mentioned sense) as a trigger factor (Passchier and Orlebeke, 1985).

THEORIES ON THE PATHOPHYSIOLOGICAL MECHANISMS OF MIGRAINE AND TENSION HEADACHE

Migraine

In some theories migraine is treated as a disorder of the vascular system, while others lay more emphasis on neural mechanisms. Most theories are based upon research on patients with classical migraine.

Wolff's vascular theory, based upon a series of experiments conducted by Wolff and others (Dalessio, 1980), is the best-known theory. Wolff divides the migraine attack into four phases. During the first phase, the so-called 'prodromal' or 'aura' phase, there is no sensation of pain. The patient often experiences feelings of restlessness, dizziness, concentration problems, reduced vision or sees flashes or zigzag lines. The blood vessels of the brain constrict during this phase, but apart from this little is known about what goes on in the body. There are also many migraine patients who do not have any subjective complaints during this phase. One or several hours later the second phase of the migraine attack sets in. This is the headache phase. This phase is characterized by severe pain on one side of the head, caused by dilatation of the extracranial vessels and a locally increased sensitivity to pain. In Wolff's opinion the vasodilation during this second phase is a reaction to the vasoconstriction of the first phase. The next, third phase is characterized by dull pain which is the result of arterial oedemata. This is followed by a fourth phase with pain caused by tension of the head and neck muscles.

An example of a neural theory is the theory that migraine is caused by a decrease in the cerebral blood flow, leading to an oxygen deficiency in the brain cells. As a result a number of biochemical and neurological processes are triggered which are associated with migraine (Lauritzen *et al.*, 1983). A different, recent theory by Sicuteri states that migraine patients have an abnormality of the central antinociceptive system in which serotonin and especially beta-endorphin play a role (Sicuteri, 1981). Endorphins are opiate-like endogenous substances that influence the sensation of pain. It appears that migraine patients have a reduced level of beta-endorphin in plasma compared to controls (Fettes *et al.*, 1985; van der Helm-Hylkema *et al.*, 1990).

It would be impossible to discuss all the remaining theories here. For a survey the reader is referred to Dalessio (1980).

Tension Headache

Compared to the large number of theories on the origins of migraine, the number of theories about tension headache is small. Originally, tension headache was supposed to be caused by too much muscular tension in shoulders, neck and head. However, the empirical basis to support this hypothesis is not very strong. Far from all tension headache patients show increased tension in the above-mentioned muscles. What is more, a reduction of muscular tension is not always accompanied by a reduction in headache—or *vice versa* (Philips, 1978). And a high tension in the above-mentioned muscles is not specific for tension headache; as a group, migraine patients show even higher tension of these muscles (Philips, 1978). In another study, no relation has been found between intensity of headache and muscular tension. The investigators assume that the pain is caused by an accumulation of tissue fluid resulting from muscular hyperactivity (van Boxtel and Goudswaard, 1984).

PSYCHOLOGICAL TREATMENT OF HEADACHE

A person suffering from recurrent headache will usually consult his or her family doctor first. Often the doctor will prescribe medicine. Medicines can be helpful, but the chronic use of pharmaca is open to objections, since these drugs all have side-effects that may vary from irksome-but-innocent to very serious. Besides, there are patients who do not find relief in drugs, or only temporarily.

In a large proportion of headache patients psychological as well as physical factors play an important role in the development of headache. It is for this reason that during the past decades headache patients have increasingly been referred for psychological treatment. Behaviour therapy and hypnotherapy play the most prominent roles in the field of psychological headache treatment. The effects of these forms of psychotherapy have been thoroughly investigated in a large number of studies.

Behaviour Therapy

In behaviour therapy the treatment of headache may consist of applying techniques aimed at changing somatic functioning, such as relaxation and biofeedback training, or of applying techniques aimed at changing behaviour patterns or cognitive styles, such as assertiveness training and/or rational emotive therapy.

Relaxation Training

In relaxation training the so-called 'relaxation response' (Benson and Klipper, 1976) is taught, which is characterized physiologically by reduced breathing frequency and muscular tone, slower heartbeat, and lower blood pressure. Relaxation training is not only effective on the physiological level but on the motor and cognitive levels as well. Everyday activities are temporarily interrupted. It is only when receiving relaxation training that many patients realize how tense and nervous they are in normal life. They are taught to relax consciously. Moreover, the patient's stream of thought is stopped when he/she is listening to the training instructions. In general, relaxation exercises provide a means of self-control that enables the patient to tackle problems more adequately.

Biofeedback Training

In the course of biofeedback experiments conducted in the laboratory of the Menninger Foundation around 1970, one of the subjects, a woman regularly suffering from migraine, discovered that an approaching migraine attack disappeared when her finger temperature was raised. This discovery led to more systematic research into the usefulness of teaching patients to warm their fingers as a treatment for migraine. The research showed that over 70% of migraine patients felt some relief after such training. Other research has since confirmed this result (Blanchard and Andrasik, 1982).

Later on biofeedback of the extracranial temporal artery was introduced in the treatment of migraine. Training is aimed at learning to reduce variations in the amplitude of pulsation in this artery. The method is based on data gathered by Graham and Wolff (Dalessio, 1980), who found that in the pain phase of a migraine attack the amplitude of pulsation in the temporal artery was extended. Administration of ergotamine, a highly vasoconstrictive substance, during the pain phase greatly reduced both the amplitude of pulsation in the temporal artery and the pain. One might say that in biofeedback training the action of ergotamine is imitated. This form of biofeedback training is more difficult to apply than finger temperature biofeedback and is therefore used less frequently.

At about the same time that temperature biofeedback was applied for the first time, another group of American researchers treated tension headache patients with electromyographic (EMG) biofeedback. In this method the patient learns to reduce the tension of the facial muscle. This method, too, was successful with a considerable number of patients in that the headache was reduced or disappeared (Blanchard and Andrasik, 1982).

Assertiveness and Rational Emotive Training

In behaviour therapy a so-called 'headache diary' is often used. In this diary the patient regularly makes notes about the presence and intensity (or the absence) of headache. Notes are also made of difficult situations, of the number of cigarettes smoked, and the amount of alcohol and medicine taken. The patient can be asked to keep the headache diary for a period before, during and after therapy in order to provide insight into the development of the headache and the effects of treatment.

Treatment can be focused on the patient's behaviour style. Many problems are in the domain of 'assertiveness': finding it difficult to express irritation, to say 'no', and to give and/or accept criticism and/or compliments. The patient is asked to describe problematic situations as accurately as possible, by answering the following questions:

What happened and who were present?
How did you react, behaviourally and emotionally?
What were the consequences?

On the basis of this information the problematic situations can be acted out in the safe surroundings of the therapist's consulting room by means of role-playing. By switching roles, the patient can gain the insight that in a special situation more adequate behaviour is possible. The patient can then adopt those elements of the new behaviour that best suit him/her.

The therapy can also be concerned with how certain situations are experienced. In that case therapists often use principles of rational emotive therapy (RET). This form of therapy, developed by Ellis, is based upon the proposition that human emotions are largely the result of thought processes (Ellis, 1958). The starting point of rational emotive therapy is that emotional problems are not primarily caused by external situations, but by irrational ideas about and interpretations of those situations. The following case illustrates this principle:

X, a 45-year-old school teacher, experiences tension particularly at school meetings. He supposes that some of his younger colleagues criticize his teaching methods, consider him old-fashioned, and do not appreciate him. These ideas, which have emerged during the past year, quickly generalize to other social situations. X is compulsively occupied by these ideas. The migraine attacks that he used to suffer once every five months have reached a frequency of once a week over the past six months. In therapy several situations are dealt with. During the sessions the irrational idea that 'they do not appreciate me because my way of teaching differs from theirs' is replaced by a more rational idea: 'There are different ways of teaching and I am happy with mine. My different way of teaching is not a reason for not appreciating me. And even if it were, it would be annoying, not terrible.' Some exercises are taped and X listens to them at home, calling the situation to mind. The compulsive behaviour disappears and the migraine gradually returns to the lower pretherapy level.

The following case is an example of a combination of relaxation biofeedback training, assertiveness training and rational emotive therapy:

L, a 10-year-old girl, is referred for behaviour therapy by her family doctor because of headache complaints that have become much more serious during the past six months. The headache is felt like a tight band around the head, is of a pricking and stinging nature, and is almost permanently present, but in particular at the end of the afternoon. Once or twice a week the headache is so bad that L has to miss school. Apart from this headache, which has to be described as tension headache, L suffers from migraine accompanied by nausea and vomiting about once every six months. L also has problems going to sleep. There are no apparent psychological problems. The therapy starts with relaxation and EMG biofeedback training of the facial muscle. L cooperates enthusiastically. After 10 sessions during a period of three months the headache has been reduced from some 21 to 10 mornings/afternoons/evenings per week. L does not have to miss school and hardly takes drugs any more. Meanwhile it has appeared from the headache diary, and from conversations with L and her parents, that there are some problems between L and her brother. In the following period various situations are gone through in the form of role-playing, in which L learns to make clear to her brother calmly but resolutely what she wants, what she does not want, and what she finds annoying about him. It appears also that L finds it hard to tolerate insecurity. To improve this situation, L is submitted to rational emotive therapy (RET) exercises, during which she is connected to an apparatus that measures the tension of the frontal facial muscle. She calls the particular situation into mind and replaces the irrational thoughts by other, more rational thoughts. She reduces any increase in muscular tension by means of images she finds pleasant, like walking in a wood and feeding the squirrels. From now on the headache disappears completely. At follow-up, one year after the therapy has ended, the improvement has been maintained.

Hypnotherapy

The application of a certain ritual induction procedure can bring a person into a hypnotic state. A hypnotic trance can be defined as a state of consciousness in which one is free from influences from the external situation and is caught up in internal experiences.

Most hypnotherapeutic procedures for headache patients consist of giving suggestions relating to muscular relaxation, improved blood flow, vascular contractions, shifting of attention, or going through difficult situations and strengthening the ego (Spinhoven, 1988). Apart from the last-mentioned element there is much analogy with the methods applied in behaviour therapy.

Results of Behaviour Therapy and Hypnosis

Results of Behaviour Therapy

During the past 15 years many investigations have been carried out on the effects of various types of behaviour therapy on headache. Most of the research concerns the influence of relaxation and/or biofeedback training. Blanchard studied the results of 48 comparable studies in the field of tension headache and 56 comparable studies in the field of migraine (Blanchard *et al.*, 1980). It appeared that as far as *tension headache* was concerned, EMG training, relaxation training, and a combination of both methods all had about the same effect (60% improvement on average). These treatments were superior to placebo procedures (35% improvement on average) and making notes in a headache diary (4.5% deterioration on average). As to *migraine*, relaxation training combined with temperature biofeedback showed the best results (65% improvement on average). Relaxation training without biofeedback resulted in 48% improvement; temperature and temporal artery biofeedback alone were clearly less effective (35% and 28% mean improvement respectively).

The analysis has led the authors to the conclusion that for *migraine* a combination of relaxation and temperature biofeedback is currently the most effective procedure. It is obvious, however, that the difference with the effects of relaxation training is not big at all. To quote Blanchard: 'The machines may be necessary some of the time' (Blanchard, 1982). For *tension headache* the authors conclude that relaxation training is as effective as biofeedback procedures.

Effect of age. Holroyd and Penzies investigated 37 comparable studies on behaviour therapy and tension headache (Holroyd and Penzies, 1986). They found that the more recent studies showed a lower percentage of success (38.8% improvement of headache on average) than the earliest studies (55.8%). From their analyses it appeared that the effects of treatment depended on client variables, especially age. On average, studies on younger patients, less than 30 years old, showed more success (55% improvement of headache) than studies on older clients (34%). Other investigators have also discovered a relation between age and therapeutic success in the same direction (Diamond and Montrose, 1984).

A follow-up study over a longer period (five years) on adult headache patients showed that after a successful relaxation/biofeedback therapy 78% of tension headache patients and 91% of migraine patients had maintained their headache improvements (Blanchard *et al.*, 1987).

With young headache patients the percentage of success of behaviour therapy is extremely high: 90% of children show a clinically significant (at least 50%) improvement of headache (Werder and Sargent, 1984; van der Helm-Hylkema *et al.*, 1990). The improvement has been maintained one year after completion of therapy (Werder and Sargent, 1984; van der Helm-Hylkema *et al.*, 1990).

Group therapy. Behaviour therapeutic methods can also be applied to groups, which saves time and consequently money. Recently we started a short group treatment of adult migraine patients which was combined with individual temperature biofeedback training. The group treatment consists of giving information about the complaints, relaxation and RET exercises, and discussing the complaints and related problems. This combination treatment brought about a reduction of headache duration that would have taken longer to achieve in exclusively individual therapy. Child migraine patients, too, showed marked improvement after a relatively short combination treatment of this kind (van der Helm-Hylkema *et al.*, 1990).

Results of Hypnosis

In a review of five studies on headache no differences were found between the results of hypnosis and biofeedback; nor between the results of hypnosis and relaxation training (Spinhoven, 1988). Unfortunately, there have been no follow-up studies of any significant size measuring the long-term effects of hypno-therapy by a more or less objective criterion, such as the headache diary. These studies should be undertaken, as there appear to be discrepancies between objectively and subjectively reported headache improvement (Friedman and Taub, 1985).

DISCUSSION

The vast literature on headache that has appeared over the past 15 years has clearly shown that both behaviour therapy and hypnotherapy can reduce headache in a considerable proportion of patients and that in the case of behaviour therapy the improvement is maintained over a longer period (Blan-chard *et al.*, 1987). Little is known about the intermediating physiological mechanisms of behaviour changes which cause symptom (headache) reduction. In the following paragraphs some data are mentioned and some hypotheses are formulated about how the effects of therapy may come about.

Relaxation Therapy and Biofeedback

Migraine patients show, both during and between attacks, increased activity of the orthosympathic part of the central nervous system (Gotoh *et al.*, 1976; Anthony, 1981). Relaxation training can reduce the level of orthosympathic activity leading to symptom reduction.

Migraine patients have a higher level of dopamine-β-hydroxylase in plasma, an enzyme indication for orthosympathic activity (Gotoh *et al.*, 1976). Kentsmith *et al.* (1976) observed a decrease of dopamine-β-hydroxylase level in a migraine patient who was successfully treated with relaxation biofeedback training. This decrease was not seen in a control subject without headache following the training.

Few are clear about the mechanisms of biofeedback procedures. One study has shown that temperature biofeedback, in which patients are taught to warm their hands, results in improvements in certain cerebral blood flows (Mathew *et al.*, 1980). This might imply reversion of the vasoconstriction that occurs in the prodromal phase of migraine. It has also been argued that temperature and vascular biofeedback work indirectly and in some patients lead to a better control and stabilization of the peripheral vascular system (Blanchard and Andrasik, 1982). However, the proposition that migraine patients show vaso-motor instability has been criticized on the grounds of methodological weakness of the studies (Morley, 1977).

Coping With Stress

When headache is reduced as a result of better coping with tension-inducing situations, one may assume that physiological changes have occurred as well. In the case of improvement of tension headache it may be assumed that the facial muscle reacts less when exposed to stressful situations. In the case of improvement of migraine the same would apply to the functioning of the temporal artery. Until now, little empirical evidence has been found to support this hypothesis (Passchier, van der Helm-Hylkema and Orlebeke, 1985). However, it should be noted that verification of the hypothesis has been carried out in a laboratory. Recent research has shown that in a naturally tense situation—an examination—migraine patients show more vasoconstriction of the temporal artery than controls (Passchier et al., 1988). In the same study a positive relation was found between emotional inhibition and vasoconstriction. As has been shown by Wolff, there is strong vasoconstriction of the temporal artery during the first phase of a migraine attack (Dalessio, 1980). Learning to cope better with difficult situations may result in a reduction of this vasoconstriction. This could be helpful to migraine patients.

In summary, to date no indications have been found of a relation between changes in physiological responses (muscular tension and vasoconstriction) and therapeutic success. It is perhaps advisable to consider other physiological mechanisms associated with headache, for instance the activity of brain neurotransmitters and hormones such as beta-endorphin.

As has been mentioned earlier, one theory states that headache is caused by a dysfunction of the brain nociceptive system. During headache the blood contains a lower level of endorphins. Pain-relieving treatment like acupuncture is found to stimulate the release of endorphins (Malizia et al., 1979). Psychological treatment of pain might have a similar affect. Empirical support for this theory is provided by two recent studies. A short behaviour therapy for children with migraine, consisting of relaxation and temperature biofeedback training as well as some RET exercises, resulted in an improvement of migraine. This improvement was accompanied by an increase in the level of beta-endorphin. Before treatment this level was low compared with that of controls. A waiting-list control group of migraine patients not receiving therapy did not show a comparable increase in endorphin, despite an improvement of headache (van der Helm-Hylkema et al., 1990). A related finding was that hypnotherapy reduced pain in arthritis patients. This was accompanied by an increased beta-endorphin level (Domangue et al., 1985).

The mechanism of the interaction between mind and brain can only be a matter of speculation. In relaxation and biofeedback training as well as in hypnosis attention is focused on somatic processes with a certain degree of dissociation from external surroundings. Possibly under such conditions a recovery of the pain system takes place, in a manner as yet inexplicable.

What is the impact of the current state of affairs on the *psychological treatment of headache patients*? Relaxation training, which in cases of migraine may be supplemented by autogenic suggestion or by temperature biofeedback to raise hand temperature, can bring relief to a considerable proportion of headache patients. Hypnotherapy can have the same effect but this is less documented. Not every headache patient needs extensive therapy. Learning to cope with difficult situations seems useful for those who indicate that the headache is caused by problems in everyday life.

NOTES

[1]Address for correspondence: H. van der Helm-Hylkema, Department of Physiological Psychology, Free University, PO Box 7161, 1007 MC Amsterdam, The Netherlands.

REFERENCES

Ad Hoc Committee on the Classification of Headache (1962). A classification of headache. *Neurology*, **12**, 378–380.

Anthony, M. (1981). Biochemical indices of sympathetic activity in migraine. *Cephalalgia*, **1**, 83–89.

Bakal, D. A. (1975). Headache: A biopsychological perspective. *Psychological Bulletin*, **82**, 369–382.

Benson, H. and Klipper, M. Z. (1976). *The Relaxation Response*. London: Collins.

Bergh, V. van den, Amery, W. K. and Waelkens, J. (1987). Trigger factors in migraine: A study conducted by the Belgian Migraine Society. *Headache*, **27**, 191–196.

Bille, B. (1987). Migraine in children. In: Ferrari, M. D., Bruyn, G. W., Padberg, G. and Zitman, F. G. (Eds) *Migraine and Other Headaches*. Boerhaave Committee for Postgraduate Education, University of Leiden, pp. 15–23.

Blanchard, E. B. (1982). Sequential comparisons of relaxation training and biofeedback in the treatment of three kinds of chronic headache, or: The machines may be necessary some of the time. *Behaviour Research & Therapy*, **20**, 1–13.

Blanchard, E. B. and Andrasik, F. (1982). Psychological assessment and treatment of headache: Recent developments and emerging issues: *Journal of Consulting and Clinical Psychology*, **50**, 859–879.

Blanchard, E. B., Andrasik, F., Ahles, T. A., Tedees, S. J. and O'Keefe, D. (1980). Migraine and tension headache. A meta-analytic review. *Behaviour Therapy*, **11**, 613–631.

Blanchard, E. B., Appelbaum, K. A., Guarnieri, P., Morrill, B. and Dentinger, M. P. (1987). Five-year prospective follow-up on the treatment of chronic headache with biofeedback and/or relaxation. *Headache*, **27**, 580–583.

Boxtel, A. van and Goudswaard, P. (1984). Absolute and proportional resting EMG levels in chronic headache patients in relation to the state of headache. *Headache*, **24**, 259–265.

Bruyn, G. W. (1983). Epidemiology of migraine: A personal view. *Headache*, **23**, 127–133.

Dalessio, D. J. (1980). Migraine. In: Dalessio, D. J. (Ed.) *Wolff's Headache and Other Head Pain*. New York: Oxford University Press, pp. 56–130.

Danby, M. (1977). *Leven met Migraine* (Living with Migraine). Assen/Amsterdam: Van Gorkum, pp. 13–32.

Diamond, S. and Montrose, D. (1984). The value of biofeedback in the treatment of chronic headache: A four-year retrospective study. *Headache*, **24**, 5–18.

Domangue, B. B., Margolis, C. G., Lieberman, D. and Kaji, H. (1985). Biochemical correlates of hypnoanalgesia in arthritic pain patients. *Journal of Clinical Psychiatry*, **46**, 235–238.

Ellis, A. (1958). Rational psychotherapy. *Journal of Genetic Psychology*, **59**, 35–49.
Fettes, I., Gawel, M., Kuzniak, S. and Edmeads, J. (1985). Endorphin levels in headache syndromes. *Headache*, **25**, 37–39.
Friedman, H. and Taub, H. A. (1985). Extended follow-up study of the effect of brief psychological procedures in migraine therapy. *American Journal of Clinical Hypnosis*, **28**, 27–33.
Gotoh, F., Kanda, T., Sakai, F., Yamamoto, M. and Takeoka, T. (1976). Serum-dopamine-β-hydroxylase activity in migraine. *Archives of Neurology*, **33**, 656–657.
Goldstein, M. and Chen, T. C. (1982). The epidemiology of disabling headache. In: Crickley, M. *et al.* (Eds) *Advances in Neurology*. New York: Raven Press, pp. 377–391.
Headache Classification Committee (1988). Classification and diagnostic criteria for headache disorders, cranial neuralgias and facial pain. *Cephalalgia*, **7**, 13–35.
Helm-Hylkema, H. van der, Orlebeke, J. F., Enting, L. A., Thijssen, J. H. H. and Ree, J. van (1990). Effects of behaviour therapy on migraine and beta-endorphin in plasma of young migraine patients. *Psychoneuroendocrinology*, (in press).
Hoelscher, M. S. and Lichstein, K. L. (1984). Behavioral assessment and treatment of child migraine: Implications for clinical research and practice. *Headache*, **24**, 94–103.
Holm, J. E., Holroyd, K. A., Hursey, K. G. and Penzies, D. B. (1986). The role of stress in recurrent tension headache. *Headache*, **26**, 160–167.
Holroyd, K. A. and Penzies, D. B. (1986). Client variables and the behavioral treatment of recurrent tension headache: A meta-analytic review. *Journal of Behavioural Medicine*, **9**, 515–536.
Kentsmith, D., Strider, D., Copenhaver, T. and Jacques, D. (1976). Effects of biofeedback upon suppression of migraine symptoms and plasma dopamine-β-hydroxylase activity. *Headache*, **16**, 173–177.
Korczyn, A. D., Carel, R. S. and Pereg, I. (1980). Correlation of headache complaints with some physiological parameters in a healthy population. *Headache*, **20**, 196–198.
Kunkel, R. S. (1976). *Mixed Headache* (Ed. O. Appenzeller). New York: Spectrum.
Lance, J. W. (1975). The different varieties of migrainous headaches. In: Saxena, P. R. (Ed.) *Migraine and Related Headaches*. Uden: Sandoz BV, pp. 15–27.
Lauritzen, N., Olsen, T. S., Lassen, N. A. and Paulson, O. B. (1983). Regulation of regional cerebral blood flow during and between migraine attacks. *Annals of Neurology*, **14**, 569–572.
Malizia, E. G., Adrencci, D., Paolucci, D., Crescenzi, F., Fabbi, A. and Fraioli, F. (1979). Electroacupuncture and peripheral beta-endorphin and ACTH levels. *Lancet*, **1**, 535–537.
Mathew, R. J., Largen, J. W., Dobbins, K., Meyer, J. S., Sakai, F. and Claghorn, J. L. (1980). Biofeedback control of skin temperature and cerebral blood flow in migraine. *Headache*, **20**, 19–29.
Morley, S. (1977). Migraine: A generalized vasomotor dysfunction? A critical review of evidence. *Headache*, **17**, 71–74.
Passchier, J., Goudswaard, P., Orlebeke, J. F. and Verhage, F. (1988). Migraine and defense mechanisms: Psychophysiological relationships in young females. *Social Science and Medicine*, **26**, 343–350.
Passchier, J., Helm-Hylkema, H. van der and Orlebeke, J. F. (1985). Lack of concordance between changes in headache activity and in psychophysiological and personality variables following treatment. *Headache*, **25**, 310–316.
Passchier, J. and Orlebeke, J. F. (1985). Headache and stress in schoolchildren. An epidemiological study. *Cephalalgia*, **5**, 167–176.
Philips, C. (1977). Headache in general practice. *Headache*, **16**, 322–329.
Philips, C. (1978). Tension headache: Theoretical problems. *Behaviour Research & Therapy*, **16**, 249–261.
Sicuteri, F. (1981). Emotional vulnerability of the antinociceptive system: Relevance in psychosomatic headache (Editorial). *Headache*, **21**, 113–115.

Spinhoven, Ph. (1988). Similarities and dissimilarities in hypnotic and nonhypnotic procedures for headache control: A review. *American Journal of Clinical Hypnosis*, **30**, 183–195.

Werder, S. W. and Sargent, J. D. (1984). A study of childhood headache using biofeedback as a treatment alternative. *Headache*, **24**, 122–126.

CHAPTER 6

Insomnia

F. M. Zwart[1]

Utrecht University, Utrecht

ABSTRACT

This chapter reviews behavioural methods in the assessment and treatment of insomnia, one of the four major types of sleep disorder (insomnia, hypersomnia, dissomnia, parasomnia). After giving some data on the epidemiology of sleep disorders, seven treatment approaches to insomnia are discussed; relaxation training, thought stopping, changes in life style, neutralizing negative expectations, systematic desensitization, changing bedroom activities, and paradoxical intentions, are all reviewed. Finally, a treatment programme is described and its results are presented. It is concluded that, despite the need for further evaluation, behavioural treatment of patients with insomnia appears to be at least as effective as pharmacological methods.

INTRODUCTION

Insomnia can be described as a deviation in the amount or character of normal sleep which results in insufficient sleep to function adequately during the daytime (Bootzin and Nicassio, 1978; Borkovec, 1982; Turner, 1986).

Since sleep is a complex phenomenon, deviations from normal sleep are related to a great number of origins. Normal sleep has a number of characteristics:

- Sleep is a state of rest of the organism
- This state emerges with a certain regularity
- The transition from waking to sleeping and back is a spontaneously occurring process that can be facilitated or hampered by certain circumstances

Behavioural Medicine
Edited by A. A. Kaptein, H. M. van der Ploeg, B. Garssen, P. J. G. Schreurs and R. Beunderman
© 1990 John Wiley & Sons Ltd.

- The transitions are not of a continuous nature, but occur abruptly
- Consciousness is changed; there is a selective exclusion of external stimuli
- Muscle tension is diminished
- Depth of sleep is not constant

Two types of sleep are known. One is 'active' sleep, that, divided over a number of periods during the night, amounts to 25% of total time asleep. The rest of the time consists of 'passive' sleep. 'Active' sleep is characterized by the occurrence of contractions of certain muscles, in particular the eye muscles, and by changes in blood pressure and respiration rate.

Passive sleep is not a steady state. Its depth varies from a light sleep, from which one is easily woken up or spontaneously awakes, to a very deep sleep that is interrupted with much more difficulty. In passive sleep four stages of increasing depth are distinguished. They are identified as 'stage 1' to 'stage 4'. After falling asleep, one's depth of sleep will increase from stage 1 to stage 4, followed by a period of active sleep. This cycle repeats itself a number of times, requiring about 90 minutes to complete and giving rise to four or five cycles during a night's sleep. The succeeding cycles differ from each other in an increasing length of the 'active' sleep period and a diminishing of the time spent in deep 'passive' sleep (stages 3 and 4).

CLASSIFICATION OF SLEEP DISORDERS

In 1979 a descriptive classification of sleep disturbances was published by the Association of Sleep Disorders Centers, ASDC (Association of Sleep Disorders Centers, 1979). One of the important objectives in the development of this 'Diagnostic Classification of Sleep and Arousal Disorders' was to gain insight into the aetiology and pathophysiology of the sleep disorders, which would ultimately lead to the development of treatment methods for patients complaining of disturbed sleep.

In the classification system four clusters of disorders are distinguished:

1. Disorders of initiating and maintaining sleep ('insomnias').
2. Disorders of excessive somnolence: 'hypersomnia'. Complaints in this cluster are undesired daytime sleepiness, an exceptional tendency to sleep, increased duration of the sleep period and difficulties in waking up fully.
3. Disorders of the sleep–wake schedule ('dissomnia'). The complaints here are not concerned with the sleep period itself, but with the rhythm whereby the sleep and wake periods alternate. In dissomnia, sleep does not occur when most needed and expected, and the waking periods are marked by drowsiness and a desire to sleep. Temporary rhythm disturbances can occur (e.g. jet lag) as well as more permanent ones.
4. Dysfunctions associated with sleep, sleep stages or partial arousals ('parasomnias'). Examples of these are sleepwalking, nightmares, night terrors, head-banging, bruxism and sleep-related enuresis.

Of these four categories of sleep disorders the insomnias are the most common complaint (Borkovec, 1982; Turner, 1986). Research in the area of sleeping problems has concentrated on this disorder. This chapter is devoted to the problem of not getting enough sleep to feel rested in the morning and not being able to function adequately during the day.

In the classification system of sleep disturbances, nine subtypes of the 'disorders of initiating and maintaining sleep' are identified by enumerating circumstances related to insomnia. They differ in the degree of association assumed between the insomnia and the 'causative' factor, varying from interpretation as a symptom of underlying psychopathology to a clear physical causation. These associated conditions are:

- Psychophysiological conditions
- Psychiatric disturbance
- The use of drugs and alcohol
- Respiratory impairment
- Myoclonus and 'restless legs' syndromes
- Environmental conditions
- 'Childhood onset' conditions
- Awakenings from active sleep or atypical EEG features
- Subjective complaint without objective findings

In concrete cases of insomnia, however, it often appears to be very difficult to identify which of the nine subtypes of insomnia prevails. In a number of cases specialized expertise and knowledge are needed that are only available in specific sleep disorder centres or sleep laboratories.

Methods of assessing insomnia are discussed by Bootzin and Engle-Friedman (1981), Cleghorn et al. (1983a) and Byerley and Gillin (1984). They all point to the importance of a thorough examination that considers the nature, intensity and frequency of the sleep disturbance as well as antecedents and possible maintaining consequences. Byerley and Gillin (1984) give an outline comprising:

- A thorough history of the complaint
- Current psychiatric status
- Marital, social and occupational history
- Past medical and psychiatric history
- Drug and medication use
- Data obtained by a 'sleep log' (sleep latency, sleeping time, number of awakenings, drug use, etc.)
- An interview with the partner

EPIDEMIOLOGY OF SLEEP DISORDERS

The incidence of insomnia has to be concluded from a number of studies that as a rule focus on specific populations within, for instance, a certain area or a certain age group. With this in mind, the estimates range from 20 to 40% of the (American) population (Bixler et al., 1979; Cleghorn et al., 1983a; Turner, 1986). A study from Western Germany concluded that 25% of the population complained about sleep (Faust and Hole, 1980). A Dutch study of a general practitioner's practice produced a similar figure (De Graaf, 1984).

Insomnia is more frequent in older persons and in women. There is also a greater incidence of insomnia complaints with patients having chronic or multiple medical problems (Byerley and Gillin, 1984).

TREATMENT OF INSOMNIA

It appears that treatment of the assumed primary cause of the disturbance will not always result in the disappearance of the insomnia (Borkovec, 1982). Apparently the complaint has a life of its own. The modification in the sleep pattern that exists in insomnia is very resistant to change. Although sleeplessness can have a number of clearly defined origins, behavioural components develop when the disturbance is of long duration. Too little sleep for too long has an influence on the daytime feeling of well-being: one becomes tired and listless. The lack of adequate sleep becomes a problem in its own right. It brings with it a preoccupation with finding means of falling asleep and a vicious circle develops: the more one tries, the less easily one falls asleep. Falling asleep will only take place of its own accord; it is a natural process that will happen without any real effort.

The most frequently practised treatment method for insomnia complaints is the prescription of medication by physicians. Not only physician-prescribed drugs but also over-the-counter preparations and alcohol are very widely used (Cleghorn et al., 1983a). Most of these remedies will not be useful for a long period. When drugs do not have the desired effects after one or two weeks, chances are small that the continuing use of the drug will be helpful in the long run. Another drawback of medication is that opiates will change the character of the sleep by influencing the normal course of the cyclic succession of the four sleep stages or suppressing 'active' sleep. Lastly, drugs may bring the problems of habituation and addiction: a diminishing of effect leads to higher doses and to noticeable consequences in the daytime, such as morning hangover effects, mental confusion and nausea (Turner and Ditomasso, 1980). In addition, they may give rise to the emergence of other sleeping disorders that are associated with the use of drugs (Association of Sleep Disorders Centers, 1979).

The preceding is not the only reason why it is important to develop behavioural treatment methods for insomnia. The effects of a chronic lack of sleep influence the daily functioning. Fatigue and numbness ensue, resulting in worry about the shortage of sleep. There is also the strong possibility of attention and concentration difficulties, which can bring on problems at home or in the work situation. In short, the quality of life will suffer from sleep disorders of long duration.

In recent years a number of articles have been published containing reviews on behavioural methods directed towards the improvement of sleep (Hyde and Pegram, 1982; Alley, 1983; Turner, 1986). An important starting point with these methods is the observation already mentioned that sleeplessness has a tendency to persist (Borkovec, 1982). If insomnia is interpreted as being secondary to underlying psychiatric, medical or environmental conditions, the initial treatment will be directed at removing these primary causes. There is, however, a behavioural component that plays a role. Insomnia can at least partly be considered as 'learned behaviour', and treatment methods should not be exclusively aimed at treatment of causes for the insomnia but also be directed towards a behaviour change.

In general, patients with insomnia will think about their complaint in causal terms. Although the establishment of clearly visible causes proves very difficult, most patients will give an obvious explanation for their sleep disturbance. They will say that their sleeplessness is caused by loneliness, or a stressful or very busy life. This attribution will make it difficult for the patient to accept any treatment that is not directed to the assumed causes. Only when insomnia is regarded as a behaviour susceptible to modification will the application of these methods become possible. This acceptance will lead to the notion that improvement can be reached by one's own efforts, instead of depending on external forces such as sleeping pills or on the removal of supposed causes. Only then will it become conceivable to accept the possibility that changing the circumstances will result in improving sleep. Against this background a number of psychological methods can be presented that may successfully combat insomnia.

Some of the methods that will be discussed are directed at relaxation. Considered are training in relaxation and methods to overcome impediments to reaching a relaxed state, such as a stream of thought that cannot be stopped or being worried when lying in bed at night. Other methods are concerned with ways to prepare oneself for a restful night, without an expectation of failing. A third behavioural approach involves stimulus control procedures that try to reassociate the bed(room) with sleep. A final method reviewed is a self-control strategy aimed at disruption of worry and rumination at bedtime: paradoxical intention.

Relaxation Training

A very important factor in the process of falling asleep is physical relaxation. This explains the emphasis on relaxation training in the treatment of insomnia. There are a number of ways to learn to relax. One of them is by getting instructions from somebody, who will explain what to do and how to do it. Voice characteristics like tone, loudness, timbre and pace partly define the effectiveness of this method of instruction, which clearly has a suggestive angle. This way of training demands as a rule individual sessions. To arrive at an acceptable level of relaxation often requires 10 or more sessions. Another manner in which relaxation training can be given is by means of audiocassettes that contain the sort of instructions used in individual training sessions as described above. The advantage of this method is the opportunity to practise intensively, and hence a shorter period of training. There are also disadvantages: there is no personal contact, the pace of the instructions cannot be adapted to the circumstances, and by repeating the same text again and again the suggestive power of the instructions will diminish. A method without a suggestive element is that of 'progressive relaxation' (Jacobson, 1938). This training is directed towards the relaxation of the body muscles. The exercises consist of a preliminary tensing of the muscle, followed by a relaxation. The training can be given in an individual session or by audiocassette, but it is also possible to use a manual outlining the steps in the exercises and the muscles involved by the use of schematic drawings.

One of the first studies on relaxation-based treatment of insomnia appeared in 1968 (Kahn, Baker and Weiss, 1968). A controlled study using progressive relaxation appeared in 1973 (Borkovec and Fowles, 1973). Turner (1986) names four representative studies that demonstrate the efficacy of progressive relaxation for the treatment of insomnia (Nicassio and Bootzin, 1974; Borkovec et al., 1979; Turner and Ascher, 1979, 1982).

Thought-stopping

Many people with insomnia complaints do not succeed in making them disappear by relaxation alone. A reason for this can be the often very long period of suffering from sleeplessness, which may give rise to a certain scepticism that in its turn prevents a really deep relaxation. Another impediment to the effect of relaxation can be the stream of thoughts going on and on when lying in bed waiting for sleep to come. This is seen by many patients as one of the causes of failure to relax sufficiently in order to fall asleep. A method known as 'thought-stopping' can be used in these cases.

Training in the method begins with instructing the patient to give free rein to his thoughts. After about one or two minutes the therapist says loudly and emphatically the word 'stop'. This same word 'stop' has to be used by the patient many times daily over a training period. Eventually this will lead to an association between saying 'stop' and an interruption of the stream of thought that is going on. To prevent this stream of thought beginning again, the patient is advised to try to visualize a peaceful situation emanating calm. This step aims to replace the active moving thoughts by a passive stationary thought with a reposeful character. By learning to use this thought-stopping method the patient can ameliorate the conditions for falling asleep. A deeper relaxation becomes possible and sleep will come easier and faster.

As a treatment for insomnia, thought-stopping has only been reported in two older case studies on anxiety-related insomnia (Taylor, cited in Wolpe, 1958; Rimm, 1973). Both authors report improvement after, respectively, four and two sessions.

Changes in Way of Life

Another improvement in the conditions surrounding the process of initiating sleep can be brought about by giving attention to the life the patient leads.

Factors may exist that tend to prevent a relaxed ending to the day. A method based on this idea formulates some rules to achieve a gradual decline in the level of arousal at the end of the day. To this end a questionnaire is used in which a number of questions assess the daily pattern of life, dealing with regularity and established habits. The answers serve to draw the patient's attention to the way he spends his days, and the role therein of routine, stress, drudgery and tempo. It may be that factors hitherto unrealized are the real inhibitors of one's ability to let go of the turmoil at the end of the day. On the basis of the completed questionnaire, changes in the way things are habitually done by the patient are discussed with the psychologist. One or two changes are agreed upon to be introduced in the week that follows. Those changes can be unrelated to the sleep problem, but have to do with altering fixed habits or doing certain things in a different way from usual.

The major reason for introducing these changes is that they let the patient experience the effects of an active intervention in the rhythm of the days that often seems unalterable. It conveys the notion to the patient that it is possible to create favourable conditions for sleep by the patient's own decision and effort.

This method builds on the notion of Coates and Thoresen (1980), who advocate the development of multicomponent treatment programmes. They stress 'the importance of changes across several dimensions of the client's life, activities and characteristic responses'.

Neutralizing Negative Expectations

After having experienced years of little or bad sleep, there often ensues a negative expectation in the patient with regard to sleep, involving an aversion to going to sleep in the evening knowing that a long period of lying awake lies ahead. A method for dealing with this anticipation tries to consciously evoke pleasing thoughts in the period just before going to bed. A questionnaire is used to assess the amount of pleasure related to a number of activities, thoughts and experiences. After that, training in visualizing those activities that were judged as pleasant follows. To facilitate the imagining of those activities at the right moment, patients are asked to make a sort of timetable of the last 30 minutes before going to bed. In this period they have to indicate a number (four or five) of easily recognizable moments that occur each evening in more or less the same manner. These can be, for instance, the locking of doors, the preparing of items for the next day, or putting out lights. It is at these recurring moments that the patient invokes one of the pleasing experiences. The purpose of this exercise is to create an atmosphere characterized not by an anticipation of the difficulties of falling asleep, but rather by a number of pleasant thoughts that can prepare for a relaxed state of mind when lying in bed.

This method, like the preceding one, is based on the self-management model formulated by Thoresen (Thoresen *et al.*, 1980), in which cognitive restructuring requires practice in replacing specific maladaptive thoughts with more adaptive and sleep-enhancing ones.

Systematic Desensitization

When lying in bed waiting for sleep to come, it often happens that thoughts of a more or less alarming character arise. They can refer to events or experiences from the remote or recent past, but can also have a more general nature. These thoughts produce an arousal that can result in anxiety, which is incompatible with relaxation.

A method that teaches how to cope with this anxiety is the behavioural technique of systematic desensitization. Its purpose is to decrease the susceptibility for anxiety-provoking thoughts or ideas. The procedure is as follows. Patients are presented with a list containing a number of topics that are often reported by people as potentially upsetting. This list comprises items like 'I worry about tomorrow', 'I hear the clock strike three', 'I will be very tired tomorrow'. Using this checklist the patient formulates those thoughts that in his or her case are responsible for a high arousal level. The statements are then rank ordered to form a hierarchy of increasing anxiety potency. The procedure of desensitization proper proceeds as follows. The patient is asked to relax. When relaxation is accomplished, he or she is instructed to imagine the situation that corresponds to the first item from the hierarchy (low arousal level). The imagined situation has to be as vivid as possible and must last for about 30 seconds. If the relaxation was disturbed by the imagining, the procedure is repeated. This goes on until the relaxation can be maintained during the imagined situation. When this goal is reached, the other items from the hierarchy are used in the same way.

This method of coping with anxiety will result in diminishing the degree to which thoughts contribute to a heightened level of arousal.

Systematic desensitization has been used as a treatment method for insomnia since 1966 (Geer and Katkin, 1966). In a review article, Ribordy and Denney (1977) conclude that the method appears to be no more effective than relaxation alone.

Changing Bedroom Activities

Chronic insomnia can entail consequences that eventually aggravate the complaints. If there is a history of recurrently lying awake at night, the bedroom may become associated with feelings of despondency arising from repeatedly and consistently failing to fall asleep. The negative anticipation and the continuous effort have a worsening effect on the ability to relax and let things go their own way to bring the needed sleep. Moreover, the bedroom will gradually change its character from a room to sleep in to a room to do all sorts of other things except sleeping. All activities one engages in when unable to fall asleep, like reading, eating or drinking, watching television and so on, will eventually be associated with the bedroom. As a result of this it will grow progressively harder to achieve the state of mind that is needed for letting the natural process of falling asleep take its course.

It will help when the bedroom regains its association with sleep. A technique that tries to realize this uses instructions to facilitate the pairing of being in bed with falling asleep (Bootzin, 1976). Those instructions include: going to bed only when feeling sleepy; avoiding non-sleeping activities in the bedroom; getting up and leaving the bedroom when not asleep within about 10 minutes; avoiding daytime naps and getting up at the same time each morning.

There are a number of studies concerning stimulus control techniques. Two recent articles show stimulus control to be more effective than no-treatment and placebo conditions, and than progressive relaxation (Lacks et al., 1983a,b).

Paradoxical Intention

A method that has also been used in the treatment of insomnia is paradoxical intention. This requires engaging in the symptomatic behaviour that is the target for treatment (Ascher and Efram, 1978; Turner and Ditomasso, 1980). It involves dismissing all effort to get to sleep. On the contrary, one has to try to stay awake as long as possible. One is not permitted to pass the time by reading or other activities or to get up from bed. This technique aims at decreasing the anxiety and worry that accompany recurrent failed attempts to get to sleep. The aim is to remain awake and therefore the 'effort to sleep' is abandoned. This will facilitate falling asleep naturally.

Reports on the effects of paradoxical intention for the treatment of insomnia are not consistent (Turner and Ascher, 1979; Lacks et al., 1983b). The procedure appears to be effective for certain individuals (Relinger and Bornstein, 1979; Espie and Lindsay, 1985). The latter advance as a possible explanation that patients experiencing considerable anxiety regarding the negative consequences of sleep loss are more likely to profit by this method than patients with high levels of physiological tension.

A TREATMENT PROGRAMME

A number of the methods mentioned were brought together to form a 'Learning to Sleep' programme that offered a group treatment to insomniacs (Zwart and Jansma, 1978). It has been in use since 1979 in different settings such as psychologists' practices, day treatment centres or social work institutions.

The programme consisted of eight weekly sessions, each of 90 minutes' duration. Six to eight patients participated. The groups were conducted by two group leaders.

In each treatment session information was supplied about sleep and sleep disturbances and a treatment procedure was explained and practised. Patients were asked to fill in a daily sleep log on sleep latency, number of hours slept, and number of awakenings. They were also asked to rate the quality of sleep and report the use of medication.

In the programme were included the methods of relaxation training, thought-stopping, changes in way of life, neutralizing negative expectations and systematic desensitization.

Results

There are data on 325 participants, 75% of whom were women. The average age was 48.7 years; 80% were aged between 25 and 65 years.

Difficulty in falling asleep was reported by 72% of the participants, frequent awakening during the night was mentioned by 38% and a short sleep duration by 29%. Two-thirds of all participants reported having more than one of these complaints simultaneously.

There was a great variation (1–55 years) in the length of time the problem had existed, the median value being 6.8 years. Regular use of sleep medication was reported by 71% of the participants.

The daily completed sleeping logs yielded some data about the effects experienced by the participants. For all parameters a significant difference (t-test, $p <$ 0.001) was found between the average values for the first and the last week of the programme. The percentage of patients reporting improvement on latency, duration and awakenings varied between 56 and 70; improvement on the quality of sleep was reported by 76%.

Investigation of the extent to which participants succeeded in keeping to the agreement made about desisting from medication showed that out of 183 persons who reported a regular use of sleeping pills in the period before the programme started:

- 43% succeeded in abstaining from the onset
- 23% succeeded by a gradual diminishing of the intake to no medication in the last week
- 8% succeeded in diminishing the dose, but did not reach total abstention
- 26% did not succeed in reducing medication use

DISCUSSION

Sleep disorders, and in particular the insomnias, are complaints afflicting many people. In contrast, knowledge about aetiology and relevant treatment methods is relatively modest. Pharmacological treatment is an obvious choice (Cleghorn et al., 1983a), but the effect achieved by medication is often only temporary (Borkovec, 1982).

In this chapter a number of behavioural treatment methods were brought together that may be used as an alternative when medication brings no further improvement.

Some of the methods reviewed have been intensively investigated. Progressive relaxation and stimulus control have been shown to be effective treatments for insomnia (Turner, 1986). Paradoxical intention does not show consistent results (Turner, 1986) and considerable variability in response to therapy was observed (Espie and Lindsay, 1985). Progressive relaxation and the other methods described were used as parts of a programme presented as 'Learning to Sleep'. The results were promising, but can only be interpreted as suggestive.

The use of a treatment package approach makes it impossible to identify the effects of separate parts of the programme. Further research is needed before it will be clear which method of treatment is suitable in a particular case of insomnia, the more so as a variability in response to the programme was observed.

NOTES

[1]Address for correspondence: F. M. Zwart, Vergiliuslaan 2, 3584 AM Utrecht, The Netherlands.

REFERENCES

Alley, P. M. (1983). Helping individuals with sleep disturbances: Some behavior therapy techniques. *Personal Guidance Journal*, **61**, 606–608.

Ascher, L. M. and Efram, S. (1978). Use of paradoxical intention in a behavioral program for sleep onset insomnia. *Journal of Consulting and Clinical Psychology*, **46**, 547–550.

Association of Sleep Disorders Centers (1979). The diagnostic classification of sleep and arousal disorders. *Sleep*, **2**, 1–137.

Bixler, E. O., Kales, A., Soldatos, C. R., Kales, J. D. and Healey, S. (1979). Prevalence of sleep disorders in the Los Angeles Metropolitan Area. *American Journal of Psychiatry*, **136**, 1257–1262.

Bootzin, R. R. (1976). Self-help techniques for controlling insomnia. In: Franks, C. M. (Ed.) *Behavior Therapy: Techniques, Principles and Patient Aids*. New York: Biomonitoring Applications, pp. 203–239.

Bootzin, R. R. and Engle-Friedman, M. (1981). The assessment of insomnia. *Behavioral Assessment*, **3**, 107–126.

Bootzin, R. R. and Nicassio, P. M. (1978). Behavioral treatments for insomnia. In: Hersen, M., Eisler, R. M. and Miller, P. M. (Eds) *Progress in Behavior Modification*, Vol. 6. New York: Academic Press, pp. 1–45.

Borkovec, T. D. (1982). Insomnia. *Journal of Consulting and Clinical Psychology*, **50**, 880–895.

Borkovec, T. D. and Fowles, D. C. (1973). Controlled investigation of the effects of progressive relaxation and hypnotic relaxation on insomnia. *Journal of Abnormal Psychology*, **82**, 153–158.

Borkovec, T. D., Grayson, J., O'Brien, G. T. and Weerts, T. C. (1979). Treatment of pseudo-insomnia and idiopathic insomnia via progressive relaxation with and without muscle tension release: An electroencephalographic evaluation. *Journal of Applied Behavior Analysis*, **12**, 37–54.

Byerley, B. and Gillin, J. C. (1984). Diagnosis and management of insomnia. *Psychiatric Clinics of North America*, **7**, 773–789.

Cleghorn, J. M., Kaplan, R. D., Bellissimo, A. and Szatmari, P. (1983a). Insomnia, I. Classification, assessment and pharmaceutical treatment. *Canadian Journal of Psychiatry*, **28**, 339–346.

Cleghorn, J. M., Bellissimo, A., Kaplan, R. D. and Szatmari, P. (1983b). Insomnia: II. Assessment and treatment of chronic insomnia. *Canadian Journal of Psychiatry*, **28**, 347–353.

Coates, T. J. and Thoresen, C. E. (1980). Treating sleep disorders: Few answers, some suggestions and many questions. In: Turner, S., Adams, H. E. and Cachoun, K. (Eds) *Handbook of Clinical Behavior Therapy*. New York: Wiley, pp. 240–289.

De Graaf, W. (1984). *Huisarts en Slaapgedrag. Waarnemingen Omtrent Slaapgedrag in de Huisartspraktijk*. Lisse: Swets and Zeitlinger.

Espie, C. A. and Lindsay, W. R. (1985). Paradoxical intention in the treatment of chronic insomnia: Six case studies illustrating variability in therapeutic response. *Behavior Research and Therapy*, **23**, 703–709.

Faust, V. and Hole, G. (1980). Zur Diagnose der Schlafstörungen. Der gestörte Schlaf (1). *Zeitschrift für Allgemeinmedizin*, **35/36**, 2423–2436.

Geer, J. H. and Katkin, E. S. (1966). Treatment of insomnia using a variant of systematic desensitization. *Journal of Abnormal Psychology*, **71**, 161–164.

Hyde, P. and Pegram, V. (1982). Sleep, sleep disorders, and some behavioral approaches to treatment of insomnia. In: Doleys, D. M., Meredith, R. L. and Ciminero, A. R. (Eds) *Behavioral Medicine*. New York: Plenum, pp. 447–470.

Jacobson, E. (1938). *Progressive Relaxation*. Chicago: University of Chicago Press.

Kahn, M., Baker, B. and Weiss, J. (1968). Treatment of insomnia by relaxation training. *Journal of Abnormal Psychology*, **73**, 556–558.

Lacks, P. E., Bertelson, A. D., Sugerman, J. and Kunkel, J. (1983a). The treatment of sleep-maintenance insomnia with stimulus-control techniques. *Behavior Research and Therapy*, **21**, 291–295.

Lacks, P. E., Bertelson, A. D., Gans, L. and Kunkel, J. (1983b). The effectiveness of three behavioral treatments for different degrees of sleep-onset insomnia. *Behavior Therapy*, **14**, 593–605.

Nicassio, P. and Bootzin, R. (1974). A comparison of progressive relaxation and autogenic training as treatments for insomnia. *Journal of Abnormal Psychology*, **83**, 253–260.

Relinger, H. and Bornstein, P. H. (1979). Treatment of sleep onset insomnia by paradoxical instruction. *Behavior Modification*, **3**, 203–222.

Ribordy, S. C. and Denney, D. R. (1977). The behavioral treatment of insomnia: An alternative to drug therapy. *Behavior Research and Therapy*, **15**, 39–50.

Rimm, D. C. (1973). Thought stopping and covert assertion in the treatment of phobias. *Journal of Consulting and Clinical Psychology*, **41**, 466–467.

Thoresen, C. E., Coates, T. J., Zarcone, V. P., Kirmil-Gray, K. and Rosekind, M. R. (1980). Treating the complaint of insomnia: Self-management perspectives. In: Ferguson, J. M. and Taylor, C. B. (Eds) *The Comprehensive Handbook of Behavioral Medicine*, Vol. 1. Jamaica, NY: Spectrum, pp. 213–234.

Turner, R. M. (1986). Behavioral self-control procedures for disorders of initiating and maintaining sleep (DIMS). *Clinical Psychology Review*, **6**, 27–38.

Turner, R. M. and Ascher, L. M. (1979). Controlled comparison of progressive relaxation, stimulus control, and paradoxical intention therapies for insomnia. *Journal of Consulting and Clinical Psychology*, **47**, 500–508.

Turner, R. M. and Ascher, L. M. (1982). Therapist factor in the treatment of insomnia. *Behavior Research and Therapy*, **20**, 33–40.

Turner, R. M. and Ditomasso, R. A. (1980). The behavioral treatment of insomnia. *International Journal of Mental Health*, **9**, 129–148.

Wolpe, J. (1958). *Psychotherapy by Reciprocal Inhibition*. Stanford: Stanford University Press.

Zwart, F. M. and Jansma, K. R. (1978). *Handleiding Slapeloosheidsbehandeling* (Manual for Treatment Program). Utrecht: Instituut voor Klinische Psychologie, Psychotherapie en Preventie.

CHAPTER 7

Cardiac Phobia

R. Beunderman[1] and D. J. Duyvis

University of Amsterdam, Amsterdam

ABSTRACT

In this chapter a survey is given of the epidemiology and symptomatology of cardiac phobia. After a description of behavioural and environmental factors that influence the development of cardiac phobia, the medical factors that influence its origin are discussed. In connection with this the problem of timely and adequate diagnostic tests is described. By means of a behavioural analysis the psychologist draws up a plan of treatment. Those factors that are potentially relevant in behavioural analysis and the consequent treatment are further discussed and explained by means of a case study.

INTRODUCTION

Patients with cardiac complaints for which no clear somatic cause can be found in a medical examination constitute an important problem in the everyday experience of a general practitioner (GP) and a cardiologist. With great persistency these patients present a range of physical complaints to the physician such as tightness, chest pain, pain in the shoulders and arms and dizziness. What is most striking is that the patients are very frightened of a reoccurrence of their complaints and frequently visit a physician to return home 'reassured' afterwards. These sudden improvements are usually shortlived, however. In order 'to make sure', extensive examinations often take place to convince the patient (and sometimes the physician as well) that 'there is nothing wrong'. When these examinations do not indicate any somatic disorder, the patient is often told that the complaints are due to 'nerves' or that they are 'psychological', and sometimes referral for psychological treatment follows. The patients are usually not

Behavioural Medicine
Edited by A. A. Kaptein, H. M. van der Ploeg, B. Garssen, P. J. G. Schreurs and R. Beunderman
© 1990 John Wiley & Sons Ltd.

quite motivated for this. They feel rejected, disappointed and cannot understand why they are suffering from complaints when no somatic disorders are found.

NOMENCLATURE

In the literature many different terms are used for the conglomerate of symptoms presented by patients suffering from cardiac phobia. As early as 1831 Forbes describes the syndrome under the name of 'functional angina'; in 1871 Da Costa speaks of 'irritable heart'. It is Freud, however, who in 1895 for the first time points out the fear that lies at the root of the patient's complaints. In this respect Freud therefore labels the syndrome as 'anxiety neurosis' (Richter and Beckmann, 1973).

After Freud, symptoms for a long time are no longer regarded as belonging to a syndrome, but are, depending on the clinician's or researcher's discipline, often seen as isolated phenomena. Thus it is possible that patients who emphasize dizziness when presenting their complaints end up with an ear, nose and throat specialist while patients who mention chest pains are often referred to a cardiologist. Not until 1947 is this syndrome described once again, this time under the name 'neurocirculatory' (Richter and Beckmann, 1973). For a survey of the many different terms that have been applied to this syndrome through the years the reader is referred to Nützinger et al. (1987).

Marks (1987) states: 'Illness phobia can be regarded as a form of focused hypochondriasis (DSM-III-R somatization disorder). In hypochondriasis the fears are diffuse and not of any particular malady (p. 297) . . . When the fear persistently focuses in a simple symptom or illness in the absence of another psychiatric disorder, the term illness phobia is appropriate' (p. 410).

Illness phobia differs from other phobias in that the stimuli that evoke fear are in the person's body rather than in his or her environment. When fear of cardiac complaints is central we speak of cardiac phobia, which is defined thus by Pfersmann, Cayrioglu and Zapotocsky (1985): the heart and its activity are in the centre of the patient's subjective experience of anxiety without there being an ascertainable organic substrate for the disturbance. Patients suffer from the constant fear that they could at any time fall victim to sudden heart death.

EPIDEMIOLOGY

Most people (84%) with cardiac phobia are aged between 21 and 48 years. Opinions differ as to division according to gender. It is estimated that 10% of a GP's list and up to some 40% of a cardiologist's practice is constituted by these patients. The prevalence of cardiac phobia in the population is estimated at 2–5% (Richter and Beckmann, 1973). It is remarkable that patients with cardiac phobia are more often married than the average population. The probability of developing cardiac phobia is independent of intelligence, education and profession. More often than an average population, patients with cardiac phobia do not partake in the labour process or function below their factual level of education (Orlemans and ten Doesschate, 1976; Marks, 1987). One often finds with people with cardiac phobia that either one of the parents or one of the children also suffers from cardiac phobia.

SYMPTOMATOLOGY

The variety of symptoms in patients with cardiac phobia is large. As an example, Orlemans and ten Doesschate (1976) review some four articles in which an extensive survey of the symptoms is given. In these articles some 75 symptoms are mentioned of which only nine occur in all four, namely, chest pain, general depression, tightness, palpitations of the heart, paraesthesia, trembling, dizziness, sleeping disorders and fear of dying. In addition, complaints like tiredness, perspiration, headache, shortness of breath, irritability and restlessness are also mentioned.

The patient's pattern of complaints may be grounds for a GP to perform extensive physical examinations which could lead to two possible results:

1. Nothing is found. Yet the patient will start to doubt even further if there is not some somatic cause ('the doctor would not examine me this thoroughly if he did not think something was wrong'). In other words, the physical examination promotes confirmation of a physical explanation of the complaints.
2. Something is found ('nothing important, but we will keep an eye on it for the time being').

In both cases the patient receives confirmation of his fears that something somatic is wrong and a process of fixation on somatic symptoms may start. In regard to the issue of keeping the influence of medical factors on the process of somatic fixation as small as possible, the question is valid as to how necessary or desirable a medical examination is for the treatment of patients with cardiac phobia. Opinions differ greatly about the value of medical examinations during the early stages of treatment. Richter and Beckmann (1973) argue that a perfunctory examination by the physician will not suffice. Orlemans and ten Doesschate (1976) on the other hand point to the danger of routine referral by a GP to a cardiologist.

One may wonder why doctors again and again perform physical examinations on these patients. One explanation for this can be found in the problems that present themselves to the GP when diagnosing symptoms of a heart attack. In practice it turns out that the symptom pattern of a patient who suffers from a heart attack at first sight strongly resembles the symptom pattern mentioned by patients with cardiac phobia. The problem then presents itself that, even after extensive specialist examination, a somatic cause cannot be found in a great many patients (Wilcox, Roland and Hampton, 1981; Todd, 1983).

Besides patterns of complaints with cardiac causes (e.g., angina pectoris and mitral valve prolapse) or another organic cause (affections of the gastrointestinal tract, respiratory tract, neurological affections, endocrinological disorders), psychophysiological causes are also possible (e.g. hyperventilation, Nützinger et al., 1987).

Though it would be better for a patient with cardiac phobia if the GP omitted extensive examination (and referral to a specialist), the opposite holds true, of course, for a patient suffering from a heart attack. For the GP not to overlook a patient with myocardial infarction is a compelling necessity. Therefore an examination should take place. Should extensive diagnostic tests be applied? Todd (1983) argues that all modern tests taken together do not with all certainty exclude a minor myocardial infarction.

It would be useful, therefore, to start from positive criteria based on actual characteristics and/or symptoms when diagnosing cardiac phobic complaints instead of diagnosing on the basis of exclusion of cardiac and/or other organic causes. To identify those criteria we undertook an investigation in the Cardiological Clinic of the Academic Medical Centre at Amsterdam. In this investigation we examined the differences and similarities between symptom patterns of patients who were classified as myocardial infarction patients and those who were classified as patients with non-cardiac chest pain. In the following paragraphs a summary of the results is given.

A Research Illustration: Patterns of Complaints in Patients with Myocardial Infarction Compared to Patients with Non-cardiac Chest Pain

In the investigation we undertook, 53 patients were interviewed who had presented at the Emergency Coronary Care Unit (ECCU) of the Academic Medical Centre at Amsterdam with symptoms of chest pain and who were classified as non-cardiac chest pain (NCCP). Their replies were compared to those of 53 patients suffering from myocardial infarction (MI) regarding symptoms they had observed during the acute phase and during the three weeks preceding the acute phase (known as the prodromal phase). It was found that patients with myocardial infarction reported pain in the centre of the chest in the acute phase more often than patients with non-cardiac chest pain. This last group of patients reported pain particularly on the left side of the chest and in the left upper arm. In Figures 7.1 and 7.2 the locations of pain symptoms are depicted as observed during the acute phase.

Significantly more often than patients with myocardial infarction, patients with non-cardiac chest pain reported (in both the acute and the prodromal phase): palpitations of the heart, paraesthesia and a 'numb feeling' in arms and legs; in the prodromal phase they also more often reported stiff and/or numb fingers (Beunderman, van Dis and Duyvis, 1987).

In a second study, 39 patients classified as angina pectoris patients were interviewed. It was found that the symptom patterns of patients with angina

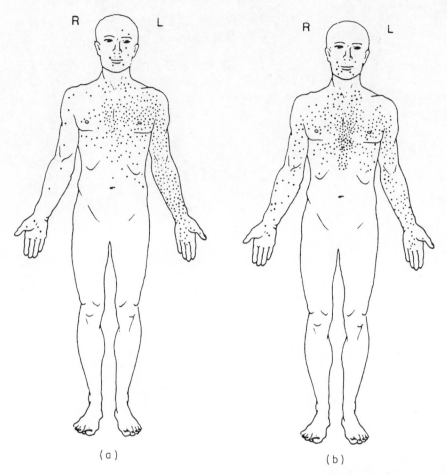

Figure 7.1. Pain symptoms during the acute phase as reported by patients (a) with functional cardiac complaints (NCCP) and (b) myocardial infarction patients. Reprinted from Beunderman, R. and Duyvis, D. J. (1983). *Psychotherapy and Psychosomatics*, **40**, 129–136. Reproduced by permission of S. Karger AG, Basel

pectoris closely resembled those of patients with a myocardial infarction (Beunderman *et al.*, 1988).

BEHAVIOURAL ANALYSIS IN PATIENTS WITH CARDIAC PHOBIA

In this section we describe a number of the most frequently occurring symptoms and behaviour (responses) of patients with cardiac phobia, the possible causes for the symptoms (stimuli), the physical factors that influence the development of complaints, and the possible consequences for the patient (and his social and medical environment). A number of factors that could facilitate the development of the complaints are identified. In the behavioural analysis the complaints are

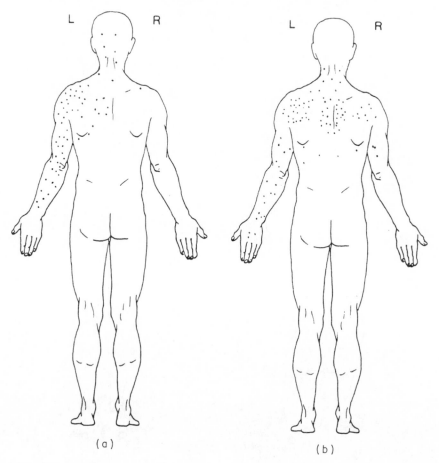

Figure 7.2. Pain symptoms during the acute phase as reported by patients (a) with functional cardiac complaints (NCCP) and (b) myocardial infarction patients. Reprinted from Beunderman, R. and Duyvis, D. J. (1983) *Psychotherapy and Psychosomatics*, **40**, 129–136. Reproduced by permission of S. Karger AG, Basel

first meticulously charted and factors are identified which possibly cause and maintain the complaints. On the basis of this analysis therapeutic measures are chosen (Emmelkamp, 1982).

Stimuli (Possible Causes for the Development of Complaints)

Though many patients describe the first attack as a 'bolt from the blue', on further exploration various events turn out to have preceded the complaints.

Stressful Events

1. Sometimes the first occasion on which the complaints occurred has been preceded by a confrontation with serious illness, impending or actual

separation from one's partner, and/or death in the patient's intimate social environment.

2. In some cases surgery has taken place. Terrifying stimuli could involve anaesthesia or unpleasant experiences when regaining consciousness after anaesthesia.

3. A period of stress may have preceded the first attack, for instance in connection with problems at work and relationships.

Perception of Physical Symptoms

4. Richter and Beckmann (1973) mention as possible causes for the occurrence of complaints alarming perceptions regarding physical sensations resulting from the use of coffee and alcohol, an allergic reaction, physical exertion or lack of sleep. Patients regard these physical sensations as the first sign of an impending heart attack, and anxiously await the next sign.

Information Concerning Heart Illnesses

5. Especially at a later stage, anything that has to do with illness and death might act as a stimulus, for example films about hospitals, obituaries, hearses, graveyards.

6. Lastly, publications in the media concerning heart illness or a doctor's advice or remark that focuses attention on the heart may induce cardiac complaints.

Responses (Behaviour and Symptoms)

Three components of complaints can be distinguished, namely, physical, cognitive and behavioural components (Orlemans and ten Doesschate, 1976; Lang, 1985; Clark, 1986; Margraf, Ehlers and Roth, 1986; Argyle, 1988).

1. Physical components include, for example, palpitations of the heart and chest pains (which the patients may describe in various ways, for instance as 'knife thrusts' or 'like a wound') and respiratory complaints (tightness, a sensation of dyspnoea, and the like). Many of the complaints can be observed in patients with the hyperventilation syndrome as well. These complaints usually occur in the form of fits.

2. Cognitive components consist of 'labelling' and 'anticipating': the patient lives in the expectation of recurrent 'cardiac complaints' or of a heart attack. As soon as certain physical sensations occur, he will immediately label these as cardiac complaints.

3. Behavioural components consist of avoidance (for instance avoidance of physical exertion) or its opposite, the 'testing of oneself' (for instance a sudden dash); the search for aid and claiming of attention (for instance the patient asks again and again for an ECG); clinging behaviour (wanting one's partner close all the time) and behaviour that tries to ensure that a partner will act in the same way (staying at home, keeping to a diet, etc.); heart control behaviour (for instance a continual taking of one's pulse).

Physical Factors that Influence the Development of Complaints

1. An important factor in the development of cardiac complaints may be faulty respiratory habits which could lead to hyperventilation. This may give rise to complaints that resemble those occurring with a heart attack.
2. Excessive use of coffee or alcohol or an influx of nicotine could cause physical sensations which are wrongly labelled as cardiac illness. The sudden giving up of smoking could also lead to physical sensations such as palpitations which are interpreted as cardiac symptoms.
3. A general condition of fatigue in a patient shortly before the first attack could play a role in the development of complaints. A patient's physical condition is also important in the period after this attack. An example of this is the patient who, after having spared himself for a long period because of 'cardiac complaints', suddenly takes up jogging and interprets the then occurring physical reactions as signs of a bad heart condition.
4. Richter and Beckmann (1973) further mention physical sensations resulting from an allergic reaction to penicillin or during recuperation from an infectious disease, sensations which are wrongly taken by the patient as being signs of a heart disease.
5. Muscular pain as a result of tension or exertion could also be interpreted by the patient as a symptom of cardiac failure.

Consequences for the Patient

Here a distinction can be made between:

1. Consequences that yield advantages to the patient, at least in the short run, such as: getting a lot of attention from intimates and physicians in the form of repeated medical examination and reassurances; control over one's environment, in particular over the partner (e.g. not wanting to be left alone)—this could be an important aspect with relational problems in particular; 'to be spared', absenteeism at work and thus possible avoidance of work for a medical (and therefore acceptable) reason.
2. Consequences which contribute to the patient's worsened condition in the long run such as: sleeping disorders—brooding, not daring to go to sleep, or simply not being tired enough (the patient spares himself during the day or thinks that he needs more sleep than is in fact the case); disorders in sexual functioning, to be found in cardiac phobics according to Richter and Beckmann (1973); accelerated exhaustion, which can be traced back to the habit of sparing oneself (not doing anything about one's physical condition) or to sleeping disorders.

Factors That Could Contribute to the Development of Complaints (Facilitating Factors)

These could be held to include:

1. Fear of illness and death. Patients often reported that talk of 'death' and anything connected with it was taboo in the parental home. One could say they have not learned to live with death, so that every thought of death is very terrifying, let alone being able to talk about it. If a confrontation is inevitable, for instance with the loss of a loved one, emotions are hidden as soon as possible, which is, however, not successful. This then leads to stress and avoidance behaviour, which eventually could lead to physical complaints.
2. Lack of social, for example interpersonal, skills. In the literature a lack of skills in both general social contact and more intimate contacts is often reported in connection with patients who have psychophysiological complaints (Marks, 1987; Nützinger et al., 1987). These findings also hold true, we believe, in the case of patients with cardiac phobia. The patients prove to have great difficulty expressing anger and grief in more personal contacts; they often give the impression of talking 'about' their feelings rather than experiencing those feelings. The lack of social skills stands out in social contacts: social contacts are often avoided.
3. Hyperactiveness. The inclination to do a lot of things at the same time is striking; patients demand an impossible much of themselves. There could be a relation to subassertiveness: difficulty in refusing, which leads them to bite off more than they can chew.

TREATMENT

Those patients that eventually end up being treated by psychologists are often not fully motivated for a psychotherapeutic approach. They feel rejected and disappointed. They have difficulty understanding why, while they have complaints, no objective somatic disorders can be found. They show a certain resistance to discussing a direct relation between physical complaints and problems.

Various treatment strategies (i.e. flooding, cognitive therapy, biofeedback, group therapy) are mentioned in the literature. The acquisition of social skills and the enlargement of opportunities to act in social situations (assertive training) can be advisable in the treatment of patients (Pfersmann, Cayrioglu and Zapotocsky, 1985; Fiegenbaum, 1986; Nützinger et al., 1987).

In the following we describe the Orlemans and ten Doesschate (1976) model where emphasis lies on a gradual transition from a very practical and supportive approach, which connects closely with what the patient reports as his physical complaints, to a form of therapy in which attention is also paid to the possible influence of psychological factors. In their theoretical model for the treatment of patients with cardiac phobia Orlemans and ten Doesschate take as their starting point the idea that cognitive factors and physical complaints (caused by hyperventilation) follow a circular process. The relation between physical complaints and fear (cardiac phobia) is established and maintained by cognitive processes, such as:

1. *Labelling*. When a patient has chest pain, it is described as an oncoming heart attack. This label then forms a source of fear which in itself may lead to a physical phenomenon.
2. *Anticipating*. When a patient does not have any complaints, he might anticipate a next attack ('if only I do not get another attack') which could in itself result in fear. This anxious anticipation could evoke complaints that are then labelled as cardiac complaints.
3. *Attention*. The processes of labelling and anticipation bring about the patient's strongly increased attention towards specific zones in his body. As a result, the level of perception is decreased and all kinds of sensations become perceptible. These sensations are then labelled as cardiac complaints. The relation can be maintained or strengthened by hyperventilation (Tyrer, Lee and Alexander, 1980).

The model of treatment that was developed with the help of the theoretical model mentioned above distinguished a step-by-step approach:

Step 1. At first the treatment is particularly focused on physical complaints. The object is to break through the circular process by changing the cognitions and tackle the hyperventilation. This is done by providing the patient with an explanation, in particular on how the process of labelling, anticipation and attention affects his anxiety and complaints. The patient also receives an explanation about the relation between fear, respiration and hyperventilation. Leaflets entitled 'Fear of serious illnesses' and 'Hyperventilation', which were written especially for the treatment of patients with cardiac phobia, are handed out. A hyperventilation provocation test as well as respiratory exercises can enhance the patient's insight into the circular process. For an extensive description of this approach the reader is referred to the chapter on hyperventilation (Chapter 11) in this book. If these interventions do not have the desired effect, one may proceed to the next step.

Step 2. The second step focuses on the patient's experience and his avoidance behaviour. If after step 1 phobia and complaints still exist, procedures are extended. Special attention is then paid to a patient's phobic avoidance behaviour and progressive relaxation is taught. What kind of behaviour is associated with fear of cardiac illness is also verified. Often the patient turns out to have become frightened of all kinds of physical exertion and because of this avoids physical exertion as much as possible. With resumption of these activities, consultation with a physiotherapist seems advisable.

Step 3. The third step aims at learning to differentiate further between psychological factors. In our opinion, steps 1 and 2 can, in principle, be performed by a physician. When these two steps have brought no results, the physician could consider referral to a psychologist. A detailed description of the way in which this therapist analyses the problems and carries out a treatment was given in the section entitled 'Behavioural analysis'.

Reassurance of the patient by relatives only controls the patient's anxiety for a short while, and prevents him or her from learning to tolerate the discomfort produced by uncertainty about physical sensations. During the treatment relatives have to learn not to be reassuring, so that the questions are not continued indefinitely (Salkovskis and Warwick, 1986; Marks, 1987).

Aside from the psychological treatment, it might be useful to arrange with the patient that he will return to the physician only at set times to discuss the physical side of the complaints. This contact is gradually diminished, depending on the results of the treatment by both physician and psychologist.

Comment

We consider it advisable that the psychologist should give extensive information about symptoms to the patient and continually check whether the patient has understood this information. Furthermore, regular contact between patient and therapist is of importance when the patient is given exercises to do at home. It will be clear that the application of steps 1, 2 and 3 demands a considerable investment of time.

CASE STUDY

Patient B is a 23-year-old man who is referred by his GP to an outpatient mental health centre because of complaints of tightness, chest pains and dizziness for which no somatic causes could be found in previous specialist examinations by a cardiologist and a specialist in internal diseases.

B has been married for two years and works in a garage. The fear of cardiac complaints and the occurrence of attacks that take place during working days, and in particular in the morning, have prevented the patient from going to work any more. His wife, who also works full time, has stayed at home for the past month in order to be with her husband in case he should have an attack. B's complaints started in a period when B had problems at work because of changes in the tasks that he was expected to perform (from general to very specialist maintenance work, in which emphasis was placed on precision). Shortly before this change at work B married, after acute problems had developed between his girl friend and her family. Marriage and the consequent move to living on his own meant to B that, as he puts it: 'I suddenly got great responsibilities towards my wife'. When B married he moved to a different neighbourhood and in this way became separated from his family, lacking his fathers' support in particular. Before, he was taken care of and he could go out freely with his friends, now he has to take care of his wife and stay at home at night. B labels the neighbourhood where he lives as dilapidated and unsafe: 'A woman cannot walk through the streets peacefully during the day, let alone at night'. Ever since B moved to this neighbourhood, he has stopped paying visits to friends and family who live out of town, because he would have to travel too far. In general, B states that he 'feels unsafe' outdoors.

Treatment began with the cognitive approach to the complaints of hyperventilation according to the model as mentioned. Besides this B also practises relaxation exercises. As the attacks occur particularly in the mornings, B is advised to omit drinking coffee in the mornings. A training in relabelling complaints also takes place here (from 'physical complaints . . . I do not know what to do' to 'physical complaints . . . let me see what is wrong').

The second step in the programme is the treatment of the phobic complaints. A decision is made to treat the fear of travelling far and to learn to perform solution strategies when stress occurs *en route*.

The third step in the programme consists of the acquisition of social skills and improvement of the circumstances in which the patient lives and works. This is done by means of role-playing, where first an analysis is made of specific problems that occur and subsequently alternative behaviour is practised.

Treatment takes place with a frequency of one session per week during the first six months. The next six months the therapy frequency is reduced sharply and treatment is stopped after one year. The patient resumes work after one month's therapy. In negotiation with his employer, the patient manages to obtain better working conditions (e.g. a rise). His wife has then been back at work for two weeks.

After the therapy has ended, B moves to a different house where he and his wife feel more at home. Fairly soon after the beginning of the treatment B resumes his social activities and dares to visit his friends and family out of town again. Due to regained confidence in driving a car, B also dares to approach his physical complaints differently, and relabelling from 'cannot be helped' to 'a nuisance, but can be handled' occurs. In follow-up after one year B reports not suffering from physical complaints or from fear of recurrence of these complaints any more.

DISCUSSION

In this chapter practically all discussion has been about the patient and not about the therapist. As far as the therapist is concerned, we believe that not only should (s)he be very patient and understanding towards the patient with a cardiac phobia, but (s)he should also learn to handle the patient's strong somatic interest. Not infrequently the patient will report that (s)he wants to have another extensive physical examination, that there are doubts about the usefulness of the treatment, or (s)he will ask whether referral to another institution is not necessary. In this way doubts are expressed concerning the possibilities of a treatment that is focused more on psychological factors.

In the light of the strong inclination to somatic fixation of the patient, we believe that close cooperation between all medical and psychological therapists involved is an essential condition. When the patient feels sufficiently reassured about the role that somatic factors play in the development of the complaints, (s)he will then learn to be accessible to the role of psychological complaints.

NOTES

[1]Addresses for correspondence: R. Beunderman, Department of Medical Psychology, University of Amsterdam, Meibergdreef 15, 1105 AZ Amsterdam, The Netherlands; D.J. Duyvis, Department of Gynaecology & Obstetrics, University of Amsterdam, Meibergdreef 15, 1105 AZ Amsterdam, The Netherlands.

REFERENCES

Argyle, N. (1988). The nature of cognitions in panic disorder. *Behaviour Research and Therapy*, **26**, 261–264.

Beunderman, R., Dis, H. van and Duyvis, D. J. (1987). Eine Vergleichsstudie somatischer und psychologischen Symptome bei Patienten mit nicht kardial bedingtem Brust-schmerz und solchen mit Myokardinfarct. In: Nützinger, D. O., Pfersmann, D., Welan, T. and Zapotocsky, H. G. (Eds) *Herzphobie*. Stuttgart: Enke Verlag, pp. 56–65.

Beunderman, R., Dis, H. van, Koster, R. W., Boel, E., Tiemessen, C. and Schippers, J. (1988). Patients with cardiac and noncardiac chest pain. In: Emmelkamp, P. M. G. *et al.* (Eds) *Annual Series of European Research in Behavior Therapy*. Lisse: Swets and Zeitlinger, pp. 231–238.

Clark, D. M. (1986). A cognitive approach to panic. *Behaviour Research and Therapy*, **24**, 461–470.

Emmelkamp, P. M. G. (1982). *Phobic and Obsessive Compulsive Disorders: Theory, Research and Practice*. New York: Plenum.

Fiegenbaum, W. (1986). Longterm efficacy of exposure *in-vivo* for cardiac phobia. In: Hand, J. and Wittchen, H. U. (Eds) *Panic and Phobias*. Berlin: Springer-Verlag, pp. 81–89.

Grol, R. (Ed.) (1982). *Huisarts en Somatische Fixatie*. Utrecht: Bohn, Scheltema & Holkema.

Lang, G. (1985). Attribution styles among patients with cardiac neurosis. Paper presented at the 15th Annual Meeting of the EABT, Munich.

Margraf, J., Ehlers, A. and Roth, W. T. (1986). Panic attacks: Theoretical models and empirical evidence. In: Hand, I. and Wittchen, H. U. (Eds) *Panic and Phobias*. Berlin: Springer-Verlag, pp. 30–43.

Marks, I. M. (1987). *Fears, Phobias and Rituals*. Oxford: Oxford University Press.

Nützinger, D. O., Pfersmann, D., Welan, T. and Zapotoczky, H. G. (Eds) (1987). *Herzphobie*. Stuttgart: Enke Verlag.

Orlemans, J. W. G. and Doesschate, R. J. A. ten (1976). Hartziektefobie: Een gedragsther-apeutisch werkmodel. *Huisarts en Wetenschap*, **19**, 323–332.

Pfersmann, D., Cayrioglu, S. and Zapotocsky, H. G. (1985). A contribution to the therapy of cardiac phobia patients. Paper presented at the 15th Annual Meeting of the EABT, Munich.

Richter, H. E. and Beckmann, D. (1973). *Herzneurose*. Stuttgart: Thieme Verlag.

Salkovskis, P. M. and Warwick, H. M. C. (1986). Morbid preoccupations, health anxiety and reassurance: A cognitive-behavioural approach to hypochrondiasis. *Behaviour Research and Therapy*, **24**, 597–602.

Todd, J. W. (1983). Query cardiac pain. *Lancet*, **1**, 330–332.

Tyrer, P., Lee, I. and Alexander, J. (1980). Awareness of cardiac function in anxious, phobic and hypochondrial patients. *Psychological Medicine*, **10**, 171–174.

Wilcox, R. G., Roland, J. M. and Hampton, J. R. (1981). Prognosis of patients with chest-pain. *British Medical Journal*, **282**, 431–433.

CHAPTER 8

Hypertension

G. Godaert[1]

Utrecht University, Utrecht

ABSTRACT

The author illustrates that hypertension is a major risk factor for cardiovascular disorders, presents some epidemiological data on hypertension, and discusses aetiological factors. Somatic, psychological and social factors are combined into a biobehavioural model of hypertension. Drug approaches have an important place in the treatment of hypertension. Behavioural methods, such as modification of life style, physical exercise, compliance improving techniques, relaxation training, and behavioural skills training, are described and illustrated by a case study. It is concluded that behavioural methods have considerable value in the treatment of hypertension, and that during pharmacological treatment of hypertension, the effects on the quality of life of patients must be taken into account.

INTRODUCTION

Usually high blood pressure is detected more or less by chance, for instance during a routine check-up or when a patient complains of headaches or feels exhausted—symptoms mostly unrelated to high blood pressure. In most cases elevated blood pressure is not noticed by the patient, so there is no prompt to pay a visit to the physician. This is rather unfortunate, as chronic elevated pressure sometimes has deleterious consequences. For this reason, hypertension is sometimes called the 'silent killer'.

When is a given blood pressure considered 'high' and when does it lead to physical sequelae? How frequently does it occur in the general population? Is

Behavioural Medicine
Edited by A. A. Kaptein, H. M. van der Ploeg, B. Garssen, P. J. G. Schreurs and R. Beunderman
© 1990 John Wiley & Sons Ltd.

'stress' one of the causes of high blood pressure? What kinds of behavioural treatments are available? Answering these questions can be helpful in directing the therapeutic endeavours of the psychologist working in a medical setting.

HYPERTENSION: RISK FACTORS, EPIDEMIOLOGY AND AETIOLOGY

Risk Factors and Epidemiology

A blood pressure increase of a few minutes or even hours may be physiologically necessary to meet the metabolic requirements triggered by physical exercise. This increase does not cause any damage to the cardiovascular system. Even a prolonged elevation of blood pressure should not be considered as a disease *per se* because it rarely provokes symptoms or clear discomfort for the patient. It is, however, an important risk factor for cardiovascular accidents. Chronic high pressure is associated with increased morbidity and mortality. More specifically, the risk for coronary infarction and cerebrovascular accidents is markedly increased in patients with hypertension. The risk is observed to rise in a continuum of 30% for each 10 mmHg increment in pressure throughout the range of blood pressures: there is no definite boundary where the surplus mortality can suddenly be noticed (Kannel and Kreger, 1981). Arbitrary boundaries are set for convenience. People with a diastolic pressure of more than 95 mmHg have a higher risk of the above-mentioned cardiovascular consequences. The incidence of coronary infarction associated with high blood pressure is higher than the sum of the incidences of all the remaining cardiovascular diseases. In comparison with a group with a diastolic blood pressure of less than 95 mmHg, the total mortality is twice as high. Essentially the same holds for systolic pressures. The idea that only the diastolic pressure is of prognostic importance is not correct; the arbitrary dividing line for systolic pressures is usually set at 160 mmHg. A chronic elevated pressure clearly is a risk factor; measures should be taken to reduce the hazards.

Epidemiology—Some Remarks

Hypertension is a major public health problem in the United States—as well as in other industrialized countries—estimated to occur in 10–15% of the general population (Hypertension Detection and Follow-up Program Cooperative Group, 1979). Garrison *et al.* (1987) compared the occurrence of hypertension between a first (1971–1975) and a second (1979–1983) examination period for both men and women. The incidence of hypertension in participants free from hypertension at the first examination increased threefold from the second to the fifth age decades in men and eightfold in women. Under the age of 40 men were twice as likely to develop hypertension, but after age 40 eight-year incidence rates were similar in men (14.2%) and women (12.9%).

Aetiology

In only 5–10% of cases with chronic blood pressure elevation can a somatic cause be found; this condition is then called 'secondary hypertension'. The remaining cases are categorized as 'primary or essential hypertensives': no specific somatic defect can be discovered that causes the elevated pressure. In multivariate analysis, adipositas, heart rate, alcohol intake and triglycerides (specific fatty substances in the blood) were found to be independent contributors to high blood pressure in one or both of the sexes. Adipositas stands out as a major controllable contributor to hypertension. Changes in body fat over eight years were related to changes in both systolic and diastolic pressure. Markedly obese women in their forties were seven times more likely to develop hypertension than were lean women of the same age (Garrison *et al.*, 1987). Other factors seem to contribute to a disruption of blood pressure regulatory mechanisms as well. Genetic and familial influences (Feinleib, 1979), salt (Mir *et al.*, 1986), and energy balance (Mancini and Strazzullo, 1986) as well as composition of the diet (Zhao *et al.*, 1986) are involved. MacMahon (1987) reviews the literature on the relation between alcohol and hypertension. Of 30 cross-sectional population studies reviewed, the majority reported small but significant elevations in blood pressure in persons consuming three drinks or more per day in comparison with non-drinkers. The maximum contribution of alcohol consumption (greater than two drinks per day) to the prevalence of hypertension was estimated to be 5–7%. Because of their greater alcohol consumption, the contribution of alcohol to hypertension in men (11%) was greater than that in women.

All these factors, however, only account for a part of the variance in blood pressure observed in a population. There is some agreement (Greenberg, 1988; Heine and Weiss, 1987) that psychological and social 'stress' factors contribute substantially. Difficult as it may be to define precisely what is meant by stress, there is accumulating evidence that 'hypertension . . . is caused by an inadequate "person–environment fit", objectively, subjectively or both, and has to be studied in its complexity with consideration of personality, behaviour patterns and stress buffering mechanisms of social support besides stressful life events' (Heine and Weiss, 1987, p. 45).

Several factors can have their share in an 'inadequate person–environment fit'. Correlations between blood pressure and stable personality characteristics such as neuroticism have been equivocal (Harrell, 1980). Behavioural style in coping with daily situations seems more related to high blood pressure (Gentry *et al.*, 1982). Subjects inhibiting overt expression of anger had a higher blood pressure. Besides this, environmental instability (areas with a high rate of criminality for example), as well as gender and race, affected blood pressure. These four risk factors were independently related to the blood pressure. Each factor increased the chance of having a blood pressure of more than 160/95 mmHg approximately 1.5 times. A white woman living in a quiet part of town openly expressing anger had a chance of 0.06 of crossing the hypertensive boundaries. A black male respondent in a socially unstable area inhibiting his anger had a chance of 0.37.

TOWARDS A BIOBEHAVIOURAL MODEL OF HYPERTENSION

How can these psychological and social factors affect blood pressure? Responses to environmental demands usually are associated with physiological activation temporarily overriding physiological homeostasis. Laboratory analogues of natural tasks show that specific task requirements activate specific physiological patterns. Active coping tasks such as mental arithmetic under time pressure mainly increase cardiac output. Tasks primarily requiring information-processing increase peripheral resistance. Cardiovascular responses to mentally challenging tasks appear to be more pronounced in the offspring of hypertensive parents (Obrist, 1980). Tuck (1986) reviews evidence for an increased sympathetic nervous system (including adrenaline and noradrenaline) involvement in cardiovascular responses to different challenges in essential hypertensive patients and in young normotensive individuals from hypertensive-prone families, as compared to normotensive subjects without a familial involvement with hypertension.

Another question is how these transient blood pressure elevations can lead to a chronically elevated pressure. Excessively demanding or long-lasting stressors are too heavy a burden for the adaptive mechanisms mentioned above, leading to more or less permanent deregulated 'stress' responses. Research with animals showed that frequent and long-lasting activations of the stress response cause structural changes in the arterial wall and lead in the long run to increased peripheral resistance and hypertension (Folkow, 1986). In humans the progression of a hyperkinetic circulation towards an increased peripheral resistance has been documented by Safar, Simon and Levenson (1984).

Relying on this type of evidence, the hypothesis has been put forward that in some hypertensive patients, blood pressure increases are associated with specific behavioural and cognitive responses to environmental demands (Obrist, 1980; Steptoe, 1981). Cardiovascular effects of 'active' coping have been most

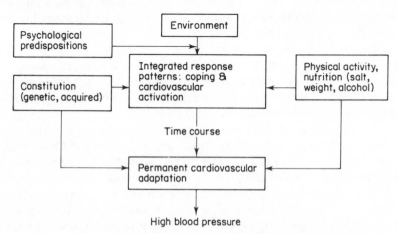

Figure 8.1. Factors contributing to essential hypertension (adapted from Steptoe, 1981)

frequently studied. Actively coping means that a subject alertly attempts to meet situational demands, and tries to control his environment. This coping is influenced by psychological predispositions such as personality traits. Active coping is accompanied by cardiovascular responses stimulated by sympathetic activation, while parasympathetic inhibition seems to be insufficient. The degree of dysregulation is affected by constitution, nutrition and physical activity. Repeated activation of these responses leads to more or less permanent haemodynamic adaptations. The process of adaptation is also influenced by constitution, nutrition and physical exercise. This process eventually results in chronically elevated blood pressure.

Interventions to be described in the following two sections can be traced back to the model outlined in Figure 8.1.

INTERVENTIONS: DRUGS AND GENERAL HEALTH MEASURES

It has been shown that drug treatment reduces morbidity and mortality due to chronically elevated blood pressure. The first intervention trials demonstrated this effect for moderate and severe hypertension (Veterans Administration Cooperative Study Group on Antihypertensive Agents, 1967, 1970). Recent trials showed that therapeutic benefit was evident in mild hypertension as well. In an Australian study (Management Committee, 1980, 1982), subjects with a diastolic pressure between 95 and 106 mmHg were treated with a placebo or active drug(s) (chlorthiazide, if necessary complemented with alphamethyldopa and propranolol). At the end of the trial, results for 2218 patients, equally distributed between the two conditions, were available. Active treatment had a beneficial effect upon the total number of cardiovascular trial endpoints. The difference was mainly due to the satisfactory effects on the incidence of cerebrovascular accidents. According to the statistical criteria of the researchers, no difference could be shown in relation to ischaemic heart problems, either fatal or non-fatal.

A similar British trial covering a population of over 17,000 has been published recently (Medical Research Council Working Party, 1985). Conclusions parallel those of the Australian trial. In the British trial, drug treatment caused a significant decrease of cardiovascular mortality due to cerebrovascular accidents: 2.6 strokes per 1000 patient years in the placebo group *versus* 1.4 in the actively treated group. Placebo and active groups did not differ in the number of recorded infarctions. Due to this, the total mortality in the actively treated group (248) was not significantly lower than in the placebo group (252). Three aspects of this intervention trial deserve further attention. First, the difference between the sum total of cerebrovascular accidents and coronary diseases in smokers *versus* non-smokers is more substantial than the difference between the active and the placebo treatment to reduce blood pressure. In other words, not smoking is more beneficial than drug treatment. In the analysis of these subgroups it emerged that drug effects were different for the two groups. The decrease of coronary events associated with the use of propranolol only occurred in subjects who did not smoke. Second, one should note the moderate *absolute* risk of people with high blood pressure: 95% of the subjects had not been affected by any cardiovascular disease. Third, annual measurements showed that between one-third and one-half of the subjects taking placebo had diastolic pressures below 95 mmHg. On the other hand, drugs can have negative side-effects that partly offset their undoubted benefits (Robertson, 1986).

Some *general therapeutic conclusions* have been drawn from these intervention trials.

1. Drug treatment of every patient with high blood pressure diminishes cerebro-vascular accidents and other complications of hypertension; this unfortunately is at the expense of a major number of low-risk patients unnecessarily treated. Drugs often have more or less serious side-effects (Medical Research Council Working Party, 1981) and are expensive. Other, non-drug treatments for lowering blood pressure should be considered and investigated. Considering the normalization of blood pressure that can be observed in a considerable proportion of patients with moderate hypertension taking placebo, a period of mere observation of blood pressure before any (drug) treatment is started seems advisable.
2. Drug treatment requires selective application. The benefits of treatment are more prominent in men than in women and in older more than in younger subjects and they are more noticeable in the extreme blood pressure range.
3. Attention should not be confined to the lowering of blood pressure by medication. Stopping smoking and reducing serum cholesterol are at least as influential in reducing coronary risk.

Blood pressure mostly can be satisfactorily controlled by medication, provided the treatment regimen is strictly followed by the patient (McClellan *et al.*, 1988). This is important, as intervention trials show that lowering of high and severe blood pressure levels reduces morbidity and mortality (Veterans Administration Cooperative Study Group on Antihypertensive Agents, 1967, 1970). A diastolic pressure of more than 115 mmHg is considered as severe hypertension that requires immediate drug treatment. A diastolic pressure of more than 100 mmHg probably requires drug treatment, especially when other risk factors such as overweight and elevated cholesterol are present. Undifferentiated use of medication in the large group of mildly elevated pressures between 90 and 100 mmHg, however, is controversial. With regard to these patients it is now recommended to first change their lifestyle, focusing on both the lowering of the blood pressure and the modification of other cardiovascular risk factors. A report of the World Health Organization recommends not starting immediately with drug therapy when dealing with a diastolic blood pressure of 90 mmHg . . . 'the first line of treatment for people with mild hypertension should be observation, perhaps combined with general health measures such as weight reduction and restriction of salt intake . . .' (WHO/ISH Mild Hypertension Liaison Committee, 1982).

Implementing behavioural interventions is not an easy task, however. Simply giving advice or recommendations often does not suffice, particularly in the long run (Wechsler *et al.*, 1983; McClellan *et al.*, 1988). How can psychologists support physicians in the important task of bringing about habit changes in hypertensive patients? When is a more specific psychological approach to be recommended, and what can be achieved?

BEHAVIOURAL TREATMENT APPROACHES

It takes years of observation on thousands of patients to document the effects of drugs on hypertension-related morbidity and mortality (see previous section). Kaplan (1985) remarks that there seems no way to provide such evidence on the efficacy of non-drug therapies for the prevention of the complications of mild hypertension. 'For that reason, the use of non-drug therapies must be accepted on the evidence that they work to lower blood pressure, are safe, and are acceptable to many patients' (p. 359). Nevertheless, Patel *et al.* (1985) show that at four-year follow-up of a controlled relaxation training study, more subjects in the control group reported having had angina and treatment for hypertension and its complications. Incidence of ischaemic heart disease, fatal myocardial infarction or electrocardiographic evidence of ischaemia was significantly greater in the control group.

In this section behavioural treatment approaches will be discussed both as to their blood pressure reducing effects and as to some ways of implementing them.

From the viewpoint of behavioural medicine several targets for intervention can be chosen. In Figure 8.1 one possibility, that of changing the environment— or helping the patient to do this—is illustrated; modification of the way of coping with the environment is another possibility. Both approaches aim to tone down the cardiovascular reactions. Changing dietary patterns, for example reduction in salt, alcohol and total caloric intake, and improving drug compliance are clearly important targets pertaining to the field of behavioural medicine. All these instances have to do with effects of behaviour on health.

First, a few interventions will be described that can be effectuated by the medical profession with some support from behavioural experts. Second, the necessity of and possibilities for a specific psychological treatment will be discussed. In Figure 8.2, a general overview of detection, surveillance and behavioural aspects of interventions in essential hypertension is presented.

A periodic check-up of the blood pressure can both preclude unnecessary drug treatment and make evident which patients need drugs or other treatment when the general health measures prove not to be efficacious.

In all the interventions to be considered, repeated measurement of blood pressure under different circumstances is of vital importance. The blood pressure taken by a doctor in a medical setting predicts forthcoming morbidity and mortality less well than readings obtained under basal conditions (Smirk, 1976) and by ambulatory measurement (Perloff, Sokolow and Cowan, 1983). Hyperreactivity of blood pressure occurring in the doctor's office (Mancia *et al.*, 1983) may be of considerable practical importance in the evaluation of patients with

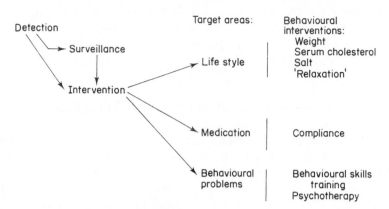

Figure 8.2. Overview of behavioural contributions to interventions in essential hypertension

mild hypertension. Recordings of blood pressure away from the medical environment—at home, at work—may be of great help (Pickering, 1987). Using ambulatory recording of blood pressure, Waeber *et al.* (1987) showed that some hypertensive patients are overtreated with drugs. There is another reason for regular (self)measurement of blood pressure. Hypertensive patients do not have 'intrinsic' information on their 'problem'. In contrast to the pain sensations for example of patients with migraine, blood pressure cannot be sensed directly and as such cannot act as an incentive to comply with therapeutic measures. Edmonds *et al.* (1985) report an increased compliance with medication after the introduction of self-measurement of blood pressure.

Changing Lifestyle: Modification of Habits

Adipositas stands out as a major controllable contributor to hypertension (Garrison *et al.*, 1987). In short clinical trials, successful *weight reduction* helped to achieve blood pressure control in obese hypertensive patients (Mancini and Strazzullo, 1986). Puddey, Beilin and Vandongen (1986) conclude that *reduction of alcohol intake* contributed to the fall in both systolic and diastolic pressure independent of weight reduction. A combination of salt restriction and reduction of overweight and alcohol intake proved to be a promising intervention for patients on drug treatment (Stamler *et al.*, 1987). In a randomized approach, one group stopped medication and was given dietary advice; the other group just stopped taking drugs. After four years a considerable proportion of the diet group decreased in overweight, and in salt and alcohol consumption; 39% still did not need resumption of the medication. In the control group only 5% were still without medication. Basler *et al.* (1987) describe a successful group-based behaviour modification programme for obese patients with essential hypertension.

Tillotson, Winston and Hall (1984) list some specific recommendations for overweight treatment of patients with high blood pressure. A number of critical conditions have to be met by the patient. Some of these are so obvious that it seems to be almost an insult to the patient to mention them: '. . . the patient acknowledges that he has high blood pressure, realizes what this can signify, accepts dietary measures as the main or adjunctive intervention for the elevated pressure . . .'. However, most hypertensive patients do not feel ill—so they easily tend to 'forget' about their condition. In everyday practice, making these assumptions explicit and repeating them periodically is of vital importance. In the coaching of medical practitioners by psychologists it is worthwhile reminding them of the basics of behavioural interventions. Personal involvement of the patient in the development and execution of a strategy for changing the nutritional habits is strongly advised. Behaviour therapy approaches to weight reduction have stressed the importance of the successive acquirement of small and very explicit steps.

Long-term success has been rated low for both weight reduction (Palgi, Bristrian and Blackburn, 1984) and moderation of alcohol intake (Wilner *et al.*, 1985). As the study of Stamler *et al.* shows, long-term effects can, however, be obtained. Of particular importance are maintenance programmes. Patients in the dietary advice group of Stamler *et al.* (1987) were followed very carefully as to their compliance with the instructions concerning weight, and their blood pressure was measured regularly. Perri *et al.* (1986) crossed two treatment conditions (behaviour therapy or behaviour therapy plus aerobic exercise) with two post-treatment conditions (no further contact or a multicomponent maintenance programme). The maintenance programme included client–therapist contact by telephone and peer self-help group meetings. At post-treatment, clients in the behaviour therapy plus aerobic exercise condition lost significantly more weight than those who received behaviour therapy only. Over an 18-month follow-up period, maintenance programme participants demonstrated significantly better weight loss progress than clients in the no-further-contact condition. The study of Robertson *et al.* (1986) shows how intensive treatment programmes may be necessary to influence alcohol consumption. Their minimal treatment condition consisted of four sessions of assessment and advice. The intensive treatment package consisted of a selection of individually tailored, cognitive-behavioural therapies lasting an average of 9.1 sessions. At follow-up (15.5 months on the average), intensively treated subjects had reduced alcohol consumption significantly more than their fellow subjects.

Attention has been paid recently to *selective dietary measures*. Kaplan (1985) gives a brief review of the contribution of sodium, potassium and the relative balance between them, magnesium, calcium, fat and fatty acids and vegetarian diets to hypertension. Amongst these, restriction of *salt intake* is one of the first dietary changes advocated both to prevent and to remediate high blood pressure (Kaplan, 1985). According to our knowledge, no programme aiming specifically at salt restriction has been published. Interestingly, an anecdote claims that providing salt sprinklers with smaller openings reduced the amount of salt used. Presumably taking simple measures can be helpful.

Some of the research reviewed by Kaplan is equivocal. If it can be proven that specific dietary components are affecting blood pressure, a new and interesting cooperative effort between dieticians and behavioural therapists should be developed.

Physical exercise is of importance in the prevention of high blood pressure. When elevated pressure is already present, moderate isotonic effort in most cases brings about a reduction; the effect declines when exercise is terminated (Cade *et al.*, 1984). Dubbert *et al.* (1984) present two case studies of behavioural control of mild hypertension with aerobic exercise. An ABAB withdrawal–reinstatement treatment design was employed, which led to essentially the same conclusions as Cade *et al.* (1984). In both subjects exercising was associated with clinically important reductions in blood pressure, independent of weight change. Cessation of exercise was systematically followed by a rapid increase in blood pressure to former, hypertensive levels.

Improving *compliance* with instructions concerning medication and other forms of treatment is of utmost importance in the treatment of high blood pressure. Treatment failures are often due to patients not—or not regularly—taking medication or not attending medical care (McClellan *et al.*, 1988). Subjects mostly do not have any direct complaints caused by an elevated blood pressure, while drugs intended to reduce blood pressure often do have unpleasant side-effects such as heart palpitations, drowsiness, impotence, nausea (Medical Research Council Working Party, 1981).

Simple measures may be helpful. Information on the drug must be clearly understood so that the patient can recall it easily. The information concerns the necessity to use the drug, the instructions for use and the possibly occurring side-effects. Medication compliance can be further supported by giving tips to remind the patient when to take the medicine ('put your pills beside your alarm clock'). Other measures can be taken to enhance habit formation ('each time you see the red sticker on your wrist watch, relax your muscles', or suggesting reinforcements to be consumed contingent upon successful completion of part of the programme) and provide feedback as to the degree of adherence by means of keeping a log on patients' daily aerobic exercises. As mentioned earlier, Edmonds *et al.* (1985) report an increased compliance with medication after the introduction of self-measurement of blood pressure. The self-recording of blood pressure increased the compliance rate in the total group from 65% at the beginning of the study to 81% at the end. In those who initially showed a poor compliance, there was an increase from 0 to 70% after self-measuring of blood pressure was introduced. Considering the practical and emotional objections involved in taking antihypertensive drugs, it is strongly recommended to work out solutions for individual problems in close cooperation with the patient (Hovell *et al.*, 1986).

Relaxation Training

Relaxation training is the most frequently used behavioural therapeutic technique in the treatment of essential hypertension (Wadden *et al.*, 1984). Relaxation exercises reduce sympathetic activation (Stone and de Leo, 1976; Hoffman *et al.*, 1982). This is important as the autonomous nervous system appears to be involved in the aetiology, respectively the sustaining of hypertension (Julius and Esler, 1975; Tuck, 1986). Wadden *et al.* (1984) summarize the effects of relaxation training and related behavioural techniques such as meditation on blood pressure as follows:

1. Relaxation training is superior to non-treatment, to blood pressure self-monitoring and to (experimental) conditions of solely giving attention to the patient.
2. Different techniques have no different effects.
3. Behavioural treatment is clearly less effective than pharmacotherapy in controlling hypertension.
4. Twenty-four-hour measurements have demonstrated generalization to different situations; long-term effects have been shown.

This positive review does not imply that no negative results have been reported (Frankel *et al.*, 1978; Surwitt, Shapiro and Good, 1978). Nevertheless, the most widely held opinion supports the use of relaxation training in a stepped-care approach, preceding or as an addition to other interventions, for example pharmacotherapy (Chesney and Black, 1986), often reducing the amount of drugs needed. As mentioned previously, relaxation training reduces other risk factors for cardiovascular disease as well (Patel *et al.*, 1985).

In a majority of cases, relaxation training cannot be considered *a priori* the exclusive treatment procedure. Especially in cases of moderate or severe hypertension, blood pressure decrease may be clinically insufficient. Relaxation training can be considered as a useful approach to help a patient change his dealing with daily life stresses (Johnston, 1986). The magnitude of blood pressure decrease varies considerably among subjects; no dependable predictors for success have been singled out (Wadden *et al.*, 1984). Relaxation training has considerable advantages, however. The technique can be readily put to use in medical settings. It can be taught in groups. Doctors or assistants with some personal affinity for this approach can be instructed relatively easily in the basic applications of relaxation techniques (Patel and Marmot, 1988). In a sense, relaxation training has 'broad spectrum effects' such as discharge of accumulated tensions and responding gradually in a more relaxed way to daily situations. Other positive effects are the reduction of anxiety and the enhancement of feelings of well-being observed in hypertensive patients besides a reduction in blood pressure (Bali, 1979; Crowther, 1983).

Several techniques have been employed to induce relaxation. Well known are progressive muscle relaxation, autogenic training, yoga and different sorts of meditation techniques (Godaert, 1981). The way in which the training programme is introduced seems to be of importance. When it was presented as a quickly working technique, an immediate decrease of blood pressure followed. When the trainees were told that it would take some time before the effects would be apparent, this indeed happened (Agras, Horne and Taylor, 1982). Instructing the patient about a technique in a direct personal contact with a trainer yields better results than the use of an audiocassette (Brauer *et al.*, 1979).

Relaxation training to reduce blood pressure has been implemented in the work setting (Chesney *et al.*, 1987) and in school (Ewart *et al.*, 1987).

Behavioural Skills Training

Many subjects qualify for a reduction of blood pressure. Therefore, initial interventions should be relatively simple to apply, as is the case with relaxation techniques. If these first interventions are not successful and (exclusive) pharmacological treatment is not indicated, more thorough diagnostic assessment is required. Psychologists are well trained for this type of work. During assessment, specific problem areas of the patient are explored. Some of these—such as violent conflicts with adolescent children or a long history of inadequate self-assertion towards one's superior—may be too complex to be handled only with broad spectrum relaxation training. In the assessment procedure, one must be careful not to jump to conclusions concerning the 'causation' of the elevated blood pressure (Kallinke, Kulick and Heim, 1982). It is not possible to rely on general statements such as 'hypertensive patients are subassertive, and therefore assertiveness training will decrease blood pressure'. In order to substantiate an hypothesis concerning the individual conditions for blood pressure increase, one can ask the patient to take blood-pressure measurements (with semiautomatic devices) along with diary notes. Alternatively, a conflict can be simulated while the blood pressure is monitored. Behavioural skills training endeavours to teach the patient adequate ways to handle specific situations which have been shown to often induce an increase in blood pressure. If one succeeds in changing these behavioural–emotional reactions, one may expect a diminution in blood-pressure responses to these situations.

Behaviour therapy has provided the psychologist with a range of structured behavioural skills trainings. Programmes for stress management training include (a) learning to discriminate sources of stress and to observe reactions to these stressors; (b) developing alternative behavioural, cognitive and emotional reactions to the stressors; and (c) bringing these skills into practice and rehearsing them over and over (Meichenbaum and Cameron, 1984). Crowther (1983) reports positive findings of stress management training and imagery on both blood-pressure and anxiety level. Charlesworth, Williams and Baer (1984) describe the application of a stress management programme conducted with hypertensive employees at the worksite. In contrast to a control group, both systolic and diastolic blood pressure were significantly reduced after a 10-week treatment period. When the former control group was then given the training, the resulting systolic and diastolic blood pressure reductions were significant. After a three-year follow-up, blood pressure was still significantly reduced.

Tailoring the technique to the specifics of the problem encountered, Ewart *et al.* (1984) experimentally treated 20 couples with communication problems. Ten of them took part in the training, 10 served as a control group. After the training, the treated group showed significantly less blood-pressure increase when confronted with communication problems with their partners. This is important because marked cardiovascular reactions are associated with the development of hypertension (Falkner *et al.*, 1981). Restriction of repeated, marked blood pressure reactions through application of learned behavioural skills might help to prevent further blood-pressure increase caused by the gradually developing structural changes in the vascular system.

Adding a form of biofeedback to therapeutic counselling (Lynch *et al.*, 1982) reveals new, interesting possibilities. During the biofeedback procedure, the patient's attention is drawn to the fluctuations in the blood pressure related to his emotional reactions to the counselling process. According to the authors, blood-pressure increases are mainly caused by psychological defensive reactions to threatening emotional contents. Assisted by the biofeedback information, patients discover which topics seem to raise their blood pressure. Helped by the therapist, they can develop new methods in their (emotional) handling of conflictual items. Needless to say, this procedure asks for psychotherapeutic qualifications in addition to technical biofeedback skills. Used as a technique by itself, biofeedback training for high blood pressure probably has little to offer in addition to general relaxation effects (Glasgow and Engel, 1987).

A CASE HISTORY

Chesney and Black (1986) advocate a step-by-step approach for the behavioural treatment of hypertension. Besides relaxation-type interventions, one should also consider other behavioural interventions. In the following case, the tailoring of a treatment programme to the peculiarities of a patient will be illustrated. In addition to the interventions mentioned in previous sections of this chapter, use is made of self-measurement of blood pressure. This procedure has some reducing effects on blood pressure (Laughlin, 1981), yields information as to which situations or problem areas are inducive of tension and/or blood-pressure increase and enhances compliance.

Mr B, 36 years old, with a systolic blood pressure of 170 mmHg and a diastolic pressure of 110 mmHg, is referred by his general practitioner to the psychologist. The patient is not taking antihypertensive medication, is 1.80 m tall and weights 117 kg. Since the age of 20 there have repeatedly been reports of 'elevated blood pressure' at physical examinations. Two years ago his physician prescribed a diuretic, following a reading of 190 mmHg systolic; this medication had no effect. His excess weight dates from his military service. For three years there have been problems concerning unemployment and social security. At present he has no job. Two years ago his handicapped daughter died. This was a terrible shock for the whole family. The physician refers this patient because he suspects that the high blood pressure is determined by unemployment problems and the inadequate working through of the loss of his child.

During the intake it becomes evident that the patient drinks a lot; 10 bottles of beer a day is no exception. He drinks to calm down when he feels tense, for example when he is reminded of the death of his child. Feelings of tensions also lead to eating between meals. Mr B mentions that he does not sleep well. He still swims and rides his bicycle, but considerably less than he used to do. We agree with the patient on the following treatment strategy:

1. Weight reduction by means of a structured programme in which the changing of eating habits in a step-by-step way is emphasized—in contrast to drastic diets with spectacular but only temporary effects.
2. Relaxation training to control tension and to consequently limit the incitement for alcohol use and eating between meals.
3. In the first treatment phase we offer the opportunity to discuss emotional problems concerning bereavement and unemployment when the patient expresses his need to do so.

During the period of four weeks preceding the training, Mr B takes his blood pressure in the morning and in the evening. Systolic blood pressure averages 156 mmHg, diastolic 106 mmHg. The completion of the programme takes eight weeks and it runs without problems. Mr B is highly motivated and conforms precisely to most of the prescribed changes in eating habits. The relaxation programme presents some problems, mainly concerning diaphragmatic breathing. After some extra training, he masters this skill as well. Mr B reports that he is feeling less tense and that he has decreased his use of alcohol. Strongly encouraged by the therapist, he spends more time on sports. From time to time he reports an occasional surge of emotions. After eight weeks he has lost 8 kg. The self-recorded pressure averages to 145/95 mmHg. A two-month period without therapeutic contacts follows; both blood pressure and weight increase somewhat. Four weekly booster sessions make up for that. At the final evaluation, Mr B reports a general feeling of improved well-being. He sleeps better, and feels tense less frequently. He feels no need for further therapeutic contacts concerning his emotional problems.

BEHAVIOURAL INTERVENTIONS IN HYPERTENSION: A SHORT OVERVIEW

If the blood pressure is repeatedly elevated, treatment should be considered. For borderline hypertensive patients (systolic blood pressure between 140 and 160 mmHg) the first step can be restricted in most cases to behavioural, non-drug interventions. At higher blood pressure levels antihypertensive medication has usually to be included; this regimen can be supported by pursuing behavioural targets.

A first behavioural step consists of advice on lifestyle and habit changes: dietary measures, increasing physical activity, stopping smoking and 'relaxing'. If medication is used, compliance should be checked regularly, and if necessary be supported by compliance-enhancing actions. Behaviourally oriented psychologists/therapists have the necessary training to coach medical professionals who oversee these first steps. Basic principles of behaviour therapy should be taken into account: the formulation of clearly defined goals divided into small successive steps so that the patient is regularly reinforced by success.

Individual counselling can be supported by group meetings of patients with similar problems, for example overweight, whether or not associated with high blood pressure. A group approach is very well suited for instruction in simple relaxation exercises focused on increasing the awareness of and changing reactions to daily life.

Eventually, behavioural problems related to the elevated blood pressure— such as obesity caused by dietary habits that have proved resistant to years of advice and diets, or seriously disturbing relational problems—will demand referral to a psychologist/behavioural therapist. The same holds for behavioural skills training and other psychological interventions; the indispensable knowledge of and practice in behavioural assessment and modification can best be provided directly by a psychologist.

Besides medical clinics, the work environment (Charlesworth, Williams and Baer, 1984; Chesney *et al.*, 1987; Patel *et al.*, 1985) and other locations (e.g. Ewart *et al.*, 1987) can be a suitable setting for interventions in high blood pressure. It will be primarily the task of psychologists to tailor intervention programmes to the population and setting chosen.

Behaviour-therapeutic support in the treatment of high blood pressure asks for rather substantial expertise and effort. The associated increase in costs can prompt the exclusive use of the 'simpler' drug treatment. In deciding between alternative treatment approaches, costs and efforts have to be weighed against the severity of the level of blood pressure and its associated short- and long-term health risks. The choices of the patient, including his or her standards for 'quality of life'—e.g. concerning the side-effects of drugs—should be seriously taken into account.

NOTES

[1]Address for correspondence: G. Godaert, Department of Clinical & Health Psychology, Utrecht University, Heidelberglaan 1, 3584 CS Utrecht, The Netherlands.

REFERENCES

Agras, W. S., Horne, M. and Taylor, C. B. (1982). Expectation and the blood pressure lowering effects of relaxation. *Psychosomatic Medicine*, **44**, 389–395.

Bali, L. R. (1979). Long term effect of relaxation on blood pressure and anxiety levels of essential hypertensive males: A controlled study. *Psychosomatic Medicine*, **41**, 637–647.

Basler, H. D., Brinkmeier, U., Buser, K., Haehn, K. D. and Moelders-Korber, R. (1987). Behaviour modification in obese patients with essential hypertension. Group treatment versus health counseling in a general practice setting. *Bibliotheca Cardiologica*, **42**, 122–129.

Brauer, A. P., Horlick, L., Nelson, E., Farquhar, J. W. and Agras, W. S. (1979). Relaxation therapy for essential hypertension: A Veterans Administration outpatient study. *Journal of Behavioral Medicine*, **2**, 21–29.

Cade, R., Wagemaker, H. *et al.* (1984). Effect of aerobic exercise on patients with systemic arterial hypertension. *American Journal of Medicine*, **77**, 785–790.

Charlesworth, E. A., Williams, B. J. and Baer, P. E. (1984). Stress management at the worksite for hypertension: Compliance, cost-benefit, health care, and hypertension-related variables. *Psychosomatic Medicine*, **46**, 387–397.

Chesney, M. A. and Black, G. (1986). Behavioral treatment of borderline hypertension: An overview of results. *Journal of Cardiovascular Pharmacology*, **8** (Suppl. 5), S57–S63.

Chesney, M. A., Black, G. W., Swan, G. E. and Ward, M. M. (1987). Relaxation training for essential hypertension at the worksite: I. The untreated mild hypertensive. *Psychosomatic Medicine*, **49**, 250–263.

Crowther, J. H. (1983). Stress management training and relaxation imagery in the treatment of essential hypertension. *Journal of Behavioral Medicine*, **6**, 169–187.

Dubbert, P. M., Martin, J. E., Zimmering, R. T. *et al.* (1984). Behavioral control of mild hypertension with aerobic exercise: Two case studies. *Behavior Therapy*, **15**, 373–380.

Edmonds, D., Foerster, E., Groth, H., Greminger, P., Siegenthaler, W. and Vetter, W. (1985). Does self-measurement of blood pressure improve patient compliance in hypertension? *Journal of Hypertension* (Suppl.), **3**, 531–534.

Ewart, C. K., Harris, W. L., Iwata, M. M., Coates, T. J., Bullock, R. and Simon, B. (1987). Feasibility and effectiveness of school based relaxation in lowering blood pressure. *Health Psychology*, **6**, 399–416.

Ewart, C. K., Taylor, C. B., Kraemer, H. C. and Agras, S. W. (1984). Reducing blood pressure reactivity during interpersonal conflict: Effects of marital communication training. *Behavior Therapy*, **15**, 473–484.

Falkner, B., Kushner, H., Onesti, G. and Angelakos, E. T. (1981). Cardiovascular characteristics in adolescents who develop essential hypertension. *Hypertension*, **3**, 521–527.

Feinleib, M. (1979). Genetics and familial aggregation of blood pressure. In: Onesti, G. and Klimt, C. R. (Eds) *Hypertension. Determinants, Complications and Interventions*. New York: Grune & Stratton, pp. 35–48.

Folkow, B. (1986). The 'structural factor' in hypertension. In: Hansson, L. (Ed.) *1986 Hypertension Yearbook*. London: Gower Academic, pp. 57–78.

Frankel, B. L., Patel, D., Horwitz, D., Friedewald, W. T. and Gaarder, K. R. (1978). Treatment of hypertension with biofeedback and relaxation techniques. *Psychosomatic Medicine*, **40**, 276–293.

Garrison, R. J., Kannel, W. B., Stokes, J. and Castelli, W. P. (1987). Incidence and precursors of hypertension in young adults: The Framingham Offspring Study. *Preventive Medicine*, **16**, 235–251.

Gentry, W. D., Chesney, A. P., Gary, H. E., Hall, R. P. and Harburg, E. (1982). Habitual anger coping styles: I. Effect on mean blood pressure and risk for essential hypertension. *Psychosomatic Medicine*, **44**, 195–202.

Glasgow, M. S. and Engel, B. T. (1987). Clinical issues in biofeedback and relaxation therapy for hypertension. In: Hatch, J. P., Fisher, J. G. and Pugh, J. D. (Eds) *Biofeedback Studies in Clinical Efficacy*, New York: Plenum.

Godaert, G. (1981). Relaxation treatment and hypertension. In: Surwitt, R. S., Wiliams, R. B. and Steptoe, A. (Eds) *Behavioral Treatment of Disease*. New York: Plenum, pp. 173–184.

Greenberg, G. (1988). Psychosocial factors and hypertension. *British Medical Journal*, **296**, 591–592.

Harrell, J. P. (1980). Psychological factors and hypertension: A status report. *Psychological Bulletin*, **87**, 482–501.

Heine, H. and Weiss, M. (1987). Life stress and hypertension. *European Heart Journal*, **8** (Suppl. B), 45–55.

Hoffman, J. W., Benson, H., Arns, P. A., Stainbroo, G. L., Landsberg, L., Young, J. B. and Gill, A. (1982). Reduced sympathetic nervous system responsivity associated with the relaxation response. *Science*, **215**, 190–192.

Hovell, M. F., Black, D. R., Mewborn, C. R., Geary, D., Agras, W. S., Kamachi, K., Kirk, R., Walton, C. and Dawson, S. (1986). Personalized versus usual care of previously uncontrolled hypertensive patients: An exploratory analysis. *Preventive Medicine*, **15**, 673–684.

Hypertension Detection and Follow-up Program Cooperative Group (1979). Five year findings of the hypertension detection and follow-up program I. Reduction in mortality of persons with high blood pressure, including mild hypertension. *Journal of the American Medical Association*, **242**, 2562–2571.

Johnston, D. W. (1986). How does relaxation training reduce blood pressure in primary hypertension? In: Dembroski, T. D., Schmidt, T. H. and Blumchen, C. (Eds) *Biological and Psychological Factors in Cardiovascular Disease*. Heidelberg: Springer.

Julius, S. and Esler, M. D. (1975). Autonomic nervous cardiovascular regulation in borderline hypertension. *American Journal of Cardiology*, **36**, 685–696.

Kallinke, D., Kulick, B. and Heim, P. (1982). Behaviour analysis and treatment of essential hypertensives. *Journal of Psychosomatic Research*, **26**, 541–549.

Kannel, W. B. and Kreger, B. E. (1981). Recent Framingham findings on morbidity in hypertension. In: Arntszenius, A. G., Dunning, A. J. and Snellen, H. A. (Eds) *Blood Pressure Measurement and Systemic Hypertension*. Breda: Medical World Press, IMS.

Kaplan, N. M. (1985). Non-drug treatment of hypertension. *Annals of Internal Medicine*, **102**, 359–373.

Laughlin, K. D. (1981). Enhancing the effectiveness of behavioral treatments for essential hypertension. *Physiology and Behavior*, **26**, 907–913.

Lynch, J. J., Thomas, S. A., Paskewitz, D. A., Malinow, K. L. and Long, J. (1982). Interpersonal aspects of blood pressure control. *Journal of Nervous and Mental Diseases*, **170**, 143–153.

Management Committee of the Australian Therapeutic Trial in Mild Hypertension (1980). The Australian therapeutic trial in mild hypertension. *Lancet*, **i**, 1261–1267.

Management Committee of the Australian Therapeutic Trial in Mild Hypertension (1982). Untreated mild hypertension. *Lancet*, Jan. 23, 185–191.

Mancia, G., Grassl, G., Pomidossi, G., Gregorina, L., Bertinieri, G., Parati, G., Ferrari, A. and Zanchetti, A. (1983). Effects of blood pressure measurement by the doctor on the patient's blood pressure and heart rate. *Lancet*, Sept. 24, 695–698.

Mancini, M. and Strazzullo, P. (1986). Energy balance and blood-pressure regulation. Update and future perspectives. *Journal of Clinical Hypertension*, **2**, 148–153.

MacMahon, S. (1987). Alcohol consumption and hypertension. *Hypertension*, **9**, 111–121.

McClellan, W. H., Hall, W. D., Brogan, D., Miles, C. and Wilber, J. A. (1988). Continuity of care in hypertension. *Archives of Internal Medicine*, **148**, 525–528.

Medical Research Council Working Party (1981). Adverse reactions to bendrofluazide and propranolol following treatment of mild hypertension. *Lancet*, **ii**, 539–543.

Medical Research Council Working Party (1985). MRC trial of mild hypertension: Principal results. *British Medical Journal*, **291**, 97–104.

Meichenbaum, D. and Cameron, R. (1984). Stress inoculation training. In: Meichenbaum, D. and Jaremko, M. E. (Eds) *Stress Reduction and Prevention*. New York: Plenum.

Mir, M. A., Mir, F., Khosla, T. and Newcombe, R. (1986). The relationship of salt intake and arterial blood pressure in salted-tea drinking Kashmiris. *International Journal of Cardiology*, **13**, 279–288.

Obrist, P. A. (1980). *Cardiovascular Psychophysiology: A Perspective*. New York: Plenum.

Palgi, A., Bristrian, B. R. and Blackburn, G. L. (1984). Two to seven years maintenance of weight loss (Abstract). *Clinical Research*, **32**, 632A.

Patel, C. and Marmot, M. (1988). Can general practitioners use training in relaxation and management of stress to reduce mild hypertension? *British Medical Journal*, **296**, 21–24.

Patel, C., Marmot, G., Terry, D. J., Carruthers, M., Hunt, B. and Patel, M. (1985). Trial of relaxation in reducing coronary risk: Four year follow-up. *British Medical Journal*, **290**, 1103–1106.

Perloff, D., Sokolow, M. and Cowan, R. (1983). The prognostic value of ambulatory blood pressures. *Journal of the American Medical Association*, **249**, 2792–2798.

Perri, M. G., McAdoo, W. G., McAllister, D. A., Laver, J. B. and Yancey, D. Z. (1986). Enhancing the efficacy of behavior therapy for obesity: Effects of aerobic exercise and a multicomponent maintenance program. *Journal of Consulting & Clinical Psychology*, **54**, 670–675.

Pickering, T. G. (1987). Strategies for the evaluation and treatment of hypertension and some implications of blood pressure variability. *Circulation*, **76** (Suppl. I), 77–82.

Puddey, I. B., Beilin, L. J. and Vandongen, R. (1986). Effect of regular alcohol use on blood pressure control in treated hypertensive subjects: A controlled study. *Clinical & Experimental Pharmacology & Physiology*, **13**, 315–318.

Robertson, I., Heather, N., Dzialdowski, A., Crawford, J. and Winton, M. (1986). A comparison of minimal versus intensive controlled drinking treatment intervention for problem drinkers. *British Journal of Clinical Psychology*, **25**, 185–194.

Robertson, J. I. S. (1986). The 1985 trials of hypertension treatment. In: Hanson, L. (Ed.) *1986 Hypertension Yearbook*. London: Gower Academic.

Safar, M. E., Simon, A. C. and Levenson, J. A. (1984). Structural changes of large arteries in sustained essential hypertension. *Hypertension*, **6** (Suppl. 3), 111, 117–111, 121.

Smirk, F. H. (1976). Casual, basal and supplemental blood pressures in 519 first-degree relatives of substantial hypertensive patients and in 350 population controls. *Clinical Science & Molecular Medicine*, **51**, 13s–17s.

Stamler, R., Stamler, J., Grimm, R., Gosch, F. C., Elmer, P. *et al.* (1987). Nutritional therapy for high blood pressure. Final Hypertension Control Program. *Journal of the American Medical Association*, **257**, 1484–1491.

Steptoe, A. (1981). *Psychological Factors in Cardiovascular Disorders*. London: Academic Press.

Stone, R. A. and de Leo, J. (1976). Psychotherapeutic control of hypertension. *New England Journal of Medicine*, **294**, 193–208.

Surwitt, R. S., Shapiro, D. and Good, M. I. (1978). Comparison of cardiovascular biofeedback, neuromuscular biofeedback and meditation in the treatment of borderline essential hypertension. *Journal of Clinical Psychology*, **46**, 252–263.

Tillotson, J. L., Winston, M. C. and Hall, Y. (1984). Critical behaviours in the dietary management of hypertension. *Journal of the American Dietetic Association*, **84**, 290–293.

Tuck, M. L. (1986). The sympathetic nervous system in essential hypertension. *American Heart Journal*, **112**, 877–886.

Veterans Administration Cooperative Study Group on Antihypertensive Agents (1967). Effects of treatment on morbidity in hypertension. I Results in patients with diastolic blood pressure averaging 115 through 129 mmHg. *Journal of the American Medical Association*, **202**, 1028–1034.

Veterans Administration Cooperative Study Group on Antihypertensive Agents (1970). Effects of treatment on morbidity in hypertension. II Results in patients with diastolic blood pressure averaging 90 through 114 mmHg. *Journal of the American Medical Association*, **213**, 1143–1152.

Wadden, T. A., Luborsky, P. C. G., Greer, S. and Crits-Cristoph, P. (1984). The behavioral treatment of essential hypertension: An update and comparison with pharmacological treatment. *Clinical Psychology Review*, **4**, 403–429.

Waeber, B., Petrillo, A., Nussberger, J. *et al.* (1987). Are some hypertensive patients overtreated? A prospective study of ambulatory blood pressure recording. *Lancet*, September 26, 732–734.

Wechsler, H., Levine, S., Idelson, R. K., Rohman, M. and Taylor, J. O. (1983). The physician's role in health providing—a survey of primary care practitioners. *New England Journal of Medicine*, **308**, 97–100.

WHO/ISH Mild Hypertension Liaison Committee (1982). Trials of the treatment of mild hypertension. *Lancet*, January 16, 149–156.

Wilner, D. M., Freeman, H. E., Monica, S. and Goldstein, M. S. (1985). Success in mental health treatment interventions: A review of 211 random assignment studies. *Journal of Social Service Research*, **8**, 1–21.

Zhao, G. S., Yuan, S. Y., Gong, B. Q., Wang, S. Z. and Cheng, Z. H. (1986). Nutrition, metabolism, and hypertension. A comparative survey between dietary variables and blood pressure among three nationalities in China. *Journal of Clinical Hypertension*, **2**, 124–131.

CHAPTER 9

Myocardial Infarction and Cardiac Rehabilitation

R. A. M. Erdman[1]

Erasmus University, Rotterdam

ABSTRACT

In this chapter attention is paid to situations with which a clinical psychologist working in a cardiology and/or cardiosurgery department may be confronted. Via the routing of the patient with a myocardial infarction, an overview is presented of the potential tasks of a psychologist at the coronary care unit and the medium care unit. The emotional problems confronting a patient upon discharge from hospital are discussed. Cardiac rehabilitation and effect measurement are covered. Finally, a concise description is given of the clinical psychologist's tasks with regard to patients with coronary bypass surgery and heart transplantation, and the education of cardiologists and nursing staff.

INTRODUCTION

Cardiovascular diseases are the major cause of death and have a high morbidity in industrialized western society (WHO, 1982). Approximately one-third of those who suffer a myocardial infarction die immediately from it. The patients who survive a myocardial infarction are usually more or less seriously handicapped in their daily functioning. This means that both physically and socially they have great difficulty in maintaining themselves at the same level as before the cardiac incident (Denolin, 1985).

In this chapter attention will be paid to situations with which the clinical psychologist working at a cardiology/cardiosurgery department may be

Behavioural Medicine
Edited by A. A. Kaptein, H. M. van der Ploeg, B. Garssen, P. J. G. Schreurs and R. Beunderman
© 1990 John Wiley & Sons Ltd.

confronted such as:

- Myocardial infarction
- Cardiac rehabilitation and effect measurement
- Coronary bypass surgery
- Heart transplantation
- Teaching

MYOCARDIAL INFARCTION AND THE PSYCHOLOGIST

Within a cardiology department there are a number of subdepartments where the assistance of a clinical psychologist will not be called in, for example the electrocardiographic (ECG) department, the catheterization department and the cardiosurgery department. However, during the last two decades the interfaces between cardiology and psychology have developed to such an extent that in 60–70% of the places where the patient gets in touch with the cardiologist and/or cardiosurgeon the psychologist will also be consulted (Doehrman, 1977; Cochran, 1984; Wiklund et al., 1985). Some typical examples are given below.

The Coronary Care Unit (CCU)

At the coronary care unit postmyocardial infarction patients may become so anxious and/or depressive that cardiologists consider the assistance of a psychologist desirable (Blanchard and Miller, 1977). When regaining consciousness at a CCU after an infarction, few patients realize that they have just escaped death. What becomes clear to the patient's mind is that there is still a life-threatening situation. The hectic-looking activities of doctors and nurses, which are mostly not understood by the patient, and witnessing the deaths of other infarction patients at the CCU may create an enormous impression and arouse latent feelings of anxiety. Therefore, the majority of CCU patients are routinely administered anxiolytics. An intensive psychological treatment at the CCU is hardly ever indicated. The patient is still too ill or too weak for this. But by means of some talks, often of an informative character, the psychologist can discuss with the patient which of these anxieties are based on real danger and which on fantasy. Because of unfamiliarity with the clinical picture and the enormous shock caused by the infarction, many patients are inclined to fantasize about permanent disablement, never being able to participate again in the labour process, and inability to function again as a fully-fledged partner or parent. Here lies a task for the psychologist. By offering the patient the opportunity to express his thoughts, which are often experienced as very embarrassing, a twofold purpose can be served: reduction of anxiety and testing the patient's fantasies against reality. In the majority of cases, especially when the myocardial infarction is less complicated, the image the patient evokes about the future is much gloomier than will appear to be justified later on. The psychologist can ask the cardiologist how serious the cardiac injury is and subsequently hear from the cardiologist how realistic the patient's anxious thoughts and fantasies are. Then the psychologist can give the patient a truer picture of the future, which will often lead to much relief and reduction of the feelings of anxiety.

Moreover, the patient can benefit from talks aiming at restoring his self-confidence. Where the patient feels weak, disabled and injured, the psychologist can emphasize that the coin also has a reverse side: 'You may have had an infarction, but apparently you are strong enough to survive it'. Such an approach may give the patient new courage and may reduce feelings of despondency and depression.

Third, the psychologist may function as an intermediary between the cardiologist and the psychiatrist. The latter is involved in the event that the feelings of anxiety or depression have become so serious that talks will no longer have the intended anxiety-reducing or antidepressant effect. If the cardiologist is in doubt or threatens to miss a psychiatric diagnosis, it is the psychologist's task to call the psychiatrist for a consultation.

Finally, at the CCU the basis can be laid for a prolonged contact with the patient, for instance if at a later stage the patient wants to discuss a change in life-style and habits because of the infarction.

The Medium Care Unit (MCU)

At the medium care unit (the department where the patient is nursed after being discharged from the CCU, which implies that there is no longer any immediate danger to life) one notices that, in addition to the feelings of anxiety and depression already mentioned, the majority of patients now begin to realize the real significance of the infarction (Wiklund *et al.*, 1985; Hackett, 1985). Apparently the feelings of anxiety at the CCU were so overwhelming and strong that they were massively denied. Some denial of feelings of anxiety during the stay at the CCU should be regarded as a healthy adjustment mechanism. Due in part to the more consciously experienced contacts with his partner and others, the patient at the MCU begins to realize that he just escaped death. Generally speaking, this may lead to two reactions.

The first is awareness of the seriousness of the situation, which often results in a wide range of feelings varying from anxiety and depression, *via* indifference, to joy because life has been preserved. In themselves the psychological phenomena just mentioned are part of the normal reaction pattern following a myocardial infarction. It would be more surprising if a patient did not pass through an anxious or depressive phase after such a direct confrontation with a life-threatening situation. If the anxiety or depressive feelings are going to preoccupy the patient too much, there is a task for the psychologist. Dealing alone with such feelings costs the patient much physical energy and may result in exhaustion symptoms. One or more talks with a psychologist who shows understanding for these problems will often lead to mitigation of the symptoms. The commonest emotional problems are:

- Anxiety over the finiteness of life
- Anxiety over unclear prospects for the future
- Feelings of powerlessness

- Dependence problems resulting in extremely regressive behaviour
- Gloominess and inclination to give up
- Emotional instability and inability to accept this
- Suppressed anger about physical vulnerability

Patients know and understand that a psychologist is not able to cure the cardiac injury. Nevertheless, they experience it as a relief to talk about their emotional problems with a positive person who is not a doctor. Where at first the feelings of anxiety impaired the patient's clear thinking and affected his self-confidence so that he threatened to disintegrate psychologically, the psychologist can reduce the chance of such a decompensation.

The next example tries to make clear exactly what is meant by the psychologist's approach. After an uncomplicated myocardial infarction, Mr A, a fifty-four-year-old bookbinder, entered a depressive state after several days spent on the MCU. Mr A felt powerless and had anxiety thoughts about his uncertain future prospects. Emotionally, Mr A became unstable: trivial matters made him cry, and this was a development he could not bear. In youth a rigid, religion-biased education had impressed on him unequivocally that men, faced with problems, do not cry. Furthermore, he was constantly apprehensive that excessive emotionality would aggravate his heart disease. In a small number of talks the psychologist was able to make clear to Mr A that (1) emotional instability is indeed a normal reaction after a myocardial infarction, (2) almost every patient (of both sexes) shows such a reaction, although none likes to exhibit it, and (3) to bottle up one's emotions is more stressful to the heart than gradually discharging one's feelings. This last argument in particular reassured the patient and his feelings of anxiety about a reinfarction decreased. To cry remained difficult for Mr A, but after three sessions with the psychologist he allowed himself to do so. His psychological suffering (especially anxiety states and depressive reactions) disappeared after five sessions. Mr A had overcome his feelings of shame about his own emotions.

The second kind of reaction relates to an euphoric state of mind. For these patients everything they have gone through is so fearful that it must be massively denied. Characteristic of this group of patients are pronouncements like 'what more can happen to me, I don't worry about such a trivial infarction' or 'when I go home tomorrow, I'll be eager to get back to work again'. The medium care patient can hardly believe that all this will be quite different back home. If in such a situation the nursing staff or the ward doctor, alarmed by the discrepancy between the patient's cardiac condition and his euphoric behaviour, should consult the psychologist, it would be an error to confront the patient at that moment with his feelings of anxiety. Apparently this particular behaviour is the patient's way of coping with life-threatening situations and the psychologist should respect this. If one tries to contradict the patient's denial, he will be made more anxious than he can bear. However, in the event of such a euphoric state of mind one should be aware of the possibility of a sudden denial breakdown (Soloff, 1977; Trijsburg et al., 1987). In order to avoid this the psychologist should visit an euphoric patient every day in order to:

1. Ascertain whether the denial of feelings of anxiety persists;
2. Support the patient's self-esteem;
3. Gradually hone the patient's sense of reality.

To illustrate this approach there follows an example for clinical practice. Mr B is a forty-two-year-old man, of Italian origin, who has been for 12 years in The Netherlands. Having spent four days on the MCU he threatened to quit the ward, because, as he said, he felt healthy and doubted if he really had an infarction (denial of feelings of anxiety). Further, Mr B stated that he could no longer neglect his pizzeria while he looked after himself. His cardiologist considered discharge from hospital at this particular stage of the recovery process strongly inadvisable. Hence, the cardiologist sought the assistance of the psychologist. Mr B gave the impression of being agitated and full of anger; he made complaints regarding his treatment and he was physically restless. In his opinion, the doctors were keeping him in hospital without good reason. During the first talk it appeared that the patient's wife during his absence managed the pizzeria. Mr B was extremely ambivalent about this. It was intolerable to him that a woman should run the show; that did not fit in with his Italian view regarding the man–wife relationship. Offended pride, anger at physical vulnerability and shame regarding (in his view) unmasculinity led to Mr B all but quitting the hospital. Just after discussing these feelings with the psychologist, Mr B's sense of reality returned; subsequently he could obey the instructions of the doctor and the nursing staff. During the discussions the psychologist emphasized the fact that Mr B over the last 10 years had built up an attractive, well-run pizzeria, an achievement he could be proud of (support of patient's self-esteem). After repeating this theme several times in different words, the patient's self-esteem increased visibly. After this stage was reached Mr B could gradually come to accept that his wife—for the time being—was in command. Later it appeared that Mr B had felt himself very much alone and abandoned, which increased his anxiety during his MCU period. A gradual release of feelings of anger and anxiety by means of talks with the psychologist increased Mr B's feelings of self-esteem and as a result his reality orientation returned.

Furthermore, experience has shown that both the nursing staff and the doctors at the medium care unit can benefit from a multidisciplinary, psycho-socially oriented weekly discussion of patients. It is advisable that the psychologist working at the medium care unit is the driving force behind such meetings, which should also include a physiotherapist, a social worker and (sometimes) a dietician, for young cardiologists in particular are seldom sufficiently trained with regard to:

1. Diagnosing anxiety and/or depressive symptoms;
2. Neurotic mechanisms;
3. Psychopathology;
4. Reducing anxiety.

The purpose of such a weekly discussion is twofold: (a) optimization of psychological care and support of the patient; and (b) *education permanente* for the other disciplines (see also later in the chapter).

When the patient is about to leave the medium care unit and prepare himself for his discharge from hospital, it is useful that he should be informed (once again) about the nature of his disease, risk factors and cardiac rehabilitation at an informative meeting. The cardiologist will inform the patient about the somatic aspects of his illness, but for the last two aspects the contribution of the psychologist is of essential importance. At the informative meeting, where the patient's partner may also be present, the psychologist will discuss the (ex-pected) emotional consequences of the infarction as well as those risk factors that, unlike the somatic ones, will have a psychosocial aetiology, such as: (1) smoking habits; (2) unhealthy eating habits; (3) type A behaviour (Suinn, 1980; Thorensen, Telch and Eaglestone, 1981); and (4) stress-handling (Johnston, 1985).

For all four psychosocial risk factors mentioned here it is particularly difficult to bring about the necessary changes in behaviour. It is the psychologist's task to emphasize the importance of changes in behaviour (with a view to secondary prevention), while he should also indicate that this is going to be very difficult. At this stage of recovery patients will not yet be motivated to undergo psychotherapeutic treatment aiming at changes in behaviour, but the psycholo-gist can still draw the patient's attention to the availability of the various (e.g. behaviour-therapeutic or insight-enhancing) psychotherapeutic facilities (Nunes, Frank and Kornfeld, 1987).

Back Home After Discharge From Hospital: Emotional Aspects

First there is the joy of meeting one's family again in familiar surroundings as well as the experience that there is still life after the infarction. But during the following weeks the confrontation with death in the past weeks will be experi-enced as an attack on life, resulting in a disturbance of the equilibrium between psychological resilience and load (Wiklund *et al.*, 1985; Hackett, 1985; Erdman *et al.*, 1986). The person of the patient is threatened. Many people believe that life-threatening accidents will happen to others rather than to themselves. When somebody suffers a myocardial infarction, he realizes that he can die prema-turely. Such a shock is attended by a multitude of emotional reactions which centre on the fear of death and/or fear of a second infarction (Trelawny-Ross and Russel, 1987). However, most patients do not speak of fear (many men avoid that word for it might be construed as weakness or unmasculinity) but of tension, nervousness or stress. Other frequently occurring forms of anxiety after a myocardial infarction are loss of concentration, sudden phobias and (at a later stage) sexual dysfunction (impotence). In addition to anxiety, the myocardial infarction is often attended by aggressive feelings resulting from the frustrations of the heart attack. For one has been found to be vulnerable and not so—limitlessly—strong as one perhaps thought or hoped. For many people, notably the hard-working ones (workaholics), the myocardial infarction is often experienced as a narcistic injury. Moreover, notably during the postmyocardial infarction stage, an infarction creates great concern over one's health, resumption of work and financial prospects. People differ as far as their frustration and uncertainty tolerance is concerned. Because of the aspects just mentioned, many postmyocardial infarction patients are more easily emotionally irritated. The (rightly) worried partner and/or the children often have to suffer for it. If the anger over the disease and the proven vulnerability cannot adequately be sublimated (transformed into socially acceptable behaviour) but is directed to one's self (the patient is then apt to describe himself as: 'I am a worrier, I always keep my feelings bottled up'), a depressive picture may arise (Hackett, 1985). Such a patient shows no initiative, is listless, complains about headaches, loses all interest in life and may become gloomy. This gamut of emotional reactions after an infarction is often accompanied by sleep disorders (not being able to fall asleep, waking up too early, nightmares) as well as emotional instability (bursting into tears, which never happened before).

The occurrence of the symptoms outlined above should be regarded as a normal reaction to a life-threatening event, in this case the myocardial infarction. If the symptoms persist for more than three to six months, other factors often play a role and psychologically there was probably something already wrong before the infarction.

Not yet mentioned are the activity fears: the fear of physical exertion. Whereas before the infarction numerous activities and actions were performed as a matter of course, there now are doubts and uncertainties about even the slightest physical exertion. Questions like: 'May I drive my car again, rake the lawn, make love, put the refuse bags outside?' etc., are frequently heard, although the patient received the cardiologist's permission to do all these things a long time ago. While the infarction patient used to be full of life, he feels in the post-myocardial infarction phase often small and dependent (on the doctors and his direct social surroundings). All this is experienced as very unpleasant and should not be underestimated. Diagnostically, the picture outlined above is described in the Anglo-Saxon literature as 'anxiety reaction' and need not necessarily be related to an infarction specifically but rather to what may happen emotionally after a traumatic event (Wiklund *et al.*, 1985; Trelawny-Ross and Russel, 1987).

When, approximately one or two weeks after being discharged from hospital, the myocardial infarction patient attends the cardiological policlinic for his first return visit, an examination by both the cardiologist and the psychologist would be the ideal situation. The latter can then observe the manner in which the patient has psychologically coped with his cardiac trauma. In order to gain a general impression of the patient's psychological make-up, the psychologist should inquire after anxiety symptoms or derivatives thereof (in reaction to the infarction), such as fear of exertion, loss of concentration, sleep disorders, phobias, sexual dysfunction and the family and work situation. On the basis of the information thus obtained it can be ascertained whether participation in or referral to a cardiac rehabilitation programme is useful.

From a psychological point of view indications for participation in such a rehabilitation programme are the occurrence or existence of:

- Feelings of anxiety and/or derivatives thereof
- Depressive feelings
- A limited social activity pattern
- Reintegration problems with regard to the work situation

Contraindications are:

- Psychopathy
- Other serious psychiatric disturbances

Not every hospital or cardiology department has the services of a psychologist and that is why the above-mentioned symptoms in postmyocardial infarction patients are not always recognized as such.

But for the majority of postmyocardial infarction patients, referral to a poli-clinic cardiac rehabilitation programme will be the optimal route for reintegration in society so that a new equilibrium can be found between psychological resilience and load (Blodgett and Pekarik, 1987).

CARDIAC REHABILITATION

In cardiac rehabilitation a distinction can be made between the psychosocial and the physical aspects. Often it is a matter of local circumstance to which kind of cardiac rehabilitation programme the postmyocardial infarction patient will be referred. It is also possible that the patient will not be referred to a cardiac rehabilitation programme (irrespective of the emotional response to the myocardial infarction) because the attending cardiologist does not see the value of rehabilitation programmes. One reason for this lack of faith is the absence of statistically significant evidence of long-term benefit in terms of morbidity and/or mortality in several randomized studies (Marra *et al.*, 1985). On the other hand, there are cardiologists who routinely refer every postmyocardial infarction patient to a rehabilitation programme, in the belief that every patient is likely to benefit from participation in such a programme. Hence participation in a cardiac rehabilitation programme depends on the attitude, the experience and beliefs of the attending cardiologist. The contribution of the psychologist (particularly his expertise in identifying anxiety states and depressive reactions) can provide a more flexible and individual-oriented reference strategy. *Physical rehabilitation programmes* are generally aimed at physical recovery and at learning to know and trust the new physical limits to be acquired. In this kind of rehabilitation programme hardly any attention is paid to psychosocial aspects of the patient. Physical exercise, circuit training and 'controlled exertion' characterize the whole programme. In the various reports of the World Health

Organization about cardiac rehabilitation this concept is described as follows: 'the entire complex of activities aimed at optimal physical, psychological and social functioning of the myocardial infarction patient' (Denolin, 1985). In *psychosocial rehabilitation programmes* emphasis is primarily placed on how to cope emotionally with the heart disease. Providing guidance with regard to the wish to resume work and information about heart diseases and/or risk factors may also be included in the goals (van Uden *et al.*, 1986). It is one of the psychologist's tasks to recommend or motivate patients whom he supposes or knows to have psychological or psychosocial problems to participate in such a cardiac rehabilitation programme.

Various 'treatments' generally come under the common title of 'cardiac rehabilitation'. Some of the commonest 'treatments' are mentioned below.

1. An introductory and informative talk at the beginning of policlinic aftercare, often together with the patient's partner and/or other myocardial infarction patients.
2. A physical activity programme with a large variety of exercises (floor exercises, circuit training, sports and games, cycling, relaxation exercises, walking, treadmill, swimming) especially aimed at enhancing self-confidence.
3. An intensive physical activity programme aimed at achieving a training effect.
4. 'Controlled' exertion, usually on the bicycle ergometer with ECG monitoring.
5. Group therapies aimed at changes in behaviour to reduce risk factors (e.g. smoking habits, stress-handling).
6. Individual psychological guidance to cope better with the cardiac incident (i.e. aimed at reducing feelings of anxiety).

One of the features of cardiac rehabilitation programmes is the multidisciplinary character of the rehabilitation team. The presence of a doctor (cardiologist, rehabilitation doctor or internist) is indispensable and a prerequisite to carry out the physical exercise programme. The physical reconditioning programme is usually carried out by physiotherapists. Additionally, depending on the nature of the problems, the assistance of the following experts is called in: nurse, social worker, psychologist, dietician and labour expert. Experience has shown that form and content of rehabilitation programmes may differ by city, region or country. These differences mainly relate to the timing of the cardiac incident, the cardiological diagnoses of the participants (myocardial infarction, bypass operation, angina pectoris, balloon dilatation), length of the rehabilitation period (varying from six weeks to years on end), age limit for admission, content of the physical reconditioning programme and the availability and nature of psychosocial aid (group and/or individual counselling, behavioural therapy and/or crisis intervention).

In reporting on the effect of cardiac rehabilitation this chapter will primarily focus on the psychosocial aspects. Formerly work resumption was used as a criterion for successful rehabilitation, but nowadays more prominence is given to other criteria.

Physical Cardiac Rehabilitation

So far investigations have shown that from a psychological point of view physical cardiac rehabilitation will sometimes have beneficial effects and sometimes not, compared with normal cardiological aftercare (Stern and Cleary, 1981; Mayou, 1983; van Dixhoorn, de Loos and Duivenvoorden, 1983; Erdman et al., 1986; Blodgett and Pekarik, 1987; Burgess et al., 1987). Stern and his research team found in 748 postmyocardial infarction patients after physical rehabilitation a decrease of depressive feelings and an increase of sexual activity; however, strangely enough, at the same time the feelings of anxiety increased in intensity. The researchers attributed this phenomenon to the fact that the greater physical exertion of the patients resulted in greater anxiety (Stern and Cleary, 1981). Increase in anxiety, in addition to an increase in feelings of well-being and a decrease in disablement perception, was found by van Dixhoorn et al. in 1983. He investigated the effect of physical training combined with relaxation exercises in a case-control study. The increase in feelings of anxiety was attributed by van Dixhoorn to the fact that as a result of the relaxation exercises, the denial of anxiety is eliminated and that emotional life is activated by such exercises (van Dixhoorn, de Loos and Duivenvoorden, 1983).

That anxiety may also decrease after participation in a rehabilitation programme was demonstrated by Erdman and his coworkers in a randomized clinical trial (Erdman et al., 1986). This investigation (of a retrospective and exploratory nature) only involved patients that suffered a myocardial infarction not longer than six months previously, were not older than 70, and had disorders such as hyperventilation, anxiety, depression and lack of self-confidence. The rehabilitation programme consisted of training in a sports hall twice a week for 90 minutes during a period of six months (warming up, running, jogging, gymnastic exercises, volleyball or badminton, and relaxation exercises, given by a physiotherapist). The responsibility for the programme was entrusted to a physiotherapist; further guidance was given by nurses, a social worker, a psychologist and cardiologists. In the event of severe psychopathology and/or severe emotional problems the psychologist was consulted. Every member of the staff joined in the activities of the patients, thus forming a close group. The cardiologists had final (medical) responsibility. Of the 64 patients eligible for this study 32 were allocated at random to the rehabilitation group and 32 to a control group. The patients from the control group received a brochure with indications about the how and why of physical training with gymnastic exercises and keep-fit recommendations for cardiac patients. They were left to the further care of 'bystanders' (relatives and general practitioner). Apart from the investigation, the patients from both groups received the usual policlinic aftercare. During the six months of the rehabilitation programme the participants were subjected twice to a psychological examination: once at the beginning, before the training, and once after six months, upon completion of the programme. The patients from the control group were also psychologically examined twice with an interval of six months. About five years later the two groups were subjected to the third and last psychological examination. For this use was made of the Heart Patient's Psychological Questionnaire (Erdman *et al.*, 1986), which measures the following four aspects of well-being: subjective well-being (lack of anxiety), disablement perception, displeasure and social inhibition. This questionnaire has been standardized on 1649 Dutch cardiac patients. In addition, inquiries were made in a structured interview about cardiological accidents, 'life events' and any changes in smoking habits and sports activities.

On average, the 32 participants in the rehabilitation programme visited three of the four training/group sessions, an attendance rate of 75%. Both groups were found to correspond in terms of the occurrence of 'life events', professional level, age and occurrence of cardiac disorders. The average age was 56 for the rehabilitation group and 54 for the control group. Compared with the control group, participation for six months in the rehabilitation programme initially led to reduced anxiety, disablement perception and smoking; the subjective feeling of well-being showed a statistically significant increase. No other statistically significant results were found. However, five years later these favourable results were no longer visible. After five years 67% of the original rehabilitation group still engaged in physical activity against 45% in the control group. From the point of view of secondary prevention this is a hopeful result. The conclusion must be that participation in a physical cardiac rehabilitation programme will only have a beneficial effect for the relatively short term. The above-mentioned results agree with the findings of Mayou *et al.* (1981) and Marra *et al.* (1985), who concluded that exercise training increased self-confidence in the early stages of convalescence but showed little overall benefit for cardiac morbidity and mortality.

Recently this finding was largely corroborated by a randomized case-control study carried out by Burgess *et al.* (1987). In their investigation, 89 postmyocardial infarction patients were randomly assigned to a physical rehabilitation programme and 91 patients received the usual cardiological aftercare. After three months the rehabilitated group was found to suffer less from feelings of anxiety, depression and stress than the control group. Furthermore, the participants turned out to be less dependent on social support from their relatives. At the follow-up meeting 13 months later these differences had disappeared (Burgess *et al.*, 1987). That participation in a physical rehabilitation programme has only a beneficial effect in the short term is in itself an important result, certainly so if it is borne in mind that feelings of anxiety, depression, insecurity and often unclear prospects for the future prevail immediately after the cardiac trauma.

For 129 postmyocardial infarction patients Mayou compared the effect of participation in three different forms of 'treatment': normal cardiological aftercare (condition 1); condition 1 plus participation in a physical rehabilitation programme; and condition 1 plus psychosocial advice. The psychosocial advice group and their wives were given, in addition to normal treatment, the opportunity to discuss any problem and received advice. The physician met the patient in the hospital and then saw couples once a week beginning after discharge from hospital. Although informative in style, discussions systematically covered symptoms and activities. Patients were encouraged to keep a daily activity diary. After three months the patients who had participated in the physical rehabilitation programme were found to be most enthusiastic about their treatment. However, there were no differences between the three groups of patients with regard to feelings of anxiety and depression, physical activities relating to work and leisure time and degree of contentment as far as social contacts were concerned (Mayou, 1983).

It should be noted that in the studies mentioned above research was invariably focused on the average effect on various psychological variables. Such a method has the drawback that it cannot be very easily deduced from the results for which individual patient the rehabilitation intervention has been successful. Meanwhile, it is sufficiently well known that physical rehabilitation is not necessary and useful for every postmyocardial infarction patient (Mayou, 1983; van Dixhoorn, de Loos and Duivenvoorden, 1983; Erdman et al., 1986). The state of the art provides no strong criteria as to which patient should be considered for participation in a rehabilitation programme. However, from the psychologist's point of view the following rule of thumb could be used as a guideline: do not refer to a rehabilitation programme a patient who persistently denies feelings of anxiety. Such patients tend to lack the motivation for effective participation in a rehabilitation programme. Those patients, however, who react to their infarction with a decrease in self-esteem, with an anxiety reaction and/or a depressive mood state are better placed to benefit from a physical rehabilitation programme.

Furthermore, researchers use different criteria for the results of their investigations; a generally accepted criterion of psychological recovery is still lacking. It is clear that individually oriented research is desirable (involving both somatic and psychosocial variables) in order to be able to determine at an early stage for which individual cardiac patient physically oriented cardiac rehabilitation is indicated.

Psychosocial Cardiac Rehabilitation

In addition, research has been conducted into the effect of psychosocial cardiac rehabilitation programmes. In this kind of intervention, emphasis is placed on counselling or on coping problems. Attention is also focused on providing information or on changes in behaviour to reduce risks. Theorell showed that providing information about physical and psychological risk factors to patients and their closest relatives reduces feelings of anxiety in postmyocardial infarction patients (Theorell, 1982). Rovario found that compared with routine cardiological aftercare, information about coronary artery disease, exercise and exercise evaluation combined with physical rehabilitation leads to better understanding of heart disease, more activity, a favourable self-image, decreased employment-related stress, more pleasure in leisure time and greater sexual activity (Rovario, Holmes and Holmsten, 1984). Finally, Friedman et al. demonstrated that type A behaviour, which is generally assumed to be 'unhealthy', can be changed and that morbidity for those whose type A behaviour is positively altered shows a statistically significant decrease (Friedman et al.,

1984). Their intervention programme consisted of 24 meetings spread over three years, which included relaxation training, cognitive restructuring, self-observation and self-affirmation. However, the underlying psychological mechanisms causing these alterations remain obscure and to what extent the intended alterations will persist in the long run is not yet known (Johnston, 1985).

Recently in The Netherlands, Falger *et al.* (1987) compared, in a case referent study, 133 male cases with first myocardial infarction from 192 hospital referents against 133 neighbourhood referents without myocardial infarction. Psycho-social risk factors, such as type A behaviour and prodromal symptoms of vital exhaustion, sleep complaints and depression (Appels, Höppener and Mulder, 1987), were assessed. All the risk indicators occurred significantly more often in myocardial infarction cases. However, to date no psychosocial cardiac rehabilitation programme has been developed with special focus on treating sleep complaints, depression and vital exhaustion. Further research is needed if this avenue is to be explored.

That the discussions about type A behaviour and the alleged 'risk' of this type of behaviour have not yet come to an end is evident from the recently published results of Ragland and Brand. These investigators found that subsequent coronary mortality in patients who had suffered a first myocardial infarction was unexpectedly lower among type A than type B patients. The simple model linking type A behaviour to coronary heart disease appears to be no longer tenable. It looks at this moment as if type A behaviour can rather be regarded as a protective factor against recurrence of a myocardial infarction (Ragland and Brand, 1988).

CORONARY BYPASS SURGERY AND THE PSYCHOLOGIST

At the cardiosurgery department the contribution of a psychologist may also be of essential importance. The patient who has to undergo coronary bypass surgery can be aided in emotionally anticipating the operation by means of psychological support and the provision of information specific to his case.

A special problem is formed by that group of patients who are on the waiting list for a bypass operation. They may have to wait for months. The aim of the information is primarily the alleviation of feelings of fear concerning the coming operation (Kendall and Watson, 1981; Anderson and Masur, 1983; Cochran, 1984; Utens, Erdman and Verhage, 1986). In the event of an operation there is always a (conscious or unconscious) fear of, for instance, the anaesthesia, pain and the result of the operation. But in the event of coronary bypass surgery another problem plays an important role. After the operation the patient has big scars both in the centre of his chest and almost over the full length of his inside left or right leg. Aesthetically this is not very attractive and by some patients (their exact number is not known) it is experienced as a real blemish, an offence to their self-esteem, so that feelings of inferiority may arise.

Although much research has been conducted into the goals and effects of information in general on recovery after an operation, only a very limited number of investigations have been made into this subject specifically directed towards coronary bypass surgery. Ramshaw and Stanley (1984) demonstrated for 23 bypass patients that the degree to which the recovery process proceeds successfully cannot be predicted so much on the basis of physical residual symptoms (postsurgical) as on the degree of neuroticism. And Hansen and Lavandero (1981) emphasized—in an investigation involving 100 bypass patients—that attention to the patient's individual needs may turn the information programme into a success. Features predictive of good postsurgical adjustment could not be identified from this investigation. Of their investigation population, 82% indicated that feelings of anxiety were reduced before the operation as a result of the multidisciplinary information programme and for that same reason 71% were able to adjust adequately after the operation according to the authors. To what extent these data can be generalized is not clear from this investigation. The researchers emphasized that close cooperation between nursing staff, physiotherapist, cardiologist and psychologist is essential for a successful information programme. What is meant by this approach will be clarified by the following example.

Mr C, a forty-six-year-old crane-driver, has to undergo bypass surgery fairly soon. During the informative, educational meeting for this kind of patient, Mr C's wife says that during the last two or three weeks her husband has been easily agitated and at times withdrawn. These are, to her, unknown aspects of his personality. During the discussion with the cardiologist, the psychologist and a member of the nursing staff, Mr C says, after some hesitation, that he sleeps very badly, anxiously imagining the forthcoming bypass operation. Then it appears (his wife was not aware of this) that some days ago Mr C had heard from a colleague at work about the kind of dangers attending such an operation ('the anaesthetic period could last much longer than planned'; 'sometimes for days after the operation'; and 'one may be given more bypasses than was decided upon'). During the discussion Mr C is able to admit for the first time that he is anxious about not coming out of anaesthesia. At this point the cardiologist informs Mr C in some detail about the anaesthetic procedures to be carried out and their more or less routine nature. Furthermore, the cardiologist explains to Mr C that though the number of bypasses needed are in general known, this is occasionally varied during the operation to achieve a better result. During this session the psychologist leads the conversation, taking into account everybody's personal feelings and circumstances. It is reassuring to Mr C to hear that other patients have similar anxieties about anaesthesia. He is further reassured by the favourable results of bypass surgery as practised in the hospital where he is to be operated on. When the cardiologist as well as the psychologist promise that they will visit Mr C during his admission to hospital before surgery to answer possible new questions his feelings of anxiety decrease visibly.

During the first three or four days after the surgical intervention the patient suffers much pain, and pain makes one insecure and anxious. Furthermore, it is striking that after the operation many patients are emotionally very unstable on the third or fourth day, which is for instance expressed in crying fits. At this stage of recovery the feelings of anxiety will be mitigated for many patients if the psychologist explains that such violent emotions are quite normal, are found in almost every patient, can be regarded as a type of adjustment and are part of finding a new equilibrium after passing through a very anxious event (Razin, 1982).

HEART TRANSPLANTATION

Heart transplantations are a relatively new development in cardiology. In this field too the psychologist has several tasks. First of all a (psychosocial) action protocol should be drawn up and later implemented. Such a protocol states for which patient psychological/psychiatric reasons are relative and/or absolute contraindications for being eligible for a heart transplantation. If it can be assumed with a fair degree of certainty that the patient will not be able to adjust to the new (postsurgical) circumstances, the transplantation should not be carried out. If the cardiologist makes such a surmise, the psychologist or psychiatrist should be consulted. The question then is always: 'Will the patient before and after the transplantation psychologically be able to adjust sufficiently to the difficult circumstances?' or, formulated otherwise: 'Will the patient be able to meet the very high demands that are made on cooperation between patient and doctor?' The patient will be faced with the following requirements for the rest of his life: (1) taking his temperature every day; (2) adhering to strict dietary rules; (3) adhering to a strict medication regime; (4) being able to stand nauseating and/or appearance-changing side-effects of medicines; (5) very frequent hospital examinations; and (6) frequent taking of biopsies.

Because of this strict regime a prediction—however hard to give—is required about the patient's adaptability. In this case special attention is paid to the patient's anxiety and frustration tolerance on the basis of his behaviour during earlier diseases or traumatic situations (Copeland, Emery and Levinson, 1987).

Moreover, in view of the severity and violence of the psychological emotions, it is the psychologist's task to offer psychosocial support both before and after the heart transplantation (O'Brien, 1985). Emotional adjustment to cardiac transplantation is a long process. The road to transplantation and beyond is divided into distinct stages, namely: (1) transplant proposal; (2) evaluation period; (3) awaiting a donor organ; (4) in-hospital phase; and (5) return home. Each stage calls for a different emotional adjustment as each stage contains a different cluster of problems. Patient adjustment is influenced by previous experience with illness and by personality factors. Before transplantation, contact with previous recipients can be of great value. Psychiatric or psychological support can greatly aid in patients with emotional adjustment problems such as anxiety states and or behavioural abnormalities (McAleer et al., 1985; Mai et al., 1986; Kühn, Davis and Lippmann, 1988).

If children are about to get a new heart, attention should not only be paid to the child's problems but also to the parents of the child. For on the one hand the parents love their child, but on the other hand it may be possible that they will reject the child to a greater or lesser extent because the heart disease upsets them, makes them anxious and calls up thoughts of death (Kris, 1984). Meanwhile, it is known from experience that a breach may arise, notably between the mother and the child. The rapidly changing appearance of the child (because of the compulsory administration of Prednison) may be a contributing factor. Sometimes intensive treatment of one of the parents calls for prolonged psychotherapeutic aid, which may extend over several years.

THE PSYCHOLOGIST AT THE CARDIOLOGY DEPARTMENT AND TEACHING

People differ in the way in which they deal with the emotions of others, and, in this case, the emotions of often very ill people. Also doctors training to be cardiologists, cardiologists and nurses have their blind spots and should therefore be aided in psychologically dealing with patients. Here too lies a task for the clinical psychologist. By means of group discussions of case studies it can be made clear to both disciplines—mostly at a cognitive level only, in fact—what emotions are, how patients express them and how these should be handled in a helpful manner. The psychologist can, for instance, elucidate the background of a patient's violent emotions and how they have developed. And the same applies to the emotional reactions of the patient's partner and/or relatives. The main themes of this kind of education invariably are the reduction of anxiety in patients and conversation technique, because without always being aware the two professional groups are daily confronted with this. With the aid of tape-recorded talks between the doctor and his patient, the psychologist can focus on conversation technical problems, such as the bad news talk, the advisory talk and the informative talk. Experience has taught that few doctors and nurses are interested in an extensive knowledge of psychological theories and/or models. They are more interested in advice directed towards clinical practice concerning the handling of—in their view—'troublesome' (read: anxious) patients. Below are three subjects that should be given prominence by psychologists in educating cardiologists and nurses about anxiety.

1. *Recognition of emotion.* In contacts with the patient it is important to have optimal cooperation between the patient and medical treatment staff in order to understand why the patient acts as he does and why he has certain wishes or demands. The same holds for the patient's thoughts, fantasies and expectations concerning his heart disease. For these reasons one should never ignore the patient's emotional life. If one does, and only places emphasis on the 'technical–somatic treatment', there will be a greater chance that feelings of anxiety will arise or persist. As in all groups, some doctors and nurses are more sensitive to the psychodynamics within the patient than their colleagues. Appreciation of this sensitivity by the psychologist is in

order as it will help increase group awareness of mental states. During the group sessions the psychologist identifies and emphasizes repeatedly those aspects of behaviour which can be interpreted as expressions of feelings. In this way the doctor and the nurses come to acquire a more psychology-orientated stance than was offered in their original training.

2. *Inquiring after feelings of anxiety.* If anxiety symptoms are recognized, such as motor unrest, fast and erratic talking and vasovegetative symptoms, it will (mostly) be experienced as a relief by the patient if the nurse or doctor asks what the feelings of anxiety are about. By means of these inquiries the feelings of anxiety may be mitigated so that they will no longer affect the patient's sense of reality. It is one of the tasks of the psychologist attached to a cardiology department to invest much time in creating learning material such as videotapes and tape-recorded talks between, for example, a psychology-minded cardiologist and his patient. For the doctor it will be useful if he is in a position to identify himself (on an unconscious level) with a sensitive colleague. In this way he could become (1) more receptive to the diagnosis of anxiety and (2) better placed to treat it.

3. *Denial of feelings of anxiety.* When the patient denies his feelings of anxiety by means of, for instance, euphoric behaviour, this should be respected in most cases. The patient will (unconsciously) show such behaviour because the seriousness of the disease is too threatening, and will be anxious to be dealt with in a different way. Psychological denial mechanisms have a function: denying (not wanting to feel) anxiety. The patient does so (at an unconscious level) because otherwise he will be overwhelmed by his feelings of anxiety. Feelings of anxiety are sometimes overlooked by doctors and/or nurses as the patient appears to have adjusted very well. It is one of the tasks of the psychologist to instruct the doctors and nurses about the function of denial (considered from a patient's point of view) and how best to cope with this defence mechanism.

CONCLUSION

This contribution demonstrates that much useful and also satisfactory work can be done by psychologists within a cardiology/cardiosurgery department. In the last two decades the cooperation between cardiologists and psychologists has intensified both with regard to treatment aspects and with regard to research. This multidisciplinary approach is expected to contribute to an improvement of the quality of life of cardiac patients.

NOTES

[1]Address for correspondence: R. A. M. Erdman, Departments of Medical Psychology and Cardiology, Erasmus University, PO Box 1738, 3000 DR Rotterdam, The Netherlands.

REFERENCES

Anderson, K. O. and Masur, F. T. (1983). Psychological preparation for invasive medical and dental procedures. *Journal of Behavioural Medicine*, **6**, 1–40.

Appels, A., Höppener, P. and Mulder, P. (1987). A questionnaire to assess premonitory symptoms of myocardial infarction. *International Journal of Cardiology*, **17**, 15–24.

Blanchard, E. B. and Miller, S. T. (1977). Psychological treatment of cardiovascular disease. *Archives of General Psychiatry*, **34**, 1402–1413.

Blodgett, C. and Pekarik, G. (1987). Program evaluation in cardiac rehabilitation I: Overview of evaluation issues. *Journal of Cardiopulmonary Rehabilitation*, **7**, 316–323.

Burgess, A. W., Lerner, D. J., D'Agostino, R. B. *et al.* (1987). A randomized control trial of cardiac rehabilitation. *Social Science and Medicine*, **24**, 359–370.

Cochran, T. M. (1984). Psychological preparation of patients for surgical procedures. *Patient Education and Counseling*, **5**, 153–158.

Copeland, J. G., Emery, R. W. and Levinson, M. M. (1987). Selection of patients for cardiac transplantation. *Circulation*, **75**, 2–9.

Denolin, H. (1985). Rehabilitation as part of comprehensive care. In: Kallio, V. and Cay, E. (Eds) *Rehabilitation After Myocardial Infarction, the European Experience*. Copenhagen: WHO, p. 24.

Dixhoorn, J. van, de Loos, J. and Duivenvoorden, H. J. (1983). Contribution of relaxation technique to the rehabilitation of myocardial infarction patients. *Psychotherapy and Psychosomatics*, **40**, 137–147.

Doehrman, S. R. (1977). Psycho-social aspects of recovery from coronary heart disease: A review. *Social Science and Medicine*, **11**, 199–218.

Erdman, R. A. M., Duivenvoorden, H. J., Verhage, F., Kazemier, M. and Hugenholtz, P. G. (1986). Predictability of beneficial effects in cardiac rehabilitation: A randomized clinical trial of psychosocial variables. *Journal of Cardiopulmonary Rehabilitation*, **6**, 206–213.

Falger, P. R. J. and Schouten, E. G. W. (1987). Welke mensen kryjen een hartinfarct? *Gedrag en Gezondheid*, **15**, 155–164.

Friedman, M., Thorensen, C. E., Gill, J. J. *et al.* (1984). Alteration of type A behavior and reduction in cardiac recurrence in post-myocardial infarction patients. *American Heart Journal*, **182**, 237–248.

Hackett, T. P. (1985). Depression following myocardial infarction. *Psychosomatics*, **26**, 23–30.

Hansen, M. and Lavandero, R. (1981). A multidisciplinary education program for patients undergoing cardiovascular surgery. *Quality Review Bulletin*, **7**, 19–24.

Johnston, D. W. (1985). Psychological interventions in cardiovascular disease. *Journal of Psychosomatic Research*, **29**, 447–456.

Kendall, P. C. and Watson, D. (1981). Psychological preparation for stressful medical procedures. In: Prokop, C. and Bradley, L. (Eds) *Medical Psychology, Contributions to Behavioral Medicine*. New York: Academic Press.

Kris, A. O. (1984). The conflicts of ambivalence. *Psychoanalytic Study of the Child*, **40**, 225–274.

Kühn, W. F., Davis, M. H. and Lippmann, S. B. (1988). Emotional adjustment to cardiac transplantation. *General Hospital Phychiatry*, **10**, 108–113.

Mai, F. M., McKenzie, F. N. *et al.* (1986). Psychiatric aspects of heart transplantation; Preoperative evaluation and postoperative sequela. *British Medical Journal*, **292**, 311–313.

Marra, S., Paolillo, V., Spadaccini, F. and Angelino, P. F. (1985). Longterm follow-up after a controlled randomized post-myocardial infarction rehabilitation programme: Effects on morbidity and mortality. *European Heart Journal*, **6**, 656–663.

Mayou, R. A. (1983). A controlled trial of early rehabilitation after myocardial infarction. *Journal of Cardiac Rehabilitation*, **3**, 397–402.

Mayou, R., Sleight, P., MacMahon, D. and Florencio, M. J. (1981). Early rehabilitation after myocardial infarction. *Lancet*, **19**, 1399–1401.

McAleer, J. M., Copeland, J. *et al.* (1985). Psychological aspects of heart transplantation. *Heart Transplant*, **4**, 234–240.

Nunes, E. V., Frank, K. A. and Kornfeld, D. S. (1987). Psychological treatment for the type A behavior pattern and for coronary heart disease: A meta-analysis of the literature. *Psychosomatic Medicine*, **48**, 159–173.

O'Brien, V. C. (1985). Psychological and social aspects of heart transplantation. *Heart Transplantation*, **4**, 229–231.

Ragland, D. R. and Brand, J. R. (1988). Type A behavior and mortality from coronary heart disease. *New England Journal of Medicine*, **318**, 65–69.

Ramshaw, J. E. and Stanley, G. (1984). Psychological adjustment to coronary artery surgery. *British Journal of Clinical Psychology*, **23**, 101–108.

Razin, A. M. (1982). Psychosocial intervention in coronary artery disease: A review. *Psychosomatic Medicine*, **44**, 363–387.

Rovario, S., Holmes, D. S. and Holmsten, R. D. (1984). Influence of a cardiac rehabilitation program and the cardiovascular, psychological and social functioning of cardiac patients. *Journal of Behavioural Medicine*, **7**, 61–81.

Soloff, P. H. (1977). Denial and rehabilitation of the post-infarction patient. *International Journal of Psychiatric Medicine*, **8**, 125–129.

Stern, M. J. and Cleary, P. (1981). National exercise and heart disease project; psychosocial changes observed during a low-level exercise program. *Archives of Internal Medicine*, **141**, 1463–1467.

Suinn, R. M. (1980). Pattern A behaviors and heart disease: Intervention approaches. In: Ferguson, J. and Taylor, C. (Eds) *The Comprehensive Handbook of Behavioral Medicine*, Vol. I. New York: Systems Interventions, Spectrum.

Theorell, T. (1982). Psychosocial interventions as part of the rehabilitation after a myocardial infarction. *International Rehabilitation Medicine*, **5**, 185–188.

Thorensen, C. E., Telch, M. J. and Eaglestone, J. R. (1981). Approaches to altering the type A behavior pattern. *Psychosomatics*, **22**, 472–479.

Trelawny-Ross, C. and Russel, O. (1987). Social and psychological responses to myocardial infarction: Multiple determinants of outcome at six months. *Journal of Psychosomatic Research*, **31**, 125–130.

Trijsburg, R. W., Erdman, R. A. M., Duivenvoorden, H. J. *et al.* (1987). Denial and overcompensation in male patients with myocardial infarction. *Psychotherapy and Psychosomatics*, **47**, 22–28.

Uden, M. M. A. T. van, Erdman, R. A. M., Zoeteweij, M. W. *et al.* (1986). Heeft hartrevalidatie effect? Een literatuurstudie. *Gedrag en Gezondheid*, **14**, 153–158.

Utens, L., Erdman, R. A. M. and Verhage, F. (1986). Het psychologisch voorbereiden van patiënten op ingrijpende medische procedures: Een literatuuroverzicht. *Gedrag en Gezondheid*, **14**, 11–18.

WHO (1982). *World Health Statistics Annual*. Geneva: WHO.

Wiklund, I., Sanne, H., Vedin, A. and Wilhelmsen, C. (1985). Coping with myocardial infarction: A model with clinical applications, a literature review. *International Rehabilitation Medicine*, **7**, 167–175.

CHAPTER 10

Asthma

W. Everaerd[1,2]

University of Amsterdam, Amsterdam

I. S. Y. Vromans

Institute of Public Health, Utrecht

and

A. M. C. van der Elst

University of Utrecht, Utrecht

ABSTRACT

Psychological factors such as fear, illness behaviour, knowledge about asthma and ability to cope with asthma might influence the course of the disease. Behaviour therapy directed at changing psychological factors seems to result in no effects on objective measures of pulmonary function and only small effects on subjective measures of complaints about asthma. The self-management approach is often seen as a means of controlling medical consumption. Its effect is probably gained through training in early recognition of bronchospasm, influencing medicine use and improving communication between patient and physician. Asthma is a complicated problem which results in considerable between-patient variation in coping with this disease. Treatment should be multilateral and fit the individual needs of the patient.

INTRODUCTION

Life ends with breathing one's last breath. A shortage of air, therefore, is a frightening experience. Asthmatic patients live with a continuous threat of

Behavioural Medicine
Edited by A. A. Kaptein, H. M. van der Ploeg, B. Garssen, P. J. G. Schreurs and R. Beunderman
© 1990 John Wiley & Sons Ltd.

sudden dyspnoea. This chapter is about asthma and its effects on the patient. Characteristics of asthma will be described, its associations with psychological factors and the results of behaviour therapy. Some remarks will be made on children with asthma. In children the course of asthma is often erratic and parents may play a special role in the manifestation of the symptoms. This places extra demands on behaviour therapy and is therefore better discussed separately.

CHARACTERISTICS OF THE DISEASE

Asthma, chronic bronchitis and emphysema are known as chronic non-specific lung diseases (CNSLD). As it is often hard to distinguish between the diseases, the term CNSLD is used; yet there are differences. In asthma, periods of dyspnoea occur at irregular intervals. In between these attacks the asthmatic patient usually has normal pulmonary function. Periods of dyspnoea vary in severity, and are mediated by spasm of the smooth muscle tissue, oedema in the mucous lining of the bronchi and excessive mucous secretion in the bronchi. Chronic bronchitis is characterized by frequent coughing and expectoration, whereas sufferers from emphysema typically complain of breathlessness in rest as well as during and after exertion.

The pathophysiology of asthma is based on bronchial hyperreactivity. In the hyperreactive bronchi of asthmatics, obstruction is induced by a large variety of stimuli. Well known are chemical compounds such as cigarette smoke and other air pollution, physical stimuli such as changes in temperature and humidity, exercise and infections. Many asthmatics are allergic; contact with allergens (e.g. pollen, animal dandruff, moulds) induces an immediate or delayed obstruction of their bronchi.

Thoughts and emotions may induce dyspnoea; many patients have commented on these associations (Rees, 1956). Breathing may be an important aspect of emotional experience: a sigh of relief, excitement causing one to gasp for breath, breathe more freely. Whether patients feel short of breath through emotions only or in fact have bronchial obstruction is not clear. In several studies emotions have been induced to measure the effects on bronchial obstruction. Emotions were induced by exposure to mental arithmetic, film and suggestions associated with the inhalation of neutral compounds (Levenson, 1979; Horton, Saruda and Kinsman, 1978; Janson-Bjerklie, 1985; Butler and Steptoe, 1986). The suggestive information supposedly induced sufficiently intense emotions and resulted in bronchial obstruction in a substantial proportion of the patients. An increase in airflow resistance measured by spirometer or forced oscillation technique led to this conclusion. Some researchers assumed that the bronchial obstruction was not mediated by suggestions but through irritation of the bronchi, because the substance was inhaled at room temperature. In a replication with the substance inhaled at body temperature, no bronchial obstruction occurred although patients reported dyspnoea (Lewis, Lewis and Tattersfield, 1984). The results of the studies into the effects of suggestive information indicate that emotions possibly induce bronchial obstruction. However, methodological shortcomings in the studies prevent a convincing conclusion.

EPIDEMIOLOGY

The incidence and prevalence of asthma are hard to measure, due to lack of a definition that is generally accepted. Therefore figures show a lot of variation. It is estimated that 3–4% of the population of the United States of America and Great Britain suffer from asthma. In a survey of several epidemiological studies, primarily among adults in Europe and the United States, the prevalence of asthma varied from 0.9 to 6.2% (Gregg, 1983). A recent study on bronchial hyperreactivity in adult rural residents in Australia showed a prevalence of asthma of 11.4% whereas only 5.9% had symptoms of asthma (Woolcock et al., 1987). Research in England showed bronchial hyperreactivity to be present in 14% of screened adults. Symptoms of asthma were not recorded. So an overestimating of morbidity caused by asthma is likely to have occurred in this study (Burney et al., 1987).

Asthma has considerable negative consequences for the patient. It causes substantial disability and necessitates medical attention. During 1980 in the United States adult asthmatics (5–15 million) were limited in their daily activities an average of 16 days, of which six were spent in bed. Asthma thus results in non-attendance at school, absenteeism from work and also social isolation. Half of the patients used medicines and over 20% had previously been hospitalized. The number of admissions of patients with asthma is rising: in 1983 there were nearly half a million hospital admissions. The death rate is probably going up also. CNSLD, of which only a part is due to asthma, nowadays is the fifth cause of death in the United States (Evans et al., 1987).

SUBJECTIVE ASPECTS

The preceding section shows the considerable social, medical and economic effects of asthma. The psychological consequences of asthma can be serious also. Patients with frequent asthma attacks are particularly hampered in their daily activities. They normally need a lot of medicines, frequently consult a GP and possibly require admission to a hospital or asthma centre.

Psychological factors seem to be closely linked to the course of disease in asthma. In patients hospitalized in an asthma centre, panic-fear disposition related to length of hospitalization, medication at discharge and rehospitalization rates (Dirks and Kinsman, 1981). In patients admitted to a general hospital, similar relations exist: disposition to anxiety, neuroticism and stigma gave a worse prognosis (Kaptein, 1982).

The relationship between psychological factors and the course of disease in asthma may be explained in several ways. Possibly neurotic or anxious people have more difficulty in coping with a disease such as asthma, just as they cope less successfully with other problems. They may suffer from tension, which perhaps induces bronchial obstruction. They also could be reacting inappropriately to their asthma. For instance, through fear or through paying too much attention to their bodily reactions, normal sensations may be misinterpreted as the beginning of an asthma attack. This can lead to excessive medicine consumption. Those patients that panic and cannot stay calm during an attack run the same risk.

On the other hand, chronic disease possibly influences one's personality. In asthma the unpredictable attacks may lead to anxiety and insecurity. In a study on 155 admitted patients, a positive correlation was indeed found between neuroticism and duration of asthma (Jones *et al.*, 1976).

It is difficult to distinguish between cause and effect of asthmatic complaints. Social isolation through avoidance of activities that could cause attacks may be an effect of asthma. However, this avoidance behaviour can also be interpreted as being due to anxiety and shame.

In the next section psychological interventions in the relief of patients' suffering will be discussed. Behaviour therapy techniques and self-management will be dealt with successively.

BEHAVIOUR THERAPY

Behavioural interventions are based on the established fact that conditioned stimuli, expectations, emotions and behaviour can cause or aggravate a bronchial obstruction. Treatment is aimed at teaching the patient to react in another way to these stimuli. The new reaction inhibits the former maladaptive reaction.

The practical approach often consists of teaching the patient to relax. The effect of the treatment is usually assessed by measuring parameters of disease features such as lung function and the number of asthma attacks. Sometimes indirect measures are used, such as daily functioning and medical consumption (e.g. use of medicines, consultations with a physician and admission to a hospital or asthma centre).

Several case reports indicate positive effects for behaviour therapy (Walton, 1960; Cooper, 1964; Moorefield, 1971; Rathus, 1973; Sirota and Mahoney, 1974; MacDonald and Oden, 1977). However, there is no certainty of a true effect because comparison with a no-treatment control group is not reported, or there is no pretest measurement and sometimes no measurement at all.

Eight controlled studies have been reported where treatment followed a fixed protocol and measurements were at least taken before and after treatment. These studies have been reviewed critically by Richter and Dahme (1982). Their conclusions to a large extent corroborate what we have found on the basis of our own review of this literature.

Treatment in each of the studies consisted of relaxation (progressive muscle relaxation or autogenic training) and in three studies this therapy was compared to a form of systematic desensitization. Six studies involved individual therapy and two group therapy. One hundred and thirty-four patients in total were treated. In seven studies the effect of relaxation therapy was scored by measuring lung function, by means of a spirometer or a peak flow meter. One study, after reanalysis by Richter and Dahme, showed a deterioration of lung function. In four studies lung function did not change and in two others it showed an improvement. In one of these two studies the claimed improvement in lung function is not supported by data. Two of the three groups showed an improvement with systematic desensitization.

Several possible explanations are offered for the meagre effects of behaviour therapy on lung function. First, incidentally recording lung function is not a valid method for measuring the course of asthma. Lung function in asthmatics is usually normal in between attacks. Periodic measurements tend to underestimate the severity of the disease by not registering all broncho-obstructive attacks, especially those occurring at night. Second, lung function measurement requires good technique and maximum effort from the patient. These factors influence the reliability of the measures. Third, it has not been proven that emotions directly cause bronchial obstruction. There is evidence for an association between emotional tension and bronchodilation, mediated by reduced parasympathic activity (Harding and Maher, 1982). However, one can imagine that relaxation would help the patient to be less troubled by broncho-obstruction by reducing fear.

Subjective asthmatic symptoms were analysed in six out of the eight studies. Four studies showed improvement. Between treatments (relaxation and systematic desensitization) no difference was found in the rate of symptom reduction. In one study relaxation was compared with placebo; here too no difference was found in reduction of complaints.

The use of medicine was measured in four studies. For one study no values have been reported, one study did not show a decrease in use of medicine for both treatments, two studies reported a non-significant decrease in use of medicine.

One study compared the rate of consultations with a physician for relaxation and placebo control. No decrease was found and no difference between the two groups.

One could easily agree with the conclusion of Richter and Dahme (1982): the results of controlled studies with behaviour therapy are not very convincing. This failure to produce improvements may be due to the use of a single standard treatment modality. These treatments apparently show a lack of flexibility with regard to the complex problems of asthma. Also, relaxation treatment can be meaningful only when tension and emotions play an important role, in comparison with other factors causing dyspnoea.

Behaviour therapy aimed at improving pulmonary function and subjective complaints should be used with discretion. Relaxation seems to be contraindicated in a number of patients, especially in those who do not experience fear or neglect their symptoms (Kinsman, Dirks and Jones, 1980).

SELF-MANAGEMENT

The self-management approach emanates from a changing view on health care, giving the patient a larger role in his own treatment than before. This change originated partly from the gigantic rise in costs to society of medical care in addition to the desire of the patient for autonomy and self-control.

Self-management approaches differ from behaviour therapy in a number of aspects. There is no *a priori* assumption that the patient is psychologically disturbed. It is postulated that the patient's way of coping with his disease is influencing the course of the disease (Burns, 1982).

Research data indicate that asthmatic patients often lack necessary knowledge and skills (Avery, March and Brook, 1980). A number of patients are unable to accurately estimate their pulmonary function. Some with severely disturbed pulmonary function feel perfect, while others with normal function feel extremely tight (Heim, Blaser and Waidelich, 1772; Rubinfeld and Pain, 1977). Some patients do not know what to do in emergencies (Dunt *et al.*, 1987), and others misuse their medicines (Lindgren, Bake and Larsson, 1987).

The goal of self-management is not to cure the disease, but to teach patients to cope with it more successfully. Success of self-management is generally measured by a reduction in medical consumption: consultations with a GP or specialist, emergency visits or admissions to hospital. Self-management is taught by provision of information and discussion and advice about the practical use of the newly acquired knowledge. Special attention will be given to the avoidance of attacks. Patients should know what typical triggers may induce asthma attacks. Screening for allergens is useful here. In addition it may be of value for the patient to keep a notebook for some time, recording complaints, circumstances and the medicines taken. Even pulmonary function as measured by a portable device may be recorded (Higgs *et al.*, 1986).

Having identified the inducing factors, avoidance may be planned. Removal of allergens often is a good solution (redecoration of the bedroom for instance) but reduction in social activities (sports, etc.) can lead to isolation of the individual, in which case it may be better to take prophylactic medication. However, the patient must be well informed about the way these medicines work in order to prevent, for instance, the taking of corticosteroids to neutralize bronchospasm. The patient and his close relatives should learn about asthma and its treatment through information transfer, preferably in a well-discussed manner. One has to keep an eye on aversion to taking prescribed medicines (out of fear of side-effects or opposition to the physician).

Attention may be given to the handling of an attack which occurs despite all precautions. Proper handling requires early recognition of the symptoms. Recording of pulmonary function may be useful here. On noting the early symptoms of an attack relaxation is recommended and the drinking of lots of lukewarm liquid to lower mucus viscosity. Medicines should be taken if these measures fail to work. The patient must be aware of how the medicines take effect and medicines must be taken in the proper way without exceeding the maximum dose. Fear and panic can be obstructive to the proper handling of an attack; relaxation exercises may give relief here too.

Most published self-management programmes concern asthmatic children and their parents. Educational programmes for children with asthma have produced improved skills in management, increased knowledge about asthma for both children and their parents, improved feelings of control of one's asthma, and fewer emergency room visits and days of hospitalization. Programmes for children have been described for different settings: outpatient clinic, school, medical office, camp programmes and in the community (Rachelefsky, 1987).

Four studies concentrate on adults with asthma. The first study (Green et al., 1977) concerns a group of 58 asthmatic patients attending the first-aid unit of a general hospital. Half of the group, 29 patients, were given one meeting where they received information and were encouraged into good self-care. The other patients functioned as the control group. For five weeks all patients kept a diary that was collected once a week by one of the researchers. At the collection visit the patients were interviewed and questions were briefly answered. For 18 weeks, visits of the patients to the first-aid unit were recorded.

After five weeks significantly more patients from the control group as compared to the meeting group visited the first-aid unit. After 18 weeks the control group had twice as many visits to the unit (98 visits vs 43 for the meeting group) and the number of patients returning to the emergency room showed the same trend (16 patients from the control group vs 10 patients from the experimental group).

Another study from the same hospital was reported two years later (Maiman et al., 1979). The effect of information was now studied in 289 asthmatic patients. In addition to verbal information half of the cases also received an information booklet. Information was given by a healthy nurse or by a nurse who herself was an asthmatic patient. The nurse with asthma disclosed her own asthma to half of the cases she informed. Information given by the asthmatic nurse proved to be effective in reducing emergency visits in the next six weeks. Disclosure of her own asthma made little difference. The booklet produced little extra effect. Patients who were instructed by the healthy nurse and had received the booklet nearly all required an emergency consultation. The researchers suggest that written information does not substitute for verbal information.

Moldofsky et al. (1979) report on a study with 79 patients. Half of this group saw information on a videotape; information on asthma and different ways of handling asthma were described and explained. The other patients only answered a list of questions and received a medical examination. Immediately after viewing the tape patients had more knowledge than their controls. At a follow-up 16 months later this difference in knowledge had disappeared. Morbidity and medical consumption were about the same for both groups.

In another study (Hilton et al., 1986) three different interventions were compared in a group of 339 patients: (1) a combination of an information booklet, a 15-minute conversation with their own physician, an audiocassette with information and prospect of a later conversation with the family doctor; (2) an information booklet; (3) no further intervention (control group).

One year later the extended package appeared to lead to greater knowledge compared to the booklet alone or no intervention. However, the groups showed no difference in self-management, compliance and asthmatic complaints. The controls even had the lowest rate of absenteeism. However, most patients from the two treated groups reported that the programme had had a positive effect on their ability to handle their asthma.

Disappointing results in the Hilton et al. and the Moldofsky et al. studies may be due to patient selection. Compared to the Green et al. and Maiman et al. studies the educational level of their patients was higher, suggesting lower benefit from the information given, as these patients had more prior knowledge of asthma. There was a further difference between the groups studied. Hilton et al.'s group consisted of patients from GP practices and they possibly had less severe asthma. With follow-up after a longer interval of time effects seem to disappear; not all studies inform us about these changes.

An important point is the ineffectiveness of impersonal ways of giving information—by only showing a videotape or giving a booklet. It appears that empathy and understanding are essential ingredients for self-management teaching.

We are at this moment conducting a study into the effects of a group format for teaching self-management. Six to eight patients meet 12 times with a team of a psychologist and a therapist with expertise on breathing techniques. The patients receive information on asthma, discuss important topics related to their illness and its management, and do relaxation exercises, rational emotive therapy and assertiveness training during the two-hour meeting. At the end of each meeting the patients receive homework, to be discussed at the next meeting. Meetings one through four are spent on strategies to deal with dyspnoea. Ample attention is paid to the emotions patients experience during an attack. In meetings five through seven the role of tensions and emotions in the development of symptoms is discussed. Meetings eight through 12 are used for learning alternative methods to handle difficult situations. Self-observations, done at home by the patients, are used continually.

CASE STUDY

Ineke, a 26-year-old patient still living with her parents, was instructed to change her coping behaviour during a period of dyspnoea at home. At the next meeting she reported that the relaxation gave her no relief. Eventually she had taken her medicines and the dyspnoea soon disappeared. However, it transpired that she had used an inhaled corticosteroid, a medicine that is not supposed to neutralize dyspnoea immediately. Further questioning revealed that she became calm the moment after taking her medicine. At that very moment she became confident that the dyspnoea would soon disappear. In the group we discussed the possibility that her belief in the effect of her medicine, more than the pharmacological effect, made her dyspnoea disappear. Ineke was not quite convinced, but promised to think about it. At the next meeting she reported that she had had another attack, but remained calm throughout. Her dyspnoea, usually lasting at least three hours, was gone in half an hour without using medicines.

Our group format follows an extensive script, including exercises, homework instructions and covering text. The preliminary positive results of our programme seem to warrant some optimism. At this moment the study is still in progress, so long-term results are not yet available.

It is appropriate to conclude that self-management as an approach to asthma reduces morbidity. Essential conditions are that information is exchanged in an active way and that an opportunity is given to discuss emotional aspects of asthma.

NOTES

[1]Addresses for correspondence: W. Everaerd, Department of Clinical Psychology, University of Amsterdam, Weesperplein 8, 1018 XA Amsterdam, The Netherlands; I. S. Y. Vromans, Institute of Public Health, Wittevrouwenkade 6, 3512 CR Utrecht, The Netherlands; A. M. C. van der Elst, Department of Pulmonary Disease, Utrecht University, PO Box 16250, 3500 CG Utrecht, The Netherlands.
[2]This chapter was prepared during research supported by the Dutch Asthma Fund (grant 82.17).

REFERENCES

Avery, C. H., March, J. and Brook, R. H. (1980). An assessment of the adequacy of self-care by adult asthmatics. *Journal of Community Health*, **5**, 167–180.

Burney, P. G. J., Britton, J. R., Chinn, S., Tattersfield, A. E., Papacosta, A. O., Kelson, M. C., Anderson, F. and Corfield, D. R. (1987). Descriptive epidemiology of bronchial reactivity in an adult population: Results from a community study. *Thorax*, **42**, 38–44.

Burns, K. L. (1982). Behavioral health care in asthma. *Public Health Review*, **10**, 339–381.

Butler, C. and Steptoe, A. (1986). Placebo responses: An experimental study of psychophysiological processes in asthmatic volunteers. *British Journal of Clinical Psychology*, **25**, 173–183.

Cooper, A. J. (1964). A case of bronchial asthma treated by behaviour therapy. *Behaviour Therapy and Research*, **1**, 351–356.

Dirks, J. F. and Kinsman, R. A. (1981). Clinical prediction of medical rehospitalization: Psychological assessment with the battery of asthma illness behavior. *Journal of Personality Assessment*, **45**, 608–613.

Dunt, D. R., Rubinfeld, A. R., Feren, P. and McClure, B. G. (1987). What patients know about their asthma. *Community Health Studies*, **11**, 125–130.

Evans, R. E., Mullally, D. I., Wilson, R. W., Gergen, P. J., Rosenberg, H. M., Grauman, J. S., Chevarley, F. M. and Feinleib, M. (1987). National trends in the morbidity and mortality of asthma in the US. Prevalence, hospitalization and death from asthma over two decades: 1965–1984. *Chest*, Suppl., **91**, 65s–74s.

Green, L. W., Werlin, S. H., Schauffler, H. H. *et al.* (1977). Research and demonstration issues in self-care: Measuring the decline of medicocentrism. *Health Education Monographs*, **5**, 161–189.

Gregg, I. (1983). Epidemiologic aspects. In: Clark, T. J. H. and Godfrey, S. (Eds) *Asthma*, 2nd edn. London: Chapman and Hall, pp. 242–284.

Harding, A. V. and Maher, K. R. (1982). Biofeedback training of cardiac acceleration: Effects on airway resistance in bronchial asthma. *Journal of Psychosomatic Research*, **26**, 447–454.

Heim, E., Blaser, A. and Waidelich, E. (1972). Dyspnea: Psychophysiological relationships. *Psychosomatic Medicine*, **34**, 405–423.

Higgs, C. M. B., Richardson, R. B., Lea, D. A., Lewis, G. T. R. and Laszlo, G. (1986). Influence of knowledge of peak flow on self assessment of asthma: Studies with a coded peak flow meter. *Thorax*, **41**, 671–675.

Hilton, S., Sibbald, B., Anderson, H. R. and Freeling, P. (1986). Controlled evaluation of the effects of patient education on asthma morbidity in general practice. *Lancet*, Jan. 4, 26–29.

Horton, D. J., Saruda, W. K. and Kinsman, R. A. (1978). Broncho constrictive suggestion in asthma. A role for airway hyperactivity and emotions. *American Review of Respiratory Diseases*, **117**, 1029–1038.

Janson-Bjerklie, S. (1985). History of emotionality triggered asthma as a predictor of airway response to suggestion. *Dissertation Abstracts International*, **45**, 2497.

Jones, N. F., Kinsman, R. A., Schum, R. and Resnikoff, Ph. (1976). Personality profiles in asthma. *Journal of Clinical Psychology*, **32**, 285–291.

Kaptein, A. A. (1982). Psychological correlates of length of hospitalization and rehospitalization in patients with acute severe asthma. *Social Science and Medicine*, **16**, 725—729.

Kinsman, R. A., Dirks, J. F. and Jones, N. F. (1980). Anxiety reduction in asthma: Four catches to general application. *Psychosomatic Medicine*, **42**, 397–405.

Levenson, R. W. (1979). Effects of thematically relevant and general stressors on responding in asthmatic and non-asthmatic subjects. *Psychosomatic Medicine*, **41**, 28–39.

Lewis, R. A., Lewis, M. N. and Tattersfield, A. E. (1984). Asthma induced by suggestion: Is it due to airway cooling? *American Review of Respiratory Diseases*, **129**, 691–695.

Lindgren, S., Bake, B. and Larsson, S. (1987). Clinical consequences of inadequate inhalation technique in asthma therapy. *European Journal of Respiratory Diseases*, **70**, 93–98.

MacDonald, W. S. and Oden, C. W. (1977). Role clarification and sanction in two cases of bronchial asthma. *Journal of Asthma Research*, **14**, 189–197.

Maiman, L. A., Green, L. W., Gibson, G. *et al.* (1979). Education for self-treatment by adult asthmatics. *Journal of the American Medical Association*, **241**, 1919–1922.

Moldofsky, H., Broder, I., Davies, G. *et al.* (1979). Videotape educational program for people with asthma. *Canadian Medical Association Journal*, **120**, 669–672.

Moorefield, C. W. (1971). The use of hypnosis and behavior therapy in asthma. *American Journal of Clinical Hypnosis*, **13**, 162–168.

Rachelefsky, G. S. (1987). Review of asthma self-management programs. *Journal of Allergy and Clinical Immunology*, **80**, 506–511.

Rathus, S. A. (1973). Motoric, autonomic and cognitive reciprocal inhibition in a case of hysterical bronchial asthma. *Adolescence*, **8**, 29–32.

Rees, L. (1956). Physical and emotional factors in bronchial asthma. *Journal of Psychosomatic Research*, **1**, 98–114.

Richter, R. and Dahme, B. (1982). Bronchial asthma in adults; there is little evidence for the effectiveness of behavioral therapy and relaxation. *Journal of Psychosomatic Research*, **26**, 533–540.

Rubinfeld, A. R. and Pain, M. C. F. (1977). Conscious perception of bronchospasm as a protective phenomenon in asthma. *Chest*, **72**, 154–158.

Sirota, A. D. and Mahoney, M. J. (1974). Relaxing on cue: The self regulation of asthma. *Journal of Behavior Therapy and Experimental Psychiatry*, **5**, 65–66.

Walton, D. (1960). The application of learning theory to the treatment in a case of bronchial asthma. In: Eysenck, H. J. (Ed.) *Behaviour Therapy and the Neurosis*. London: Pergamon, pp. 188–189.

Woolcock, A. J., Peat, J. K., Salome, C. M., Yan, K., Anderson, S. D., Schoeffel, R. E., McCowage, G. and Killalea, T. (1987). Prevalence of bronchial hyperresponsiveness and asthma in a rural adult population. *Thorax*, **42**, 361–368.

CHAPTER 11

Hyperventilation Syndrome

B. Garssen[1]

University of Amsterdam, Amsterdam

and

H. Rijken

Utrecht University, Utrecht

ABSTRACT

The hyperventilation syndrome consists of a number of complaints that are in the main induced by hyperventilation. Another symptom-producing factor seems to be the tensing of the thoracic muscles. In the long run the increased muscle tension will lead to unpleasant sensations such as breathlessness, a tight feeling in the chest, or even precordial pain. We have suggested that the tendency to hyperventilate often develops in reaction to these annoying symptoms. Because of the abundance and variety of symptoms which are in themselves distressing and threatening, tension and worry often occur and new attacks are anxiously anticipated. In a number of patients this fear induces avoidance behaviour in the form of agoraphobia or social phobia.

Treatment should be arranged in accordance with the seriousness and duration of complaints, and the role of these complaints in daily life. In many patients the illness condition is self-perpetuating: the situations that once elicited symptoms no longer play an important role, while fear of the frequent reappearance of complaints has become the dominant factor. In those cases it is important to focus treatment on the deviant breathing behaviour and the fear of bodily sensations. To this end some treatment methods have been described, namely: explanation of the role of hyperventilation in symptom production, the use of a bag as an emergency measure, the voluntary provocation of a hyperventilation attack, and relaxation and breathing instructions. This approach is

Behavioural Medicine
Edited by A. A. Kaptein, H. M. van der Ploeg, B. Garssen, P. J. G. Schreurs and R. Beunderman
© 1990 John Wiley & Sons Ltd.

sufficient for a number of patients. Sometimes (other) psychological problems are so serious that they should be dealt with in therapy. As an example a case history has been presented.

INTRODUCTION

In 1937 the first comprehensive clinical description of the hyperventilation syndrome (HVS) was published by Kerr, Dalton and Gliebe. Afterwards reviews regularly appeared (Weimann, 1968; Lum, 1976; Magarian, 1982; Brashear, 1983; Garssen and Rijken, 1986). Only recently, however, has the HVS become generally known among patients, psychologists, general practitioners and medical specialists. At the present time the syndrome seems to occur more frequently, but probably this only appears to be so. Patients who are now classified as belonging to the category of the HVS would once have been seen as cases of neurocirculatory asthenia, Da Costa syndrome, anxiety neurosis, or 'nervous breakdown'. Because of earlier ignorance among medical specialists, the syndrome was often overlooked and patients were sent from one specialist to another. Present common knowledge has definite advantages. Patients with hyperventilation complaints are now seen less as 'exaggerating' or 'hysterical'. Patients can be reassured by means of information that has been gathered by scientists and clinicians and disseminated by medical cases and publications in popular magazines. Different forms of therapies have been developed and unnecessary medical examinations and inadequate treatments can be prevented. However, this familiarity also has some negative aspects. Sometimes patients are too easily categorized under the heading HVS. The diagnosis HVS is also used as a disguise for a doctor's ignorance or uncertainty. When no somatic basis has been found, the patient is sometimes put off with the simple statement that the complaints are caused by hyperventilation. This information alone is of no help to patients.

This chapter describes the clinical picture—epidemiological data and the pattern of complaints—and diagnostic procedures. A great deal of attention is also devoted to treatment.

The HVS is more than the occurrence of episodic or chronic hyperventilation and its consequent complaints, although this is the core of the syndrome. Another symptom-producing factor that probably plays a role in the HVS is a prolonged increase in muscle tension, especially in the muscles of the chest. This may induce the characteristic symptoms of feeling of tightness in the chest, breathlessness, and precordial pain (Friedman, 1945). These sensations are certainly not caused by hyperventilation; they are more likely the antecedents of an increase in ventilation.

Other elements that form an essential part of the HVS may be summarized under the heading 'anxiety'. In rare cases hyperventilation is induced by somatic causes such as brain damage or metabolic acidosis (a decreased pH because of metabolic factors such as inadequate kidney functioning), but if these are the main inducing factors the term 'HVS' is not appropriate. 'Anxiety' seems to be the most important factor in the HVS, that is: (a) the experience of stressful events that are not adequately coped with and (b) the interpretation of somatic complaints as threatening, leading to anxious anticipation of new attacks and avoidance behaviour. Consequently 'anxiety' may be both a causative factor and a consequence of hyperventilation. Anxiety and avoidance are sometimes present to such an extent that the condition is called an 'anxiety disorder'.

EPIDEMIOLOGY

Data on the incidence of the HVS in the general population are lacking. The occurrence of the HVS among medical patients is 4–11%, according to estimates in various groups of patients: an internal medical practice, a cardio-ambulatory service, emergency cases of an outpatient clinic and a neurology practice (Rice, 1950; Yu, Yim and Stanfield, 1959; Dölle, 1964; Pincus, 1978). In these studies two to seven times more female than male HVS patients are found (Yu, Yim and Stanfield, 1959; Dölle, 1964; Enzer and Walker, 1976; Weimann, 1968; Pincus, 1978). The study of Lum (1975) is exceptional in finding a ratio of 1 : 1. Most HVS patients range in age between 15 and 55 years. The syndrome does also occur among younger people, though these cases are rare (Enzer and Walker, 1976; Herman, Stickler and Lucas, 1981).

DESCRIPTION OF COMPLAINTS AND DIAGNOSTIC PROCEDURES

The HVS is a group of complaints the majority of which are produced by hyperventilation. Hyperventilation is a higher degree of ventilation—brought about by an increase in respiratory frequency and/or amplitude—than necessary to meet the demands of the body. This excessive ventilation results in a decrease in alveolar and arterial carbon dioxide pressure (PCO_2) and an increase of arterial pH (respiratory alkalosis). Secondary physiological changes are induced if hyperventilation is sufficiently great. The most important are:

1. Constriction of cerebral arteries
2. Increased neural excitability
3. Increased production of lactic and pyruvic acid
4. Lowering of phosphate level in arterial blood

Complaints often mentioned by HVS patients are:

- Respiratory complaints: breathlessness, tightness round the chest, increased frequency and/or depth of respiration, frequent sighing
- Tetanic symptoms: tingling (most frequently in the fingers, but also in the arms, round the mouth and sometimes elsewhere), stiffness of muscles, trembling of the hands

- Cerebral complaints: dizziness, blurred vision, faintness, headache
- Cardiac sensations: tachycardia, palpitations, precordial pain
- Temperature sensations: cold hands or feet, shivering, warm feeling in the head
- Gastrointestinal complaints: sickness, abdominal distention or pain
- General complaints: tension, anxiety, panic, fatigue, insomnia

For the diagnosis HVS the following criteria must be fulfilled:

- There are various, frequently occurring (at least once a week) somatic complaints
- These complaints are not induced by a somatic factor, apart from hyperventilation
- Several of these complaints are produced by voluntary hyperventilation and are recognized by the patient as similar to the complaints in daily life

For the assessment of complaints the Nijmegen Questionnaire (van Dixhoorn and Duivenvoorden, 1985) may be used. This questionnaire, presented in Figure 11.1, asks how often 16 complaints occur and is scored on a five-point scale, ranging from 0 (never) to 4 (very often). Scores are added and the sumscore thus ranges between 0 and 64. Though the HVS cannot be diagnosed on the basis of reported complaints alone, a high score is indicative. If the patient's sumscore exceeds the value of 22, she or he is probably an HVS patient (Garssen *et al.*, 1984).

The respiratory pattern of the patient may provide additional indications. An irregular sighing pattern is described as characteristic for the patient with HVS. However, other breathing patterns do occur. Some patients demonstrate a rapid, shallow, and very regular pattern without any sighs. A systematic study into how often both patterns occur has not been conducted. The alveolar CO_2 tension is sometimes lowered during baseline measurements (that is, when no particular instructions are given with regard to the breathing pattern). However, normal alveolar CO_2 values are certainly not exceptional. HVS patients may only hyperventilate during attacks, while having a normal respiratory pattern in between. If the alveolar CO_2 tension is lowered on repeated measurements, the patient apparently hyperventilates chronically. To conclude, only exceptional breathing patterns may give indications for the diagnosis HVS. However, their absence does not exclude the diagnosis.

Though claims have been made that either the acute or the chronic form of hyperventilation predominates, accurate data are lacking. A distinction between the acute and the chronic form can be made with respect to the occurrence of hyperventilation, but also with respect to the frequency of occurrence of complaints. Mixed forms may occur: some complaints may only arise during attacks, while other symptoms are chronically present. If so, the chronic complaints such as headache and nausea are often less clearly related to hyperventilation, while attackwise occurring symptoms, such as breathlessness, dizziness and tingling, bear a clear relation to hyperventilation.

Date : ....
Name : ....
Age : ....
Sex : male / female

Below is given a list of complaints which are possibly appropriate to your case. Please complete by circling one of the vertical strokes opposite each question.

	Never	Rarely	Sometimes	Often	Very often
1. Pain in the chest	⊢————+————+————+————+————⊣				
2. Tension	⊢————+————+————+————+————⊣				
3. Blurred vision	⊢————+————+————+————+————⊣				
4. Dizziness	⊢————+————+————+————+————⊣				
5. Confusion, losing normal contact	⊢————+————+————+————+————⊣				
6. Breathing faster or deeper	⊢————+————+————+————+————⊣				
7. Breathlessness	⊢————+————+————+————+————⊣				
8. Tightness around chest	⊢————+————+————+————+————⊣				
9. Stomach feels blown up	⊢————+————+————+————+————⊣				
10. Tingling in fingers	⊢————+————+————+————+————⊣				
11. Inability to take a deep breath	⊢————+————+————+————+————⊣				
12. Stiffness of fingers or arms	⊢————+————+————+————+————⊣				
13. Stiffness around mouth	⊢————+————+————+————+————⊣				
14. Cold hands or feet	⊢————+————+————+————+————⊣				
15. Pounding heart	⊢————+————+————+————+————⊣				
16. Anxiety	⊢————+————+————+————+————⊣				

Figure 11.1. Nijmegen HVS Questionnaire

HVS patients are often mentally and somatically tense and agitated, as can be seen from their rigid posture, restless movements, or tics. A high thoracic respiratory pattern can often be observed by looking at the patient.

To be certain about the diagnosis, a provocation test should be performed. The patient is asked to breathe as fast and as deeply as possible for 1.5–3 min. In doing this the alveolar CO_2 tension has to be lowered to at least 20 mmHg. Afterwards the patient is asked about symptoms experienced during or shortly after this period of voluntary hyperventilation. If the patient considers them as similar to his complaints in daily life, a diagnosis of HVS is made.

To draw up a provisional strategy for handling a patient's problems it is often sufficient to have the data on the questionnaire on somatic complaints, a medical examination, and information from an anamnestic interview. This interview should be focused on the following topics:

- What are the main complaints?
- Did stressful situations occur before the onset of the first attacks?
- Are there any stressful circumstances that aggravated the complaints in the course of time?
- Did the complaints lead to worry, anxiety, or tension?
- Does the patient avoid certain situations for fear of new attacks?

THE DEVELOPMENT OF THE HYPERVENTILATION SYNDROME

It is often stated that HVS is caused by 'stress'. What is meant is the stress of being exposed to serious life events and/or the lack of sufficient skills to cope with problems. This explanation seems to be correct, though insufficient. In an earlier study (Garssen, van Veenendaal and Bloemink, 1983) we asked 26 HVS patients if they could remember important events that happened before the beginning of their complaints. The following situations were mentioned (only situations are given that have been reported by more than one person; many persons mentioned more than one event): death of a relative, eight; conflicts with the partner, divorce, seven; financial problems, problems at work, six; quarrels with parents (in law), four; problems related to pregnancy, four; involuntary childlessness, three. Only one out of the 26 patients did not report any problematic situation. These data seem to indicate a causative role for stressful life events in the development of HVS. However, this explanation is insufficient in that a high frequency of such events increases the likelihood of occurrence for all kinds of somatic complaints (Rahe, 1974).

In support of the 'stress hypothesis', experimental studies may be mentioned that have demonstrated hyperventilation to occur in normal subjects when exposed to arousing conditions. However, closer inspection of these results shows that the degree of hyperventilation in these normal subjects is less severe than in HVS patients during an attack (Garssen and Rijken, 1986). So, this line of research does not provide a sufficient explanation either. We would suggest that HVS is the result of a learning process, starting with the tendency to tense the muscles of the trunk in response to threatening situations. This is a general stress response, but some people seem particularly inclined to manifest this response and to sustain it even when the eliciting situation has ended. Movements of the diaphragm are transferred to the abdominal wall and to the lower part of the chest wall. Tensing the muscles of the trunk impedes these diaphragmatic movements. Diaphragmatic activity contributes most to ventilation and its obstruction has to be compensated by an increased participation of the intercostal muscles. Prolonged overactivity of these thoracic muscles will result in unpleasant sensations, such as a feeling of tightness, breathlessness or even sensations of suffocation. In the same way pain in the heart region may develop, as was demonstrated in an experiment by Friedman (1945).

Hyperventilation may occur as a reaction to these sensations, leading to more complaints such as dizziness, faintness, tingling, and tremors. The regular, rapid, and somewhat shallow respiratory pattern is probably the consequence of the increased muscle tension. The incidence of bursts of deep inhalations may be seen—at least in the beginning—as a more or less voluntary reaction to the build-up of tension in the chest. However, in some patients the feeling of tightness will be continually interrupted by sighs, leading to the irregular sighing pattern.

The advantages of this theory are that (a) an explanation is offered for the respiratory behaviour of HVS patients and (b) the occurrence of symptoms that are not caused by hyperventilation itself, such as the chest complaints mentioned above, is made plausible. Moreover, the theory agrees with certain clinical impressions. There are patients who have complaints that are also found in HVS patients. Yet these patients do not fulfil the strict criteria for the HVS. If the theory is correct, this subgroup of patients have passed through the first stage—the maintenance of a prolonged increase in tension of the trunk muscles—but do not hyperventilate in reaction.

RELATION WITH ANXIETY DISORDERS

Once complaints have occurred, the further course depends on how these complaints are interpreted by the patient. If the first attack was a baffling phenomenon to the patient or was attributed to a serious disease, such as cancer or heart disease, anxious anticipation of new attacks will develop. This anxious anticipation will lead to physiological activation, thereby increasing the chance of new attacks occurring, resulting in the circular process illustrated in Figure 11.2. This vicious circle is further elucidated in the chapter on heart disease phobia in this book (Chapter 7).

The continual reappearance of attacks, or the continuous presence of complaints, may lead to changes in behaviour such as irritation, bursts of anger, drawing back into oneself, or avoidance of specific situations. If a person is seriously hindered in his daily activities because of the tension, anxiety and/or avoidance behaviour, an anxiety disorder as described in the DSM-III-R (American Psychiatric Association, 1987) has developed. Of particular importance here are the categories agoraphobia, panic disorder and—to a lesser degree— generalized anxiety disorder. The occurrence of attacks is often especially feared when alone, in situations from which escape might be difficult, and when many strangers are present, that is, in situations such as: being far away from home, crowded shops or department stores, elevators, or travelling alone by train or bus. If such situations are systematically avoided, the syndrome of agoraphobia has developed. It appears that somewhat more than 60% of agoraphobia patients also meet the criteria for the HVS (Garssen, van Veenendaal and Bloemink, 1983).

There is a striking similarity between panic attacks as described in the DSM-III-R and hyperventilation attacks. Therefore a considerable overlap is plausible

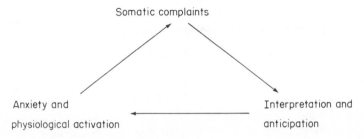

Figure 11.2. Vicious circle of anxious anticipation

between HVS and the category panic disorder in the DSM-III-R (Bass, Kart-sounis and Lelliot, 1987). Actual data on this subject are, however, lacking at the present moment. The relation between both diagnostic categories appeared from a study by Hibbert and Pilsburgh (1988) in a few patients with panic attacks and agoraphobia. When these patients indicated that they experienced panic, the arterial CO_2 tension appeared to have been reduced considerably. In another study, a low alveolar PCO_2 was found during baseline measurements in patients with panic attacks (Rapee, 1986). In addition, more complaints were induced by voluntary hyperventilation in these patients compared to a control group, and 80% of the patients with panic disorder experienced their complaints as similar to the complaints during spontaneous panic attacks. In two therapy evaluation studies, it was found that a treatment aimed at controlling hyperventilation complaints led to a reduction in panic attacks, anxiety and avoidance behaviour in psychiatric outpatients (Bonn, Readhead and Timmons, 1984; Clark, Salkovskis and Chalkley, 1985).

TREATMENT

To what degree hyperventilation complaints interfere with daily activities differs from patient to patient. When one talks to HVS patients some of them readily indicate one or more sources of stress. Ventilation of their worries often has a relieving effect. In these patients the somatic complaints themselves and the fear of these complaints then disappear into the background. However, especially if the complaints continue for some time, the frequent reappearance of complaints may become the central theme. For these patients emotional problems—depressed mood, anxiety, and worry—seem to be more a consequence than a cause of the somatic complaints. The next section focuses on this category of patients.

Though treatment should be adjusted to individual demands, two objectives are generally set in a behavioural treatment for HVS patients:

1. Learning to cope with hyperventilation and the fear of new attacks.
2. Learning to cope with stressful situations in general

Learning to Cope with Hyperventilation Complaints

With respect to complaints the following components should be distinguished: a physiological component (physical tension and abnormal respiratory behaviour), a cognitive component (attention, attribution, and anticipation) and a behavioural component (such as looking for reassurance by means of regular visits to the general practitioner or specialist; avoidance of certain situations). For therapy to be successful, all three components should be given attention. How can they be dealt with?

Information

The first step in the treatment is to give an easily understood explanation about (1) the physiological causes of the somatic complaints and (2) the relationship between stressful life events and the appearance of complaints. An oral explanation may be supported by written material. Correct information about the somatic cause gives the patient the first opportunity to ascribe his complaints no longer to a serious disease but to a particular way of breathing and to excessive tensing of certain muscles.

Coping with Hyperventilation Attacks

If a patient suffers from violent hyperventilation attacks, breathing into a bag may be advised as an emergency measure. However, clinical experiences made us aware that patients packed off home with the mere advice 'Use a plastic bag if necessary' do not follow this advice, or they put it into practice incorrectly. The instruction will be more effective if the therapist demonstrates how to use and hold the bag: over the nose and mouth, and not necessarily totally closed. Furthermore, it is important that the patient breathes quietly into the bag for at least five minutes. If attacks are greatly feared, their voluntary provocation and abatement with the help of a plastic bag is a useful therapeutic measure. The patient can thus see that attacks no longer happen to her or him, but that she or he is in control of the attacks.

Relaxation and Breathing Exercises

For most HVS patients it is necessary to learn specific skills to prevent attacks. Because patients are often generally tense and have bad breathing habits, treatments aimed at general relaxation and methods directed at changing respiratory behaviour may be useful. Vlaander-van der Giessen and Lindeboom (1982) compared the effect of breathing exercises (a programme of practice in slow breathing and learning to use abdominal wall movements more in breathing) and relaxation training with the changes in a no-treatment group. The treatment consisted of eight sessions of one hour each. Breathing instructions as well as relaxation training appeared to be more effective than no treatment. Compared with the control group, the frequency and intensity of attacks decreased significantly. Only with respect to intensity of attacks did specific breathing instructions work better than general relaxation. At a one-year follow-up the post-treatment effects remained. The majority of patients still had some complaints but could cope with them better.

With regard to relaxation, two methods we successfully taught were the shortened versions of the progressive relaxation method of Jacobson and the autogenic training of Schultz (self-suggestion method). We found it better to start with the more active and physically oriented method and to turn to a more suggestive method afterwards, especially in patients who find it difficult to concentrate and are afraid of experiencing bodily sensations and loss of control.

A high thoracic breathing pattern seems to be characteristic for many HVS patients. Intercostal muscles are thereby stiffened and diaphragmatic movements are impeded. Patients have to learn to relax the upper chest muscles and to make greater use of their diaphragm. It seems that the latter cannot be achieved directly, for instance by increasing abdominal movements (Wade, 1954), but the indirect method of relaxing the chest muscles, which will allow the diaphragm to move more freely, will be effective.

The direct and positive effects of slowing down the breathing have been demonstrated in experiments on healthy subjects. A lower respiratory rate resulted in a diminution of subjective and physiological responses to stressful stimuli (McCaul, Solomon and Holmes, 1979). In HVS patients slowing down the respiratory rate is also effective because it disrupts the pattern of high thoracic breathing. It is mainly the expiratory phase that is lengthened with a decrease in rate of respiration (Bendixen, Smith and Mead, 1964). This makes it difficult to maintain a high inspiratory level of breathing. Therefore, when breathing instructions are given special attention should be paid to the lengthening of expiration. Counting will be helpful, for instance: IN, 1–2, OUT, 3–4–5–6–7. Humming is another method for increasing expiration time. In addition, patients should be made aware of any faulty breathing habits, such as frequent sighing or the tendency not to pause when speaking.

By the method developed by Grossman, de Swart and Defares (1985), the patient can practise a slow breathing pattern using a small portable instrument which produces sound signals in a breathing rhythm. The patient is requested to follow this pattern three times a day for 10 minutes. Changes were measured over a 10-week treatment period. In comparison to a control group the experimental group had improved substantially, as was evident from a significantly greater reduction in number of complaints and in anxiety. Moreover, breathing resting frequency was lower and recovery of respiration after voluntary overventilation was faster.

It is important to discuss with the patient when and how these skills are to be practised in daily life. Many HVS patients are inclined to run from one activity to another without taking breaks, even for practising exercises. Patients often comment: 'If I sit still, I start to concentrate on my body and that is the moment when symptoms appear'. In such cases it is recommended to discuss the vicious circle of attention focusing, labelling and appearance of complaints. Patients should not, of course, continually observe their own breathing behaviour. A middle course has to be adopted between obsessional engagement in bodily symptoms on the one hand and avoiding paying any attention to them on the other.

The methods described above can be applied by a clinical psychologist or a general practitioner. For the teaching of relaxation and breathing exercises the aid of a physiotherapist may be called in. It is important that the physiotherapist understands the problems of patients with hyperventilation complaints and is willing to let a patient see that he can do something to cope with complaints. If this general approach does not produce satisfactory results, it will be necessary to analyse in more detail the factors that induce and maintain complaints and to apply a more specialized treatment, as presented below.

Learning to Cope with Stressful Life Situations

In terms of a functional analysis of the patient's complaints (see Chapter 1), the behaviour therapist will make an inventory of which coping skills are in the patient's repertoire and which are lacking. If the patient systematically avoids certain situations, a programme is designed to teach the patient to gradually expose himself to these situations. Sometimes specific overwhelming situations are the occasion for the development of hyperventilation symptoms, for instance the loss of a beloved person by death or divorce. In such cases negative emotions such as grief or anger have to be dealt with in therapy. The patient may also be chronically burdened by—often unspoken—lingering conflicts with the partner, the family, or in the work situation. Depending on the specific problems, treatment will involve interventions directed at relieving social anxiety, at improvement in communication with the partner or the family, or at improving more general problem-solving skills.

The frequent occurrence of somatic complaints and panic attacks may lead the patient to repeatedly seek support and reassurance from his relatives or his general practitioner. Such patients, who act both in a dependent and a demanding way, are often seen on the medical circuit. The behaviour therapist, the general practitioner or consulting physician and the patient should make explicit arrangements about whether or not medical examinations will be carried out and whether medication will be prescribed.

The dependant and demanding behaviour with respect to the partner can best be discussed in his or her presence. It is our experience that partners of HVS patients often feel very uncertain about how to react to the patient's complaints.

There is a group of patients in whom no precipitating events are found for their complaints. They are often permanently tense and they follow a hectic lifestyle. These patients want to do many things at the same time, while making high demands upon themselves. To give an example: a woman who brings up three schoolchildren, assists her husband in administrative tasks and in between takes care of an older, invalid neighbour. Despite the occurrence of stress symptoms her motto is: 'A young woman of 35 should be able to manage all these things'. It is useful to let the patient make notes of all daily activities for some weeks and to discuss in treatment what demands are set when engaging in these activities. Such a survey can be illuminating for the patient and will form a starting point for a better scheduling of activities with more breaks and more relaxing activities, and may lead to less extreme standards being set.

A CASE HISTORY

As has been stated above, patients are sometimes adequately helped by a treatment aimed at a better control of the hyperventilation symptoms alone. In the therapy of Mr A, described below, it turned out to be necessary also to pay attention to his agoraphobic avoidance behaviour and to problems in the relationship with his wife.

Mr A, a man of nearly 40, was referred by his general practitioner because of vague somatic complaints such as fatigue, breathlessness and dizziness, and frequent panic attacks. In the course of the year preceding his referral, the area he was able to move freely about in had become smaller and smaller; he only dared to drive his car in his own village.

The patient was a mechanic with an installation business. He took pride in the fact that nobody could ever find fault with his work. However, if he had to do a job outside his home village, he tried to avoid it. He was afraid of panicking on the way. Some of his colleagues and his boss were informed about his problems and made fewer demands on him for a long time. The direct cause of his asking for help was a discussion with his boss, who had told him in a friendly but decisive way that the situation could no longer be tolerated.

A said that he had often been anxious as a child and had suffered from nightmares. As a boy of 10 he had been suddenly confronted with his grand-mother lying in state in a funeral parlour. He had been very attached to her and the image of her dead body had obsessed him for a long time. His grand-mother's death could not be discussed at home. Even now A blamed his parents for not having noticed what obsessed him in those days.

About two years previously his wife had to undergo a serious operation and had been admitted to hospital for several months. He had managed to carry on rather well during his wife's stay in hospital. His symptoms had appeared after her return. At that time he often visited his general practitioner, who could not find any somatic basis for his complaints, and advised him to take a rest for a while. As this brought no improvement, A was referred to a behaviour therapist.

After two assessment sessions it was decided—in accordance with A's wishes—to get to grips first with the severe panic attacks and agoraphobic complaints. The hyperventilation provocation test was positive and the meaning of this outcome was fully discussed. A had occasionally heard of hyperventila-tion, but thought it irrelevant to his case. He was given an information sheet with the instruction that he and his wife should read it through carefully at home. Next, some treatment sessions were spent on relaxation and breathing exercises. Together with A, a programme was devised for him to practise in situations that were difficult for him, such as shopping alone and driving his car outside the central part of his village. The results were quite good: A's range of action had considerably enlarged, though he had to be stimulated regularly to carry on.

During treatment A revealed that he had a terrible fear of dying during panic attacks. Death was a central theme in his life. He was encouraged to speak about the times he had been confronted with death, and about his feelings of sorrow and abandonment. He felt this as a great relief. At about the twentieth session, A revealed that he had difficulty in discussing these topics with his wife. For some time he had been a member of a religious fellowship where he had found help with these questions about life and death. His wife strongly opposed this and found religious matters rubbish. Because A wanted to avoid quarrels with his wife, he had given up attending church. He also remarked that his wife seemed to be more and more jealous of his going out. Some therapy sessions were arranged with the couple to reopen their communication about such themes as religion and jealousy. Therapy could then be finished with reasonable success: panic attacks and agoraphobic behaviour had disappeared almost completely. Only when A felt oppressed did hyperventilation symptoms trouble him now and then. However, these no longer caused fear.

NOTES

[1]Addresses for correspondence: B. Garssen, Department of Medical Psychology, University of Amsterdam, Meibergdreef 15, 1105 AZ Amsterdam, The Netherlands; H. Rijken, Department of Psychiatry, Utrecht University, PO Box 85500, 3508 GA Utrecht, The Netherlands.

REFERENCES

American Psychiatric Association (1987). *Diagnostic and Statistical Manual of Mental Disorders-III-Revised*. Washington DC: APA.

Bass, C., Kartsounis, L. and Lelliot, P. (1987). Hyperventilation and its relationship to anxiety and panic. *Integrative Psychiatry*, **5**, 274–291.

Bendixen, H. H., Smith, S. M. and Mead, J. (1964). Pattern of ventilation in young adults. *Journal of Applied Physiology*, **19**, 195–198.

Bonn, J. A., Readhead, C. P. A. and Timmons, B. H. (1984). Enhanced behavioural response in agoraphobic patients pretreated with breathing retraining. *Lancet*, Sept. 22, 665–669.

Brashear, R. E. (1983). Hyperventilation syndrome. *Lung*, **161**, 257–273.

Clark, M. D., Salkovskis, P. M. and Chalkley, A. J. (1985). Respiratory control as a treatment for panic attacks. *Journal of Behavior Therapy and Experimental Psychiatry*, **16**, 23–30.

Dixhoorn, J. van and Duivenvoorden, H. J. (1985). Efficacy of Nijmegen Questionnaire in recognition of the hyperventilation syndrome. *Journal of Psychosomatic Research*, **29**, 199–206.

Dölle, W. (1964). Hyperventilation und Hyperventilationssyndrom. *Medische Klinik*, **59**, 695–699.

Enzer, N. B. and Walker, P. A. (1976). Hyperventilation syndrome in childhood. *Pediatrics*, **70**, 521–532.

Friedman, M. (1945). Studies concerning the etiology and pathogenesis of neurocirculatory asthenia. *Heart*, **30**, 557–567.

Garssen, B., Colla, P., Dixhoorn, J. van, Doorn, P. van, Folgering, H. T. M., Stoop, A. P. and Swart, J. C. G. de (1984). Het herkennen van het Hyperventilatie Syndroom. *Medisch Contact*, **35**, 1122–1124.

Garssen, B. and Rijken, J. M. (1986). Clinical aspects and treatment of the hyperventilation syndrome. *Behavioral Psychotherapy*, **14**, 46–86.

Garssen, B., Veenendaal, W. van and Bloemink, R. (1983). Agoraphobia and the hyperventilation syndrome. *Behavior Research and Therapy*, **21**, 643–649.

Grossman, P., Swart, J. C. G. de and Defares, P. B. (1985). A controlled study of a breathing therapy for treatment of hyperventilation syndrome. *Journal of Psychosomatic Research*, **29**, 49–58.

Herman, S. P., Stickler, G. B. and Lucas, A. R. (1981). Hyperventilation syndrome in children and adolescents: Long-term follow-up *Pediatrics*, **67**, 183–187.

Hibbert, G. A. and Pilsburg, D. (1988). Hyperventilation in panic attacks: ambulant monitoring of transcutaneous carbon dioxide. *British Journal of Psychiatry*, **153**, 76–80.

Kerr, W. J., Dalton, J. W. and Gliebe, P. A. (1937). Some physical phenomena associated with the anxiety states and their relation to hyperventilation. *Annals of Internal Medicine*, II, 961–992.

Lum, L. C. (1975). Hyperventilation: The tip and the iceberg. *Journal of Psychosomatic Research*, **19**, 375–383.

Lum, L. C. (1976). The syndrome of habitual chronic hyperventilation. In: Hill, O. W. (Ed.) *Modern Trends in Psychosomatic Medicine 3*. London: Butterworths, pp. 196–230.

Magarian, G. J. (1982). Hyperventilation syndromes: Infrequently recognized common expression of anxiety and stress. *Medicine*, **61**, 219–236.

McCaul, K. D., Solomon, S. and Holmes, D. S. (1979). Effects of paced respiration and expectations on physiological and psychological responses to threat. *Journal of Personality and Social Psychology*, **37**, 564–571.

Pincus, J. H. (1978). Disorders of conscious awareness. Hyperventilation syndrome. *British Journal of Hospital Medicine*, **19**, 312–313.

Rahe, R. H. (1974). Life change and subsequent illness reports. In: Gunderson, E. K. E. and Rahe, R. H. (Eds) *Life Stress and Illness*. Springfield, Illinois: C. C. Thomas, pp. 58–78.

Rapee, R. (1986). Differential response to hyperventilation in panic disorder and generalized anxiety disorder. *Journal of Abnormal Psychology*, **95**, 24–28.

Rice, R. L. (1950). Symptom patterns of the HVS. *The American Journal of Medicine*, **8**, 691–700.

Vlaander-van der Giessen, C. J. M. and Lindeboom, I. (1982). De behandeling van patienten met hyperventilatieklachten. *Gezondheid en Samenleving*, **3**, 73–78.

Wade, O. L. (1954). Movements of the thoracic cage and diaphragm in respiration. *Journal of Physiology*, **124**, 193–212.

Weimann, G. (1968). *Das Hyperventilationssyndrom*. Munchen: Urban & Schwarzenberg.

Yu, P. M., Yim, B. J. B. and Stanfield, A. (1959). Hyperventilation syndrome. Changes in the electrocardiogram, blood gases and electrolytes during voluntary hyperventilation; Possible mechanisms and clinical implications. *Archives of Internal Medicine*, **103**, 902–913.

CHAPTER 12

Outpatient Management of Anorexia Nervosa

W. Vandereycken[1]

University Psychiatric Center St Jozef, Kortenberg

ABSTRACT

The outpatient management of anorexia nervosa is described according to four levels of approach: identification, information, intervention, and intensive treatment. On the first level, emphasis is laid upon early detection and positive diagnosis of anorexia nervosa by focusing on behavioural and attitudinal features of the patient. In mild or benign cases confrontation and information may suffice to induce a rapid reversal of the symptoms. This second level includes (confronting or reassuring) medical clarification and general educational instruction in order to allow the parents to handle the problem themselves. A considerable number of patients, however, require more specific interventions—the third level of problem management. A concrete procedure involving the patient and the family in a directive, problem-specific and contractual approach is presented. Finally, several patients need an intensive and mostly multifaceted treatment programme. On this level, the limits of outpatient therapy must be seriously questioned.

INTRODUCTION

The guidelines in this chapter cannot be read as a detailed script for everyday clinical practice because of three forms of inevitable abstraction. First of all, it reflects the viewpoint of the author with his preference for a behavioural–interactional approach. Secondly, it is addressed to the average clinician and imagined reader whose skills and experience are unknown. Finally, the typical textbook case of anorexia nervosa is a rarity. In this respect, we will use, for

Behavioural Medicine
Edited by A. A. Kaptein, H. M. van der Ploeg, B. Garssen, P. J. G. Schreurs and R. Beunderman
© 1990 John Wiley & Sons Ltd.

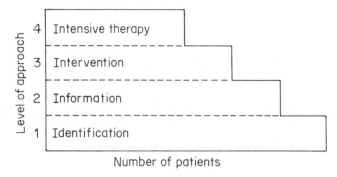

Figure 12.1. The four I or eye levels in problem management

practical reasons, the female pronouns when speaking about the anorexic patient, which does not imply that the approach would be essentially different for male patients (Vandereycken and Van den Broucke, 1984).

For didactic reasons, we have structured this chapter according to different levels of outpatient management. This is inspired by the model of Annon (1976) for the management of sexual dysfunctions, which may serve as an illustration of a rationale for the sequential utilization of various treatment approaches following a hierarchy of interventions—from simple patient education and advice to a complex intensive treatment strategy. In this conceptual scheme, one can move from an initial level of problem difficulty, where perhaps only reassurance is required, to a final level of difficulty where intensive, multimodal treatment is needed. Each level requires a different degree of therapist skill and competence. A close linkage between assessment and treatment is necessary in order to determine the (possibly changing) level of intervention needed. We translated this model into a scheme of four 'I' levels by which the clinician may choose to approach the problem (Figure 12.1). With each patient, the clinician has to start at the first level (problem identification or diagnosis) but whether or not he will engage in a higher level may depend on several factors, amongst which an important one relates to the clinician himself, especially if he is working in a private practice or in a setting with limited therapeutic possibilities or resources. Then he has to question his own position and whether he is the right person to treat this patient, recognizing the limits of his experience and/or his treatment potential. In general, when faced with an anorexia nervosa patient, the clinician is advised to seek outside consultation with a psychiatrist or psychologist before starting a comprehensive treatment plan (Loro, 1982). Management of eating disorders at the third and fourth level (specific interventions or intensive treatment) might be too difficult unless the clinician is specially trained in psychotherapeutic methods and has enough experience.

IDENTIFICATION

The issue of (differential) diagnosis is discussed elsewhere (Nussbaum *et al.*, 1985). Here we will only mention specific ideas about the diagnostic process in anorexia nervosa. The main aim of the identification phase is early detection, with emphasis upon positive diagnosis and special attention to psychosocial assessment. *Early detection* is certainly the first and crucial step in secondary prevention because it enables early intervention, which is generally associated with good outcome (Vandereycken and Meermann, 1984b). But recognition of (mild forms of) anorexia nervosa may be hampered by the patient, who usually conceals the problem, and/or by the family, who unwittingly collude with this until the disorder becomes severe. The patient's indifference toward physical symptoms of starvation can mislead clinicians, who are attuned to hearing complaints, into ignoring them (Casper, 1982). In fact, it is the contrast between the 'abnormal' physical appearance (emaciation and symptoms of starvation) and the attitude of 'normality' (reflected in professional, intellectual or athletic functioning) which must raise the suspicion of anorexia nervosa. All too often clinicians tend to proceed according to a 'negative' diagnostic process which is primarily aimed at excluding somatic causes. Pursued by the nagging fear drummed into him as a medical student of missing something, a stream of differential diagnoses will run through the clinician's mind. If he is not aware of the many physiological (metabolic and endocrinological) abnormalities that may be associated with malnutrition, he will be tempted to ask for more and more extended technical investigations which only reveal more confusing abnormalities linked with an endless list of differential diagnoses! Such a diagnostic procedure would not only result in a series of unnecessary investigations but above all in a delay before therapy could begin.

With some basic knowledge of the psychological peculiarities of anorexia nervosa it should not be that difficult to reach a *positive diagnosis* based on the behavioural characteristics of the syndrome (as emphasized in DSM-III). Instead of focusing on appetite or body weight, the clinician should pay attention to the patient's attitude towards eating and body shape, and he will find that she expresses a pursuit of thinness or a weight phobia. When this positive diagnosis has been made, a limited number of technical investigations are necessary to document the physiological status of the patient. Usually a laboratory check-up (red and white blood count, electrolytes, liver parameters, total protein) and an electrocardiogram will suffice. The clinician will then realize that the physiological abnormalities are signs of malnutrition and will usually return to the normal range with weight gain. Indeed, another pitfall is treating the physical sequelae of starvation instead of the starvation itself, for example prescribing sleeping medication for sleeplessness, laxatives for complaints of constipation, or hormones for amenorrhoea (Casper, 1982).

Finally, the clinician has to widen his medical diagnostic scope to a kind of *psychosocial assessment*. First of all, he will quickly learn that information from the patient's relatives (especially the parents) may reveal much more than X-rays and endocrinological tests. Furthermore, the family's perception of the problem may have important therapeutic implications. We already mentioned the patient's denial of illness (Vandereycken and Vanderlinden, 1983) as a crucial stumbling block. This implies that the attitude of the parents will influence the referral process. Especially in young adolescents, parental attitudes may serve as impediments to treatment (Andersen, 1985):

Denial or recognition failure. The parents fail to recognize the seriousness of their child's eating disorder, perhaps because they admire her self-mastery, physical appearance/performances or intellectual productivity; the child's problem then mirrors a collusion with one or both parents.

Uncertainty or confrontation failure. The parents do recognize the problem but assume a wait-and-see attitude because they fear that any intervention may only aggravate the problem or lead to disruptive family conflicts; often this attitude reflects the parents' lack of agreement on how to approach their child.

Impotence or intervention failure. These parents want to solve the problem on their own; although they fail to handle it (mainly because of lack of joint authority), seeking professional help is viewed as an admission of their inadequacy or is felt as threatening because it might reveal other intrafamilial problems they prefer to keep concealed.

In each of these cases, self-protection or protection of the family is the main motive for the delay in seeking professional help or for the refusal of (some types of) treatment.

In recent years, the burgeoning popular and scientific interest in anorexia nervosa risks promoting the fashionable aspect or special attractiveness of this 'modern' disease. This may lead to an overidentification both on the part of the family and the health care professionals. Both parties may be too easily alarmed when faced, for instance, with a child who sometimes refuses to eat. Anorexia nervosa means a lot more than periodic food refusal or a tendency to be slim. But, in general, the clinician more often encounters resistance on the part of the family. Besides those described above, it usually concerns parents who are alarmed by the weight loss or related signs of anorexia such as amenorrhea but who believe their child is the victim of a strange somatic illness. In fact, they are reluctant to face up to the psychological implications of anorexia nervosa. Here, the clinician has the advantage of being more easily accepted by the family as a medical specialist than, for instance, a psychiatrist. He has to be careful, however, not to reinforce the parents' conceptualization of the 'illness', for example by carrying out too many technical investigations before reaching a positive diagnosis as discussed earlier. The clinician must use instead his authority towards the parents in a confrontational approach we will now describe (see also Vandereycken, Kog and Vanderlinden, 1989).

INFORMATION

The physical examination of the patient is not merely a diagnostic observation procedure but the first step towards treatment if used as a means of confronting both the patient and the family with the seriousness and psychological nature of the disorder. The clinician should inform the patient of the physical dangers of starvation, vomiting or laxative/diuretic abuse. Usually, parents welcome this injection of reality and authority and experience considerable relief when the clinician decides to intervene and, in effect, take over responsibility for the identified patient (Stern *et al.*, 1981). Although it is essential to avoid a purely authoritarian role, the clinician must win and sustain the confidence of both the patient and the parents in order that collaboration rather than contention becomes the basis and keynote of treatment. The patient should not leave after the first appointment with a feeling she has encountered an adversary, but someone who could turn into an ally. Therefore, the anorexic must be persuaded that treatment will be aimed at increasing rather than diminishing her own autonomy (Welbourne and Purgold, 1984).

Changing the patient's denial and resistance (in fact, fear of 'imposed' change) into her being prepared to contemplate real change in herself is often a difficult task (Crisp, 1980). If the clinician tries to speak the anorexic's language, he may get in touch with the experiential world of the patient. 'The aim is to convert the patient from someone exercising extreme resistance and denial to someone who can acknowledge "the price she is paying" for her illness and move her from an egosyntonic position to that of a patient' (Kalucy, 1978, p. 200). The first thing to do then is to convince the patient and her family that they should participate in a treatment programme. In doing this it is important to emphasize the *benefits of treatment*, first of all for the patient herself. She can be told, for instance, that with treatment she can expect: (1) a decrease in the obsessive thoughts she has about food and body weight that interfere with her ability to concentrate on other matters; (2) a resumption of more normal eating patterns so that she will feel more comfortable socializing with peers; (3) a relief from insomnia and depressive symptoms or mood swings so that she will feel less irritable; and (4) a restoration of her previous activity level, especially if she now feels she no longer has the energy to be active (Halmi, 1983).

An alliance can be established by addressing the patient's emotional isolation and unhappiness and by emphasizing that treatment is aimed at helping her resume a normal life. The patient must experience the clinician's true concern for her future emotional and physical well-being for which a normal weight is a natural prerequisite (Casper, 1982). Moreover, it is only during weight restoration or after the patient has reached a normal body weight that she will reexperience the conflicts which led her to adopt an anorexic 'solution'. But the pitfall here is that the focus on weight gain may convey the message that the clinician is not interested in the person of the patient but only in her body weight and physiology. 'It is making a fundamentally "anorexic" mistake; it treats weight as a magical quality, allowing numbers on the dial to take over from reality. This is really the difficulty with all approaches to treatment which lay down rigid rules about weight gain' (Lawrence, 1984). One has to avoid the patient's body becoming the object of struggle and confrontation between herself and those who are trying to help her.

The *parents' support* is essential for the clinician and considerable time should be spent explaining the rationale and purpose of treatment in order to help ensure their continued cooperation. But in several cases, the parents must be first convinced of the seriousness of the disorder. The question of how to get the parents to comply with the diagnosis and/or the need for treatment will depend particularly on their conceptualization of the problem ('illness') and their attitude (fears, expectations) towards eventual treatment. Sometimes a direct confrontation with the severity of the condition must be deliberately exaggerated and dramatized as a kind of 'horror' technique in order to frighten seemingly unconcerned parents (e.g. by quoting statistics on the mortality of anorexia nervosa). In other cases of overanxious parents, the opposite must be done: clear factual information is given to reassure the parents or restore the confidence in their educational skills. The clinician must be aware that most parents are inclined to feel guilty about their child's problem although this might be concealed behind a series of defence mechanisms described above. All too easily, the clinician may be tempted to act as a 'superparent' who has to repair what the real parents have done wrong. Therefore, one has to avoid blaming directly or indirectly the parents for being the cause of the disorder (in anorexia nervosa the traditional scapegoat is the mother). A related mistake is to interpret each case of anorexia as a sign of family pathology. Causal hypotheses related to a so-called typical 'anorexogenic' family are still to be critically tested and, as yet, must be considered unproven generalizations (Kog and Vandereycken, 1985).

A final remark concerns *laymen literature and self-help organizations*. There is a vast amount of recent popular literature on anorexia nervosa and related eating disorders: vulgarized scientific, general guidance or self-help and (auto)biographical material (Vandereycken and Meermann, 1984a). This literature may be helpful both for patients and relatives to get a clearer picture of the disorder (e.g. its psychological nature associated with a complex disturbed physiology) and its treatment (e.g. the need for and the several forms of therapy). Reading such books may also have certain disadvantages: patients, for instance, may learn new tricks (e.g. vomiting) in order to enlarge their anorectic behaviour repertoire (Chiodo and Latimer, 1983); it may reinforce certain myths about anorexia (e.g. the 'disturbed' family); it risks inducing untoward effects through the appealing image of this fashionable disease. These risks also apply to self-help organizations, which, on the other hand, may provide an effective means of support, information and motivation for both patients and relatives. Many appear to be well informed in the advice and guidance they offer, not least because they draw on the experiences of the patients and those living with them. Self-help groups complement professional treatment by serving as a bridge for people who are discouraged by their therapy or who are not quite ready to step into treatment. Through supportive consciousness-raising experiences, these groups may help patients or parents become ready for or sustain the effort during treatment. Many organizations act as a 'go-between' in this respect and provide channels through which expert help can be sought.

INTERVENTION

We know little or nothing about the 'natural' course of anorexia nervosa in its various forms and degrees of severity. When faced with early or mild forms of eating disorder, the question arises whether or not they represent transient stages of distress which may disappear completely without any therapeutic intervention. This means that in some cases no treatment may be the prescription of choice (Frances and Clarkin, 1981). The clinician must question his 'indispensability' and be aware that the greater the rescue fantasies he has, the greater the risk of ill-considered therapeutic activism. It is a basic principle that the patient herself can be or has to become the main agent of change. Moreover, the patient can turn to significant persons in her social milieu in order to get support or help. This implies that the clinician, after the identification and information/confrontation process, may decide to give the patient the opportunity to reverse her problematic situation on her own. It is advisable then to schedule some follow-up appointments aimed at evaluating the patient's progress.

In a great number of patients, however, specific therapeutic interventions are wanted or urgently needed. We prefer a behaviourally oriented family approach including a consistent and lucid strategy that:

- Emphasizes the patient's responsibility for taking care of her own health;
- Provides the parents with something concrete to do at home and thus decreases their anxiety and helplessness in dealing with an anorectic child;
- Is aimed at avoiding self-defeating power struggles by neutralizing the problem of food refusal or threatening weight loss.

Such an approach is best characterized as 'a collaborative effort directed and catalyzed by the therapist and carried out by the patient and her family in their daily lives. The therapist needs to be actively engaged in the process of treatment, at times being patient and understanding and, at times, being challenging and insistent' (Sargent and Liebman, 1984). We will now describe briefly the outpatient strategy which, according to our clinical experience, has a very favourable cost/benefit ratio (Vandereycken and Meermann, 1984a).

No causal explanations are given with regard to the anorexic problems, following the axiom that we cannot change the past but can try to avoid repeating its unfruitful experiences. Two basic rules are explained: the family has to restore its normal living pattern and the patient has to restore her health. Weight restitution is the patient's own and primary responsibility, but her fear of losing control over eating and becoming overweight impede cooperation. Therefore, assurance must be given, time and again, that the therapist will take care that the patient's weight will be restored to a normal age-appropriate level, i.e. fluctuating within reasonable minimum and maximum limits. A contract is made regarding minimal weight gain required (depending on the patient's physical condition but usually a minimum of 500 g and a maximum of 3 kg a week, the latter limit in order to avoid overeating). If the patient does not meet this condition after a certain period (e.g. less than 1.5 kg after three weeks) some consequences will follow with an increasing degree of severity (e.g. limitation of physical activity, interdiction of working or studying, hospitalization). All these consequences are decided upon, in agreement with the parents, before treatment starts. The patient has to eat in a separate room at the usual dinner times, and she is free to eat what and how much she likes within this rule. However, she has access only to the same food the other family members are eating at the same time. Moreover, she is not allowed to eat in other rooms or at other times, to buy or hoard food, to interfere with cooking or with her mother's choice of menu. No family member is permitted to control her eating or to make comments about it; the same applies to her weight, which is only controlled by the therapist.

The rationale of this approach is twofold. (1) Anorexia nervosa patients have difficulty eating with others and the more they are controlled, the less they eat; even if the other family members do not make any comments on her eating behaviour while eating together, she will still feel non-verbal control on what is happening with her plate, therefore it is easier for her to start learning to eat normally again while alone. (2) The family has to learn to resume normal mealtimes as a social event; this means that they have to return to their usual eating habits with no special menu (low-calorie diet) for one member and without controlling each other's eating behaviour. Moreover, instead of talking about food or body shape, they have to resume normal dinner-table talk so that dining may again become a pleasant family meeting. The patient may rejoin the family during mealtimes once she can eat properly for her age (but the therapist must be careful about allowing this too soon).

It is the family's responsibility to see that these rules are respected and that eventual consequences of the contract will be carried out. We often explain here to the worried parents that, in order to prevent cardiovascular complications, it is far more important to be concerned about hyperactivity ('exhaustion of a weak body') than about the patient's eating behaviour. 'It is easier for you to achieve a decrease of her physical activity than an increase in her food intake.' In this way we are deflecting attention onto a symptom which is less disruptive for family interactions. In other words, we ask the parents to be concerned in a constructive way. It would be an impossible and perhaps even an unhealthy task for parents (though many clinicians appear to expect this from them) not to pay any attention whatsoever or to relinquish all concern. On the other hand, we ask the patient to report any interference of a family member with her eating or weight.

Such a restructuring of the interactional nature of non-eating within a family context may soon have a great impact, especially if the parents are following the rules. Therefore, in the beginning their cooperation is much more important than the patient's, who will usually test out the strictness of the contract by non-compliance or partial collaboration. If the parents do not comply, this can be used as a confrontation with the therapist's 'growing evidence that there must be something wrong in this family'. This might bring the parents closer to compliance or closer to the decision to hospitalize the patient. Indeed, although they seek help, some parents do not give up their own ineffective efforts to fatten the patient and they cannot admit having failed in this respect. Others sabotage the treatment or undermine the contract with the (unexpressed) intention or hope that the 'expert' himself will fail too! *Crisis induction* is a strategy aimed at bringing the parents to the point of admitting failure or impotence. The lunch session described by Minuchin, Rosman and Baker (1978) is partially directed toward the same purpose. The family is invited to have lunch with the therapist, who allows them to repeat their usual unsuccessful attempts to get the patient to eat. The therapist underlines their failure as strongly as possible and tries to get the parents to acknowledge that the patient has 'won' again. Our contract system may be used in a similar way. In a case where we feel that outpatient treatment is almost impossible for any chance of success, but the parents or the patients wish one last chance, we go along with their wish and design a time-limited (3–4 weeks) contract with strict rules as mentioned above. If they fail to reach the goal of a minimal weight gain within the prearranged timespan, we label it as too difficult a condition to be treated on an outpatient basis. Usually the parents are more likely then to accept hospitalization or even ask for it themselves. On the other hand, when the outpatient contract works, the changing family atmosphere and the patient's weight gain will reinforce the therapist's credibility to such an extent that he may shift the focus gradually from eating to interpersonal issues.

The further steps are usually centred around the particular attachment–autonomy problems in families with adolescent children. The aim is that the individual can achieve the next developmental step and that the family can allow this. We want to stress here that the so-called symptom-oriented approach we presented suffices in many cases to bring about by itself a considerable reestablishment of a 'normal' family functioning without engaging in specific family therapy. Whether the latter is really needed or not (or whether other interventions are needed, e.g. individual psychotherapy) will depend upon the functional analysis of the anorexic symptoms and related intra- and interpersonal functioning during treatment. Therapy, even when focused on symptomatic behaviour, is the best means for analysing a problem and testing hypotheses with regard to its aetiology and, in particular, its maintaining factors. This is another reason for our plea not to waste valuable time on complex diagnostic examinations, but rather to try out some therapeutic intervention as soon as possible. An early or final conclusion of this procedure can be that a more specialized, intensive approach to treatment is necessary.

INTENSIVE THERAPY

An undetermined number of anorexia nervosa patients need a specific and intensive long-term multimodal treatment to induce and maintain significant changes in their life pattern. In many cases, this implies that several professionals are involved at the same time in the therapy of the anorexic and/or her family. Most common is the intentional splitting of different therapeutic functions; for instance, the clinician takes care of the physical condition and the weight restoration, while a psychotherapist tries to get a grip on the patient's inner psychological and interactional experiences. Close contact must then exist among the therapists involved so that they are functioning as a unified team in order to avoid the danger of being played off against one another. The discussion on the content and form of specialized and mostly inpatient treatment of anorexic patients goes beyond the scope of this chapter (it is treated elsewhere in Powers, 1985). But what does concern the clinician is the decision for hospitalization.

With the exception of medical emergency indications, the decision to hospitalize an anorexia nervosa patient is usually based on a combination of criteria (Vandereycken, 1987):

1. *Medical criteria* which concern, in particular, a serious and potentially life-threatening deterioration of the patient's health:
   - severe acute or unremitting extreme weight loss (e.g. more than 30% below normal weight);
   - dangerous alterations in vital signs (postural hypotension, bradycardia, hypothermia) and electrolyte imbalance (hypokalaemia);
   - intercurrent infection in a cachectic patient;
   - suicidal tendencies or attempts, and psychotic reactions.
2. *Psychosocial criteria* referring to a seriously disturbed life situation that may be, at the same time, cause and consequence of the eating disorder and thus create a vicious circle in which the patient is imprisoned:
   - marked family disturbance inaccessible to treatment;
   - abnormal social isolation with avoidance of interpersonal contacts or inability to engage in study or work.
3. *Psychotherapeutic criteria*, especially in patients with a poorer prognosis (longer duration of illness, late onset of disease, occurrence of bulimia, vomiting or purging):
   - previous treatment failures, lack of motivation or even refusal to engage in outpatient therapy;
   - the need for an intensive psychotherapeutic milieu which can induce a change process that otherwise would take a long time to achieve.

The decision of hospitalization and its execution must be placed in a constructive therapeutic context instead of being the result of a power struggle the clinician feels he is losing. In the latter case, referral for hospitalization disguises the clinician's counteraggression and frustrating helplessness: he is only interested in 'winning' the battle by punishing the 'stubborn' patient (or family) while keeping his own peace of mind. Whilst admission to hospital might make the situation safe for a while, it may represent 'a counterproductive retreat from confrontation with certain life difficulties and signify confirmation of sick role in the eyes of relatives who then dissociate themselves from active participation in therapy (Morgan, Purgold and Welbourne, 1983, p. 286). As Liebman, Sargent and Silver (1983) rightly stress, it is necessary to prevent the family from using hospitalization to reinforce the patient's role as the symptom-bearer for the family, as well as to prevent the parents from perceiving the admission as further acknowledgement of their personal failure as parents.

When there is no doubt about the need for hospitalization, the question arises of where the patient should be admitted. Some prefer a medical setting because it is less threatening and avoids the stigma of a mental hospital (Hodas, Liebman and Collins, 1982). In our opinion (Vandereycken, 1987) this is only partially valid. First of all, the family's attitude must be taken into account. For example, if the parents conceive the eating disorder as a somatic illness, this idea may be reinforced by a hospitalization in a purely medical setting. Moreover, we believe the major aim of the clinician's work with anorexics and their family is to help them over whatever treatment barrier exists. It is not so much a question of medical *versus* psychiatric hospitalization but rather of whether a particular hospital unit has sufficient experience with the treatment of eating disorders.

CONCLUSION

When faced with an anorexia nervosa patient, the clinician plays an important role in the secondary prevention of the disorder. By making an early positive diagnosis, he avoids the still too frequent situation that patients are burdened by too many technical examinations and that valuable time is wasted before treatment begins. According to the degree of complexity of the disorder as well as to his own clinical experience and treatment potential, the clinician must choose the appropriate level of outpatient management. It is a leading principle that outpatient therapy should be tried unless emergency situations force the hospitalization of the patient or unless there are solid reasons for preferring inpatient management. The clinician is justified in attempting outpatient therapy on the condition that he regularly evaluates its costs and benefits both with respect to the patient and the family involved. The best guarantees for success are a constructive patient/family–therapist relationship and an explicit and consistent treatment plan based upon a multidimensional problem analysis.

NOTES

[1]Address for correspondence: W. Vandereycken, University Psychiatric Center St Jozef, B-3070 Kortenberg, Belgium.

REFERENCES

Andersen, A. E. (1985). *Practical Comprehensive Treatment of Anorexia Nervosa and Bulimia*. Baltimore: Johns Hopkins University Press.
Annon, J. (1976). *The Behavioral Treatment of Sexual Problems*. New York: Harper & Row.
Casper, R. C. (1982). Treatment principles in anorexia nervosa. In: Feinstein, S. C. (Ed.) *Adolescent Psychiatry*, Vol. X. Chicago: University of Chicago Press, pp. 431–454.
Chiodo, J. and Latimer, P. R. (1983). Vomiting as a learned weight-control technique in bulimia. *Journal of Behavior Therapy and Experimental Psychiatry*, **14**, 131–135.
Crisp, A. H. (1980). *Anorexia Nervosa—Let Me Be*. London, New York: Academic Press, Grune & Stratton.
Frances, A. and Clarkin, J. F. (1981). No treatment as the prescription of choice. *Archives of General Psychiatry*, **38**, 542–545.
Halmi, K. A. (1983). Treatment of anorexia nervosa: A discussion. *Journal of Adolescent Health Care*, **4**, 47–50.

Hodas, G., Liebman, R. and Collins, M. J. (1982). Pediatric hospitalization in the treatment of anorexia nervosa. In Harbin, H. T. (Ed.) *The Psychiatric Hospital and the Family*. Jamaica, NY: Spectrum, pp. 131–141.

Kalucy, R. S. (1978). An approach to the therapy of anorexia nervosa. *Journal of Adolescence*, **1**, 197–228.

Kog, E. and Vandereycken, W. (1985). Family characteristics of anorexia nervosa and bulimia: A review of the research literature. *Clinical Psychology Review*, **5**, 159–180.

Lawrence, M. (1984). *The Anorexic Experience*. London: The Women's Press.

Liebman, R., Sargent, J. and Silver, M. (1983). A family systems orientation to the treatment of anorexia nervosa. *Journal of the American Academy of Child Psychiatry*, **22**, 128–133.

Loro, A. D. (1982). Treatment for eating disorders. In: Boudewyns, P. A. and Keefe, F. J. (Eds) *Behavioral Medicine in General Medical Practice*. Menlo Park: Addison Wesley, pp. 217–236.

Minuchin, S., Rosman, B. and Baker, L. (1978). *Psychosomatic Families. Anorexia Nervosa in Context*. Cambridge: Harvard University Press.

Morgan, H. G., Purgold, J. and Welbourne, J. (1983). Management and outcome in anorexia nervosa. A standardized prognostic study. *British Journal of Psychiatry*, **143**, 282–287.

Nussbaum, M. P., Shenker, I. R., Shaw, H. and Frank, S. (1985). Differential diagnosis and pathogenesis of anorexia nervosa. *Pediatrician*, **12**, 110–117.

Powers, P. S. (1985). Inpatient treatment of anorexia nervosa. *Pediatrician*, **12**, 126–133.

Sargent, J. and Liebman, R. (1984). Outpatient treatment of anorexia nervosa. *Psychiatric Clinics of North America*, **7**, 235–245.

Stern, S., Whitaker, C. A., Hagemann, N. J., Anderson, R. B. and Bargman, G. J. (1981). Anorexia nervosa: The hospital's role in family treatment. *Family Process*, **20**, 395–408.

Vandereycken, W. (1987). The management of patients with anorexia nervosa and bulimia; Basic principles and general guidelines. In: Beumont, P. J. V., Burrows, R. C. and Casper, G. D. (Eds) *Handbook of Eating Disorders, Vol. I. Anorexia Nervosa and Bulimia*. Amsterdam: Elsevier/North Holland.

Vandereycken, W., Kog, E. and Vanderlinden, J. (1989). *The Family Approach to Eating Disorders*. New York: PMA Publications.

Vandereycken, W. and Meermann, R. (1984a). *Anorexia Nervosa. A Clinician's Guide to Treatment*. Berlin, New York: de Gruyter.

Vandereycken, W. and Meermann, R. (1984b). Anorexia nervosa: Is prevention possible? *International Journal of Psychiatry in Medicine*, **14**, 191–205.

Vandereycken, W. and Van den Broucke, S. (1984). Anorexia nervosa in males. *Acta Psychiatrica Scandinavica*, **70**, 447–454.

Vandereycken, W. and Vanderlinden, J. (1983). Denial of illness and the use of self-reporting measures in anorexia nervosa patients. *International Journal of Eating Disorders*, **2**, 101–107.

Welbourne, J. and Purgold, J. (1984). *The Eating Sickness: Anorexia, Bulimia, and the Myth of Suicide by Slimming*. Brighton: Harvester Press.

CHAPTER 13

Bulimia Nervosa

W. L. Weeda-Mannak[1]

Free University, Amsterdam

ABSTRACT

Bulimia nervosa has recently emerged as a condition of recurrent episodes of overeating, followed by vomiting, use of laxatives or diuretics, dieting or exercise. The syndrome predominantly occurs among females of adolescence and young adulthood with high needs for achievement. Diagnosis and management of bulimia nervosa is difficult, since multiple factors are involved in the onset and maintenance of the disorder. Attention is given to the medical complications of the eating and purging behaviour. The different diagnostic and therapeutic interventions are outlined and clinically illustrated.

INTRODUCTION

Bulimia nervosa refers to the condition of recurrent episodes of gross overeating (bulimia), followed by self-induced vomiting, use of laxatives or diuretics, intensive dieting or excessive exercise in order to control weight. Bulimic eating patterns were first identified by Stunkard (1959), who used the expression 'binge eating syndrome' to describe similar behaviour in a minority of obese patients. Over the past decade evidence has accumulated indicating that bulimia also occurs in subjects who are severely underweight and suffer from anorexia nervosa (Casper, 1983). The notion that bulimia may occur in individuals with normal body weight has contributed to the delineation of bulimia as a distinct disease entity. Until recently, considerable controversy existed concerning the diagnostic criteria for bulimia. To a large extent this debate has been resolved with the introduction of the DSM-III-R criteria (American Psychiatric Association, 1987) for bulimia nervosa. Identification of bulimia nervosa has been

Behavioural Medicine
Edited by A. A. Kaptein, H. M. van der Ploeg, B. Garssen, P. J. G. Schreurs and R. Beunderman

hampered by the lack of specific physical symptoms, while management has been complicated by the fact that eating disorders are multidetermined and require a multifaceted treatment. The historical development of bulimia towards the distinct syndrome 'bulimia nervosa' will be briefly summarized in this chapter. The biological, psychological and social factors contributing to the onset and maintenance of bulimia nervosa will be illustrated by presentation of a clinical report. The different diagnostic steps and therapeutic interventions involved in the management of a patient with bulimia nervosa will be described. Aspects of the multidisciplinary and multifaceted treatment will be outlined.

THE EMERGENCE OF BULIMIA NERVOSA AS A SYNDROME

Bulimia as a Symptom of Obesity

Bulimia literally means 'ox hunger', and refers to episodes of rapid consumption of large amounts of food in discrete periods of time. Stunkard (1959) identified this type of eating behaviour in a minority (5%) of obese patients. He noted that their eating behaviour alternated between periods of normal eating and periods of overeating. The pattern of overeating was observed to occur more frequently in times of emotional stress. Since Stunkard's report, a number of studies have appeared indicating that alternating periods of uncontrollable overeating and periods of normal food intake commonly occur in obese patients, exceeding the frequency of 5% mentioned by Stunkard (Edelman, 1981; Marcus and Wing, 1987). Bruch (1974) used the term 'thin fat people' to refer to the subgroup of obese patients who lost weight and displayed periods of overeating.

Bulimia as a Symptom of Anorexia Nervosa

Gull (1874), in his classic paper on anorexia nervosa, originally mentioned overeating as a symptom in a female patient with anorexia nervosa: 'occasionally for a day or two the appetite was voracious' (p. 22). Up to 1940 a few clinical reports described the occurrence of overeating in relation to cases of anorexia nervosa (Casper, 1983). The absence of systematically recorded signs of bulimia is surprising, as since 1980 several studies have accumulated indicating that a significant proportion of patients with anorexia nervosa suffer from bulimic eating episodes. Probably, the diagnostic term 'anorexia nervosa', implying that appetite is absent, may have led to neglecting the systematic observation of bulimic eating behaviour in anorectic patients. Of all case studies since 1940 that have appeared concerning overeating, Binswanger's (1944) study of Ellen West may be the most illustrative one. This patient, mistakenly diagnosed as a case of schizophrenia, gave a detailed account of her desperate struggle against 'the constant desire for food'. Since fasting and overeating could occur intermittently in the same individual, several authors considered bulimia and anorexia nervosa to be extreme poles of one continuum of disturbed eating behaviour instead of being two separate diagnostic entities. Diagnostic names such as 'hyperorexia', 'dysorexia' (Guiora, 1967) or 'bulimarexia' (Boskind-Lodahl, 1976) are illustrative examples of this latter point of view.

Bulimia as an Ominous Variant of Anorexia Nervosa

In 1979 Russell published a study of 30 patients whose symptoms could be characterized by: (a) the presence of intractable urges to overeat, followed by (b) various attempts to counter the fattening effect of food by inducing vomiting, abuse of laxatives or diuretics or by starvation, and (c) a morbid fear of becoming obese. These patients shared the morbid fear of fatness with patients suffering from anorexia nervosa, but contrary to anorectic patients, overeating, and not starvation, was found to be the most predominant symptom. Russell (1979) considered this condition to be an ominous variant of anorexia nervosa and named it 'bulimia nervosa'.

Bulimia as a Distinct Diagnostic Entity

Bulimia as a symptom may occur in individuals suffering from anorexia nervosa and obesity. However, accumulating empirical evidence has indicated that bulimia could also occur in individuals with a normal body weight (Wardle and Beinart, 1981). This evidence has significantly contributed to the differentiation of bulimia as a distinct clinical disorder separate from anorexia nervosa, as defined in the DSM-III (American Psychiatric Association, 1980). The presence of previous anorexia nervosa served as a criterion to exclude a present diagnosis of bulimia. Garner, Garfinkel and O'Shaughnessy (1985), in their study comparing bulimia patients of normal weight to anorexia nervosa patients with and without bulimia, have advocated abandoning previous weight as a criterion for the diagnosis of bulimia. Anorexia nervosa patients with bulimia were found to be more similar to bulimia patients with normal weight than to anorexia nervosa patients without bulimia. Hence, their data did not validate the diagnostic distinction of the DSM-III criteria (American Psychiatric Association, 1980) of anorexic *versus* normal weight bulimia patients. Recently, the controversy concerning the most appropriate set of diagnostic criteria for bulimia and bulimia nervosa has been resolved to a large extent with the introduction of the DSM-III-R criteria (American Psychiatric Association, 1987) for bulimia nervosa (Table 13.1).

Table 13.1. Diagnostic criteria for bulimia nervosa (DSM-III-R)

A. Recurrent episodes of binge eating (rapid consumption of a large amount of food in a discrete period of time)
B. A feeling of lack of control over eating behaviour during the eating binges
C. The person regularly engages in either self-induced vomiting, use of laxatives or diuretics, strict dieting or fasting, or vigorous exercise in order to prevent weight gain
D. A minimum average of two binge eating episodes a week for at least three months
E. Persistent overconcern with body shape and weight

THE CORE ELEMENTS OF BULIMIA NERVOSA

According to the DSM-III-R criteria the core symptoms of bulimia nervosa are: (a) a feeling of loss of control over eating with accompanied consumption of a large amount of food and (b) the use of various methods of weight control such as fasting, self-induced vomiting, the taking of laxatives and/or diuretics and excessive exercising. In contrast to the previous criteria for bulimia, the revised criteria emphasize the concern over weight and shape. Thus the revised criteria exclude those individuals whose eating behaviour is disturbed but who do not fear gaining weight. Fairburn (1987) has recently provided operational diagnostic criteria for bulimia nervosa based upon the DSM-III-R which can be applied for clinical and research purposes.

PREVALENCE OF BULIMIA NERVOSA

Epidemiological studies on the prevalence of bulimia nervosa have provided very diverse results. In a questionnaire survey at the State University of New York, Halmi, Falk and Schwartz (1981) found the highest prevalence rate for bulimia. No fewer than 35% of the female students considered themselves to be 'binge eaters'. When confined to the total student population, 13% of the male and female students could be classified as 'binge eaters'. Pyle et al. (1983) found a less high prevalence figure: 4.5% of the female freshman college students suffered from bulimia, whereas 1% compensated for the binge eating by inducing vomiting. A similar rate of 5% for bulimia associated with self-induced vomiting has been found by Johnson et al. (1984) in a population of high-school girls.

Bulimia nervosa predominantly occurs in female subjects. Halmi, Falk and Schwartz (1981) found that 87% of the bulimic individuals were female. Pyle et al. (1983) also found that bulimia nervosa occurs four times more frequently in females than in males. Recent results indicate that bulimic behaviour of clinical severity, satisfying the more restricted diagnostic criteria for bulimia nervosa, occurs in approximately 5% of females in adolescence and young adulthood (Freeman, Henderson and Henderson, 1988).

THE ONSET AND COURSE OF BULIMIA NERVOSA

The onset of bulimic eating behaviour usually follows a period of voluntary dieting and accompanying weight loss. The loss of weight may be related to various circumstances, such as unintended weight gain, an increased interest in the opposite sex, stressful life events such as loss of or separation from a significant person, confusion about sexual role or identity, and occupational or developmental stress.

Since the overeating is preceded by caloric restriction, several investigators have assumed that the restriction of food significantly contributes to the onset of eating binges. Herman and Polivy (1980) have proposed that restrained eating behaviour could easily dysregulate the intake of food. Pyle, Mitchell and Eckert (1981) have found that over 80% of their bulimic patients suffer from these intractable urges to overeat after a period of dieting and weight loss.

Empirical support for the postulation that caloric deprivation contributes to the onset of bulimia has also been found in the starvation study of Keys *et al.* (1950). They examined a group of males who volunteered to participate in a starvation experiment. Prior to participating, all subjects had been physically and mentally investigated and were considered to be 'healthy, both mentally and physically'. After a period of significant restriction of their food intake, the subjects suffered from intractable urges to overeat. These eating binges, absent prior to the starvation experiment, lasted long after the food intake had been restored. Bulimic anorexia nervosa patients have also indicated that their eating binges began after a considerable period of food restriction and weight loss (Garfinkel, Moldofsky and Garner, 1980). The onset of bulimic episodes followed a period of dieting and weight loss and has been related to the loss of a physiologically programmed body-weight level 'set point' (Keesey, 1980). Besides the physiological factors, Herman and Polivy (1980) have found that other factors such as anxiety, depression and the intake of alcohol also tend to augment overeating in dieting individuals.

The onset of bulimia appears to be correlated with the occurrence of a great number of potentially stressful events for bulimic anorexia nervosa patients (Strober, 1984) as well as for normal weight bulimia patients (Lacy, Coker and Birtchnell, 1986). However, a recent study of Shatford and Evans (1986) has indicated that environmental stressors such as life events and daily hassles are not directly related to bulimia. Their model of stress as a process indicated that coping skills were an important mediating variable. They showed that the coping strategies used by bulimic patients tended to be ineffective in handling stress. Consequently, the stress is more apt to result in the expression of bulimic or other disordered behaviour.

The frequency and severity of behaviours to counter the effect of binge eating has been found to be positively related to the duration of the bulimic eating disorder (Johnson and Larson, 1982).

One may conclude from these findings that early identification and intervention of bulimia nervosa may contribute to favourable prognosis. However, feelings of shame about their loss of control over eating behaviour commonly lead patients to delay presenting themselves for medical care. If they do seek medical care, they may do so because they are concerned about their physical well-being rather than because of their disturbed eating behaviour (Mitchell *et al.*, 1987). The onset and maintenance of bulimia nervosa is usually associated with serious psychological and physical morbidity. The medical complications related to bulimia nervosa will be discussed later in this chapter.

CLINICAL FEATURES

Body Weight

The majority of patients with bulimia nervosa have weighed within the normal range for their height, age and sex (10% below or above standard body weight for age and height). Often the reason for dieting is not actual, but perceived overweight. The percentage of bulimia nervosa patients with past unequivocal anorexia nervosa has been found to vary considerably over different studies, ranging from 14% (Pyle, Mitchell and Eckert, 1981) to more than 50% (Russell, 1979). It has been suggested that this variation may reflect sampling biases rather than the true incidence of anorexia nervosa in bulimia (Gandour, 1984).

Eating Behaviour

The frequency and duration of eating binges varies across samples. Rates of eating binges differ from two times a week to six times a day. The intensity of overeating is usually described in terms of energy intake, that is, the amount of calories ingested. The amount of calories ingested during a binge has ranged from 3500 calories up to 20,000 calories (Russell, 1979). During eating binges the person almost invariably resorts to food which she usually does not allow herself to eat because of the fattening effects. The food preferred may be ice cream, chocolate, bread, cookies, marmalade or puddings or so-called 'junk food'. The mean duration of an eating binge is approximately one hour. The food is rapidly consumed without tasting what is eaten. Bulimic patients prefer to be alone while overeating. Most eating binges occur later in the day after work or school, or late at night. In some cases overeating may also take place during the day.

The overeating frequently follows in a chain reaction fashion after ingestion of just a small amount of 'forbidden' food. Feeling she has already failed to conform to the prescribed standard, the individual reacts in the manner 'Since I just failed, I may as well completely fail'.

Negative interpersonal factors are the major triggers of bulimic episodes (Wilson and Smith, 1987). The binge eating itself or the vomiting brings temporary relief from the negative emotions. However, it also occurs that depressive moods and anxiety follow the overeating and sometimes lead to suicidal thoughts or acts (Abraham and Beumont, 1982). After having overeaten, the patient commonly promises herself that binge eating is never going to happen again, and she usually puts herself on a strict diet again.

Methods to Prevent Weight Gain

The DSM-III-R criteria (American Psychiatric Association, 1987) now require the presence of compensating behaviour for the diagnosis of bulimia nervosa by fasting, vomiting, use of laxatives and/or diuretics and excessive physical exercising. Self-induced vomiting is facilitated by the intake of fluids. Initial vomiting usually takes place after the consumption of a large meal, or by hearing from others that vomiting is a method employed to control weight.

Methods to induce vomiting include inserting fingers into the mouth and throat and inducing a gag reflex. Sometimes the handle of a toothbrush or spoon is used to induce vomiting. It also happens that a patient vomits by contracting her abdominal and thoracic muscles. The frequency of vomiting may vary from twice a week to 15 times a day.

The taking of laxatives and diuretics is also aimed at preventing the consequences of overeating. The quantities of laxatives ingested range from 10 pills to hundreds a day. Such large quantities usually grow steadily. Patients with bulimia nervosa may also engage in excessive exercises, use of amphetamine tablets and diuretics to prevent weight gain.

Recent studies have indicated that the omission of insulin is used to induce glycosuria in female patients with insulin-dependent diabetes mellitus. This method is a novel and life-threatening way of preventing weight gain after overeating (Hudson, Wentworth and Hudson, 1983).

Medical Complications

Several medical complications have been reported to occur in connection with bulimia nervosa (Mitchell *et al.*, 1987). Directly related to the gross overeating is abdominal fullness and abdominal pain; more serious consequences, for instance gastric dilatation or gastric rupture, have also been reported (Mitchell, Pyle and Miner, 1982). The combination of overeating and starvation may result in menstrual irregularities or in some cases the cessation of menstruation. A significant proportion of all patients have reported at least one episode of amenorrhoea (Gandour, 1984). The onset of amenorrhoea was related to emaciation, although the weight loss may not be severe. Other physical consequences frequently reported are swelling of the parotid or salivary glands, sore throats,

Table 13.2. Medical complications associated with bulimia nervosa

Binge eating/restriction	Vomiting	Purging
Gastric dilatation	Electrolyte	Dehydration
Gastric rupture	disturbances	
Menstrual disorders	Hypokalaemia	
Salivary gland enlargement	leading to:	
	renal failure	
	heart failure	
	tetania	
	epileptic seizures	
	lethargy	
	Sore throat	
	Dental disorders	

calluses over the dorsum of the hand caused by using the hand to stimulate the gag reflex mechanically, and dental problems (Russell, 1979; Abraham and Beumont, 1982; Mitchell *et al.*, 1987).

Vomiting and purging leads to loss of fluids and electrolyte disturbances (Mitchell *et al.*, 1987). For example, the loss of potassium, leading to hypokalaemia may result in severe somatic complications. Omission of insulin, to prevent weight gain after overeating in patients with insulin-dependent diabetes mellitus, commonly results in poor metabolic control (Hudson, Wentworth and Hudson, 1983; Rodin, Johnson and Garfinkel, 1986) and an early onset of diabetic complications (Steel *et al.*, 1987). Table 13.2 presents the medical complications associated with the disturbed eating patterns of bulimia nervosa patients.

Psychological Characteristics of Patients with Bulimia Nervosa

The search for characterizing psychological features in bulimia nervosa has been hampered by methodological weaknesses; pre-illness personality features have been mostly assessed after the onset of illness. Most psychological variables have not been operationally defined; instruments have been poorly validated. Most studies lack the comparison with appropriate control groups. According to the results of recent studies, one may conclude that the bulimic personality is that of an individual with a high need for achievement and recognition, but whose anxiety and lack of impulse control will make achievement of her goals particularly difficult (Dunn and Ondercin, 1981; Weeda-Mannak *et al.*, 1983; Weeda-Mannak and Drop, 1985).

The most important and distressing psychological consequence of caloric deprivation is the mental preoccupation with food. Depressive moods have frequently been found in patients with bulimia nervosa. The relationship between bulimia and depression, however, still remains unclear. In most cases depression has been considered to be a consequence of the disturbed eating behaviour.

DIAGNOSIS AND MANAGEMENT OF BULIMIA NERVOSA

Bulimia nervosa can be associated with serious psychological and physical morbidity. Hence diagnostic and therapeutic measures from somatic and behavioural disciplines should be interrelated and integrated.

The initial consultation serves a vital function in a treatment programme. It presents the clinician with difficult tasks (Johnson, 1985): (a) to obtain sufficient information to make a diagnosis and (b) treatment recommendations and (c) to establish a trusting relationship with the patient.

In order to facilitate the development of a trusting relationship, it is crucial to be frank and open from the start. This involves the clinician being open about the diagnosis and the treatment programme, as well as the therapeutic procedures.

The Establishment of a Trusting Relationship

Many patients with bulimia nervosa are reluctant to discuss their symptoms with their physicians (Mitchell *et al.*, 1987). If they seek medical treatment they usually do so because of concern about their physical health. Binge-eating and self-induced vomiting are surrounded with feelings of guilt and secrecy (Fairburn and Cooper, 1982). Such feelings of shame and embarrassment may interfere with the establishment of a trusting relationship.

Frequently reported characteristics of patients with bulimia nervosa are a high need for approval and control (Dunn and Ondercin, 1981), a strong drive to achieve (Russell, 1979), less impulse control (Johnson and Larson, 1982; Dunn and Ondercin, 1981), anxiety and depression.

The strong need for control may also contribute importantly to the difficulty of the formation of a working alliance. For a bulimic patient, seeking treatment usually implies admitting that she has a problem for which she has failed to find a solution. Treatment means that she has given away the control and responsibility for her own life. As a consequence of this she may be totally disappointed if therapeutic interventions do not produce immediate relief of her symptoms (Herzog and Copeland, 1985). She may feel then that the therapist is not worth trusting. Since the therapeutic relationship with patients suffering from bulimia nervosa should be characterized by trust and support, it inevitably requires from the therapist the ability to cope with feelings of intense emotions and frustration (Cohler, 1977). A warm, caring, although distant ('fact-finding') relationship has been advocated (Bruch, 1978). A fact-finding type of therapeutic relationship may be facilitated by providing objective information to the patient in order to obtain subjective data. Examples of appropriate questions are: 'We know from recent studies that . . . (this) . . . may occur' or, 'Other patients have reported suffering from . . . have you had similar experiences?'.

The Initial Interview

Several arguments have been advanced to conduct a structured, instead of an unstructured interview with patients suffering from bulimia nervosa. Johnson (1985) has stated that one of the most important advantages of a structured interview is that it allows the clinician to demonstrate his awareness of some of the characterizing aspects of eating disorders.

The interview begins with a question concerning the specific reason(s) that the patient is seeking treatment. The purpose of this inquiry is to obtain information on how long she has been suffering from her problems, what her expectations are and whether she is seeking medical care voluntarily or has been forced by friends, family or other relatives.

It is important to inquire whether she has ever talked with anyone about her eating difficulties, and who is informed about her seeking treatment.

At the end of the interview, when talking about treatment recommendations, these topics should be brought under discussion again.

During the interview the following topics should be investigated:

1. History of weight and the relationship with menstruation and events. Questions are posed about the patient's highest and lowest weights (starting with the onset of puberty), the course of her weight and significant weight fluctuations. Weight fluctuations must be investigated within the context of menstrual irregularity and important life changes. Patients should be informed about the importance of obtaining information on these issues. By informing her about the possible relationship between changes in weight and menstruation as well as situational stress the patient is encouraged to think about her symptoms in a more rational way. She may discover behaviour patterns as a way to adapt to situational changes and events.

   It is important to detect when bulimia occurred for the first time and to inquire about the particular reason for weight loss. Did she start dieting after an unexpected weight gain, after a critical remark concerning her appearance, after specific life events or after a change in her lifestyle or living conditions? Or has the initial weight loss been due to a specific illness?

   If the patient had lost weight due to voluntary dieting, at what weight did she feel 'alright'? Does she consider a professional career to be the reason for her striving to be thin?

2. Eating habits and eating behaviour. What is the frequency of her eating binges? How does she compensate for her eating binges? By fasting, self-induced vomiting, using laxatives and/or diuretics, excessive exercising? What kind of food is consumed during an eating binge? At what times does she binge? At the end of a day? After she feels that she has eaten something she should avoid? When she feels tense, anxious, disappointed or lonely? What does she do to prevent herself from bingeing? Does she only vomit after a binge, or after each ingestion of forbidden food? What other methods does she use to prevent weight gain?

   Does she know that food restriction increases the risk of binge-eating? Does she know that vomiting may maintain the overeating? Is she aware of the risks of vomiting and the use of laxatives and/or diuretics?

3. Menstrual history and sexual history. As menstrual irregularities commonly occur in women with bulimia nervosa, it is important to inquire about the presence of regular menses. At what time did the menarche occur? Have her cycles been regular since then? Has she suffered from (periods of) amenorrhea? Is she using or has she ever used oral contraceptives?

   Clinical findings suggest that eating disorders occur more frequently in women with premenstrual syndromes (Gladis and Walsh, 1987); therefore it is important to obtain information about whether the eating problems vary according to the menstrual cycle.

   Bulimic women, in contrast to patients with other eating disorders like anorexia nervosa, usually report a full range of sexual interest and behaviour up to frank promiscuity (Johnson, 1985).

4. Life adjustment. The purpose of this topic is to assess the quality of daily life of the patient. What kind of study or occupation is she engaged in? Does the eating disorder affect her daily occupational or study activities? Does she

have interpersonal and/or sexual relationships? How does she perceive the quality of these relationships? Does the eating disorder interfere with her interpersonal and sexual life? What are the possible effects of her symptoms? Has she told anybody about her eating problem? Does she hide her symptoms from her social environment?

Diagnostic Conclusion and Treatment Recommendations

The patient should be informed about the preliminary conclusions, which are based upon the data obtained from the interview. Information concerning the vicious cycle of binge eating and fasting must be provided. It allows the clinician to ask the patient whether she is willing to break this cycle by stopping compensating for her eating behaviour and to accept the probable consequence of weight gain.

It is also important to question the patient about her expectations of treatment: for example, does she expect an immediate relief of her symptoms, does she expect a sudden, positive change in her life? It is necessary to provide her with information about the facts and common experiences during treatment. Social support is important during and after treatment (Schwartz, Barrett and Saba, 1985); it is therefore important to encourage the patient to think about relatives, friends or others with whom she prefers to talk about her eating problem and to provide a safe context for experiencing new behaviours.

Physical Examination

Knowledge concerning the medical consequences of bulimia nervosa has accumulated in recent years. Mitchell *et al.* (1985) have examined 275 bulimic patients. Systematic questioning of these patients revealed that weakness, abdominal fullness and swelling of the parotid or salivary gland were commonly reported. However, for a clinician who is not familiar with the treatment of patients with eating disorders, there are only few, if any, observable signs of bulimia nervosa, such as skin changes or lesions over the dorsum of the hand, enlargement of parotid or salivary glands and dental enamel erosion (Herzog and Copeland, 1985). An overview of other physical signs indicative for bulimia nervosa has been given in Table 13.1. Physical examination should also include assessment of height and weight.

Laboratory Testing

The methods used to prevent weight gain—vomiting, excessive exercise, abuse of laxatives and diuretics—may all result in loss of sodium and potassium (Mitchell *et al.*, 1987). Electrolyte disturbances must be excluded by laboratory testing as a matter of routine. In cases of amenorrhoea endocrine testing may be indicated. In bulimic patients with insulin-dependent diabetes mellitus parameters of glycaemic control must be assessed.

Additional Information

Towards the end of the first interview all patients are informed about the rationale for monitoring their eating behaviour and are instructed how to monitor their behaviour. Monitoring sheets are then provided. Despite some variation in the sheets that are used, the purpose of self-monitoring invariably is to ascertain under which circumstances eating takes place and under which circumtances eating problems arise. The patient is taught to keep the time units of recording as short as possible. Since the eating behaviour is linked to feelings of shame it is important to emphasize that the patient will not be evaluated in terms of 'good or bad', but that factual acknowledgement of the eating problem is one step towards solving the problem and regaining control.

Other additional information on past physical appearance and/or weight can be obtained by requesting the patient to bring some photographs of herself from the time prior to, after and during the course of her dieting.

BEHAVIOURAL MODELS IN THE TREATMENT OF BULIMIA NERVOSA

Four behavioural models have been applied in the treatment of bulimia nervosa: (1) the eating-habit control model; (2) the anxiety-reducing model; (3) the cognitive behavioural model; and (4) the interpersonal stress model. The treatment procedures described in this chapter include elements of these therapeutic approaches.

1. The eating-habit control model has been described by Johnson and Brief (1983). The disturbed eating pattern of patients with bulimia nervosa results from the patient's attempt to lose weight by an unrealistic diet. When she fails to keep her unrealistic, strict dietary rules, she may rebound and binge. She then tries to compensate subsequently by intensifying her diet. Once confronted with her inability to escape from this cycle, she may resort to vomiting or the use of laxatives, which in turn starts a new vicious circle.

   According to the eating-habit control model, the bulimic patient is treated by helping her to resist the eating binges using behavioural methods and to set realistic goals for her weight and weight control by providing information.
2. The anxiety reduction model has been developed and applied by Leitenberg *et al.* (1984). They have proposed the view that in order to gain control over the bulimic disorder, the problem must be attacked from the vomiting rather than from the overeating side. Since the fear of gaining weight after overeating is temporarily reduced by vomiting, the vomiting or purging in bulimia nervosa has an anxiety-reducing function. In cases where vomiting was prevented, bulimic patients did not binge.

   Hence they postulated the following. Since the vomiting has been established as an escape response, vomiting maintains the bingeing rather than bingeing inducing the vomiting. In fact, vomiting is so effective in relieving negative feelings that it may not be necessary for a bulimic person to resist her urges to overeat. Vomiting rather than binge-eating becomes the 'primary mechanism for tension regulation'.

Johnson and Brief (1983) have also found that binge-eating becomes more severe as vomiting occurs and that in the presence of vomiting binge-eating increases in frequency. In accord with their theoretical model, Rosen and Leitenberg (1985) have advocated a treatment model of exposure to the feared food and prevention of the habitual escape (vomiting) for patients with bulimia nervosa. In line with behavioural treatments of other anxiety-based disorders, they found that repeated exposure to feared stimuli (eating without vomiting) leads to both decreased anxiety while eating as well as an increased ability to eat normal amounts of food (Leitenberg *et al.*, 1984).

3. The cognitive behavioural model has been developed and described by Fairburn (1985). Fairburn assumes that the binge-eating results partly from faulty beliefs about weight and shape and partly from inadequate coping behaviour. He distinguishes three stages of cognitive behavioural intervention.

   The purpose of stage 1 is to disrupt the habitual binge-eating, vomiting and laxative abuse. Specific advice, such as the prescription of a regular eating pattern, provision of information about the physical consequences of binge-eating, vomiting and laxative abuse, the 'effectiveness' of compensative methods as well as the importance of regular weighing, is given. Once the bingeing is on an intermittent basis, attention is then directed to factors maintaining the overeating and to the modification of eating behaviour.

   Stage 2 is aimed at the identification of the circumstances that tend to result in binge-eating and of helping the patient to develop more effective coping strategies. Treatment is also cognitively oriented: thoughts, beliefs and assumptions that perpetuate the eating behaviour are identified and modified.

   Stage 3, the final stage, is aimed at maintaining the behavioural change and the prevention of relapse.

4. According to the interpersonal stress model (Abraham and Beaumont, 1982) binge-eating is triggered by stressful events. Negative feelings of deprivation, depression, anxiety, anger and interpersonal problems involving loss and rejection trigger the urge to binge. The overeating temporarily reduces the stress in the absence of alternative coping strategies. From this perspective binge-eating has the function of regulating negative emotions. According to this model, the bulimic patient is helped in resisting her eating binges in times of stress and in developing other stress-reducing behaviours.

The treatment of bulimia nervosa requires an examination of the 'function' of overeating and vomiting. The treatment procedures have to be in line with this functional analysis of the eating and purging behaviour. Usually the treatment programme consists of diverse behaviour modification strategies: the self-monitoring of eating and purging behaviour, the provision of information on consequences of these behaviours, modification of faulty beliefs and thoughts, exposure to feared stimuli (eating without vomiting), and, in addition, training in adequate coping behaviour. These behavioural interventions can be conducted on an outpatient basis. Only in cases of significant risk of suicide or the presence of a life-threatening situation (severe electrolyte disturbances, or the excessive use of laxatives and diuretics) will hospitalization be indicated. To illustrate the multifaceted aspects of a multidisciplinary treatment programme, a patient with bulimia nervosa is represented and therapeutic interventions are outlined.

MULTIFACETED THERAPY: A CASE DESCRIPTION

The patient, B, is a 15-year-old girl suffering from bulimia nervosa.

She was treated earlier in three therapeutic settings: two treatment programmes were on the inpatient basis and one on an outpatient basis.

The first time the patient was hospitalized in a centre with much experience in the treatment of eating disorders. She was dismissed after six weeks when she was free of her symptoms. After returning home her bulimic symptoms had started again, precipitated by the stressful event of loss of her only friend. She was hospitalized again in another hospital familiar with the treatment of patients with eating disorders and dismissed after she was considered 'recovered'. She was then referred to a family therapist for follow-up treatment. Because of the lack of progress, which was probably related to the therapist's unfamiliarity with the treatment of eating disorders, the patient was then referred to our hospital.

Weight and the Relationship with Menstruation and Events

The patient's height was 1.65 m, her highest weight 51 kg and her lowest weight 42 kg. She began to lose weight two years ago, as a result of her wish to live a life of asceticism. She therefore began to discipline herself with respect to her eating behaviour, but also with respect to her intellectual and physical activity. She always tried to exceed her limits.

At the first interview in the hospital, she reported that she was feeling completely 'out of control'. Her menses had ceased early in the course of initial weight loss. Her actual weight was 44 kg.

Eating Habits and Eating Behaviour

Her first binge occurred after the family moved to Holland. Frightened to gain weight, patient B began to vomit and to use laxatives after bingeing. The eating binges usually occurred at home, at the end of the day, when she returned from school. The frequency of these eating binges ranged from four to seven times a day and were followed by self-induced vomiting.

Having conflicts with her mother from an early childhood made her dependent on others (outside the home) to provide her with the respect, attention and love she needed. As a result of the move to Holland she was confined to her family and therefore having to repress her feelings of anger and misunderstanding. Unable to find the support from friends she had had previously, she became tense, insecure and isolated. On making a new friend who provided her with attention and respect, her negative emotions were relieved. When her new friend moved to another country, her feelings of loneliness and the fear of rejection again were triggered once more.

She used to be a bright student, excelling in intellectual, music and sporting activities, which gave her the social involvement she wanted. Now she felt socially isolated, especially during the lunch-hour at school, the opportunity for all students to meet their friends.

When her friend left school, patient B avoided the social contacts with other students during lunchtime. Withdrawing, she then began to binge and vomit. Afraid of these moments that triggered her bingeing and of not resisting the urge to binge, B began to miss school. When she stayed home her mother blamed her for not being strong and avoiding her problems at school. B's eating binges and vomiting increased. At the time of the interview at admission she was bingeing and vomiting several times during the day.

Menstrual and Sexual History

Menarche occurred when she was 12 years old. She always had irregular menses. Her weight was always relatively low and she was engaged in intensive sporting activities. During initial weight loss, she ceased to have menstrual cycles. She had had no sexual experiences and was not interested in boys or dating.

Life Adjustment

Life for the family had significantly changed after the move to Holland: they had lost a safe social and material world. In addition, for B the move abroad implied she had lost her way of dealing with the conflicts at home.

Performances and achievements were very important to gain social acceptance from the environment she used to live in. The familiar ways she employed to gain social approval were no longer effective in Holland. Her excellent performances in sport could not be demonstrated, as the teams had already been selected for the trimester. Intellectual performance was considered of less importance than wearing the right clothes and shoes. Wearing the right outfit was not possible due to the sudden unfavourable change in financial conditions. Her bingeing and vomiting behaviour were ineffective ways of coping with her situation and prevented her from getting into social interaction with her peers. Hence her fear of rejection increased. Unable to break this vicious circle, she had begun to avoid school, which in turn had led to an increase in the bingeing and vomiting.

Diagnostic Conclusions and Treatment Recommendations

The diagnosis of bulimia nervosa was confirmed. Both the patient and her parents were informed of the consequences of dieting, especially the loss of a physiologically regulated body weight ('set point') which resulted in an increased risk of binge-eating. Other precipitating factors of bulimia, such as negative emotions and interpersonal stress, were also emphasized. Information about the medical consequences of bulimia nervosa was provided and the patient as well as her parents was advised to see the internist.

They were advised to inform the headmaster of the school about the problems and that she had sought treatment. The patient was also asked if she was willing to break the vicious circle of bingeing and vomiting by (a) attending school again, (b) following the prescription of regular meals, (c) preventing vomiting and accepting a possible weight gain. No other homework assignment was given other than to monitor her eating behaviour as well as the circumstances to which the eating had been linked.

Additional Information from Laboratory Testing

The consultation with the internist, especially the laboratory testing of blood samples, revealed the presence of hypokalaemia. The self-monitoring indicated that bulimia was related to conflicts in the family as well as to feelings of anger, loneliness and rejection. For this reason recommendations for individual treatment of the patient as well as family therapy for the parents and the children were made.

DISCUSSION OF CASE REPORT: OUTLINE OF A MULTIFACETED TREATMENT OF BULIMIA NERVOSA

The treatment programme for this patient was based upon the functional analysis of her eating behaviour and consisted of the following components:

1. Establishment of a working therapeutic relationship.
2. Provision of information and education.
3. Breaking the vicious circle of isolation–overeating–vomiting–isolation.
4. Developing interpersonal and problem-solving skills with the patient and the family. This includes arranging adjuvant family therapy.

The Establishment of a Working Therapeutic Relationship

It was made clear to the patient and her parents that the therapist had a working relationship with the patient and that the contacts between the therapist and the parents were only aimed at creating an understanding, supportive social environment (for instance by providing information about treatment plans). They were also informed about the role of family conflicts that precipitated and perpetuated the bulimic behaviour. For this reason adjuvant family therapy was recommended and arranged.

Provision of Information and Education

The patient was provided with information on the effect of food restriction, the physical consequences of binge-eating, self-induced vomiting and/or laxatives, the 'effect' of vomiting as a perpetuating factor of bingeing, and the importance of having a regular schedule for eating and attending school.

Breaking the Vicious Circle

To break the vicious circle of overeating and vomiting, a regular eating pattern was prescribed. The patient was advised to rejoin the family or the peer group while eating. In order to break the circle of social isolation–overeating–vomiting–social isolation, B was encouraged to find alternative ways of coping with interpersonal stress. Faulty cognitions and beliefs such as 'I do not satisfy their standards' were identified and modified into alternative ways of thinking—'I may not wear the same sweater, but it does not imply that my self-esteem should be less'. B was also encouraged to find alternative ways to contact her peers than during lunchtime, such as joining the sports team to watch the matches or accompanying a person or group she liked to a concert or movie.

Developing Interpersonal and Problem-solving Skills

The patient was instructed to use the social skills she had already developed in her previous social surroundings, such as expressing positive emotions to other people. She was also informed that the acquisition of new (cultural-bound) social skills might be necessary to develop new interpersonal contacts. Acquisition of these skills could take place during individual therapy sessions by using behaviour modification methods.

In order to resolve family conflicts, the family was referred to a family therapist.

THE EFFECTIVENESS OF PSYCHOLOGICAL INTERVENTION IN BULIMIA NERVOSA

Data on the outcome of bulimia nervosa are scarce. The lack of empirical evidence to determine the long-term efficacy of short-term treatment is related to the relatively recent identification of the syndrome. Herzog, Keller and Lavori (1988) recently reviewed the results of seven studies on the outcome of bulimia nervosa. Twenty-nine to 87% of the subjects continued their bulimic eating behaviour at least occasionally at follow-up; only 33% of the patients were found to be abstaining from binge-eating after one year (Mitchell et al., 1985). Vomiting behaviour was found to occur at least occasionally in 28–77% of the patients, while 33% of the subjects were still abusing laxatives at follow-up. The efficacy of multimodal treatment of bulimia nervosa was found to be related to the presence or absence of affective disorders.

CONCLUSIONS AND RECOMMENDATIONS

Bulimia nervosa, like other eating disorders, is a multidetermined disorder requiring a multifaceted treatment programme. The treatment of patients with bulimia nervosa entails several delicate and difficult tasks for the clinician. Among these are (a) the need to develop a trusting relationship; (b) the need to cope with vulnerable elements of this relationship like the patient's disappointment if therapeutic interventions do not produce immediate relief; (c) the necessity of dealing with disturbed eating behaviour and the possible resulting medical complications; and (d) the need to be open about these matters without using them as a method to press the patient towards therapeutic change.

The clinician will be able to perform such tasks if he is aware of and has an understanding of the most crucial aspects of eating disorders.

NOTES

[1]Address for correspondence: W. L. Weeda-Mannak, Division of Reproductive Endocrinology and Fertility, Free University Hospital, 1007 MB Amsterdam, The Netherlands.
The author acknowledges the support of A. J. M. Donker.

REFERENCES

Abraham, S. F. and Beumont, P. J. (1982). How patients describe bulimia or binge eating. *Psychological Medicine*, **12**, 625–635.

American Psychiatric Association (1980). *Diagnostic and Statistical Manual of Mental Disorders*, 3rd edn. Washington, DC: APA.

American Psychiatric Association (1987). *Diagnostic and Statistical Manual of Mental Disorders*, 3rd revised edn. Washington, DC: APA.

Binswanger, L. (1944). Der Fall Ellen West. *Schweizerisches Archiv für Neurologie und Psychiatrie*, **53**, 255–277.

Boskind-Lodahl, M. (1976). Cinderella's stepsisters: A feminist perspective on anorexia nervosa and bulimia. *Journal of Women in Culture and Society*, **2**, 342–356.

Bruch, H. (1974). *Eating Disorders*. London: Routledge & Kegan Paul.

Bruch, H. (1978). *The Golden Cage: The Enigma of Anorexia Nervosa*. Cambridge, MA: Harvard University Press.

Casper, R. C. (1983). On the emergence of bulimia nervosa as a syndrome: A historical view. *International Journal of Eating Disorders*, **2**, 3–16.

Cohler, B. (1977). The significance of the therapist's feelings in the treatment of anorexia nervosa. In: Feinstein, S. C. and Giovacchini, P. L. (Eds) *Adolescent Psychiatry*. New York: Aronson, pp. 352–384.

Dunn, P. K. and Ondercin, P. (1981). Personality variables related to compulsive eating in college women. *Journal of Clinical Psychology*, **37**, 43–49.

Edelman, B. (1981). Binge eating in normal weight and overweight individuals. *Psychological Reports*, **49**, 739–746.

Fairburn, C. G. (1985). Cognitive-behavioural treatment. In: Garner, D. M. and Garfinkel, P. E. (Eds) *Handbook of Psychotherapy for Anorexia Nervosa and Bulimia*. New York: Guilford Press, pp. 160–191.

Fairburn, C. F. (1987). The definition of bulimia nervosa: Guidelines for clinicians and research workers. *Annals of Behavioral Medicine*, **9**, 3–7.

Fairburn, C. G. and Cooper, P. J. (1982). Self-induced vomiting and bulimia nervosa: An undetected problem. *British Medical Journal*, **284**, 1153–1155.

Freeman, C. P., Henderson, M. and Henderson, A. (1988). Incidence and prevalence of bulimia nervosa. Paper presented at the Third International Conference on Eating Disorders, April 22–24, New York (Abstract).

Gandour, M. J. (1984). Bulimia: Clinical description, assessment, etiology, and treatment. *International Journal of Eating Disorders*, **3**, 3–38.

Garfinkel, P. E., Moldofsky, H. and Garner, D. M. (1980). The heterogeneity of anorexia nervosa: Bulimia as a distinct subgroup. *Archives of General Psychiatry*, **37**, 1036–1040.

Garner, D. M., Garfinkel, P. E. and O'Shaughnessy, M. (1985). The validity of distinction between bulimia with and without anorexia nervosa. *American Journal of Psychiatry*, **142**, 581–587.

Gladis, M. M. and Walsh, B. T. (1987). Premenstrual exacerbation of binge eating in bulimia. *American Journal of Psychiatry*, **144**, 1592–1595.

Guiora, A. Z. (1967). Dysorexia: A psychopathological study of anorexia nervosa and bulimia. *American Journal of Psychiatry*, **124**, 391–393.

Gull, W. W. (1874). Apepsia hysterica: Anorexia nervosa. *Transcripts of the Clinical Society of London*, **7**, 22–28.

Halmi, K. A., Falk, J. R. and Schwartz, E. (1981). Binge-eating and vomiting: A survey of a college population. *Psychological Medicine*, **11**, 697–706.

Herman, C. B. and Polivy, J. (1980). Restrained eating. In: Stunkard, A. J. (Ed.) *Obesity*. Philadelphia: W. B. Saunders, pp. 208–225.

Herzog, D. B. and Copeland, P. M. (1985). Eating disorders. *New England Journal of Medicine*, **313**, 295–303.

Herzog, D. B., Keller, M. B. and Lavori, P. W. (1988). Outcome in anorexia nervosa and bulimia nervosa. *Journal of Nervous and Mental Disease*, **176**, 131–143.

Hudson, M. S., Wentworth, S. M. and Hudson, J. I. (1983). Bulimia and diabetes (Letter). *New England Journal of Medicine*, **309**, 431–432.

Johnson, C. (1985). Initial consultation for patients with bulimia and anorexia nervosa. In: Garner, D. M. and Garfinkel, P. E. (Eds) *Handbook of Psychotherapy for Anorexia Nervosa and Bulimia*. New York: Guilford Press, pp. 19–51.

Johnson, C. and Larson, R. (1982). Bulimia: An analysis of moods and behavior. *Psychosomatic Medicine*, **44**, 341–351.

Johnson, C., Lewis, C., Love, S., Lewis, L. and Stuckey, M. (1984). Incidence and correlates of bulimic behavior in a female high school population. *Journal of Youth and Adolescence*, **13**, 15–26.

Johnson, W. G. and Brief, D. (1983) Bulimia. *Behavioral Medicine Update*, **4**, 16–21.

Keesey, R. E. (1980). A set point analysis of the regulation of body weight. In: Stunkard, A. J. (Ed.) *Obesity*. Philadelphia: W. B. Saunders.

Keys, A., Brozek, J., Henschel, A., Mickelsen, O. and Taylor, H. L. (1950). *The Biology of Human Starvation*. Minneapolis: University of Minnesota Press.

Lacey, J. H., Coker, S. and Birtchnell, S. A. (1986). Bulimia: Factors associated with its etiology and maintenance. *International Journal of Eating Disorders*, **55**, 475–487.

Leitenberg, H., Gros, J., Peterson, J. and Rosen, J. C. (1984). Analysis of an anxiety model and the process of change during exposure plus response prevention treatment of bulimia nervosa. *Behavior Therapy*, **15**, 3–20.

Marcus, M. D. and Wing, R. R. (1987). Binge eating among the obese. *Annals of Behavioral Medicine*, **9**, 23–27.

Mitchell, J. E., Hatsukami, D., Eckert, E. D. and Pyle, R. L. (1985). Characteristics of 275 patients with bulimia. *American Journal of Psychiatry*, **142**, 482–485.

Mitchell, J. E., Pyle, R. and Miner, R. (1982). Gastric dilatation as a complication of bulimia. *Psychosomatics*, **9**, 96–97.

Mitchell, J. E., Seim, H. C., Colon, E. and Pomeroy, C. (1987). Medical complications and medical management of bulimia. *Annals of Internal Medicine*, **107**, 71–77.

Pyle, R. L., Mitchell, J. E. and Eckert, E. D. (1981). Bulimia: A report of 34 cases. *Journal of Clinical Psychiatry*, **42**, 60–64.

Pyle, R. L., Mitchell, J. E., Eckert, E. D., Halverson, P. A., Neuman, P. A. and Goff, G. M. (1983). The incidence of bulimia in freshman college students. *International Journal of Eating Disorders*, **2**, 75–85.

Rodin, G. M., Johnson, L. E. and Garfinkel, P. E. (1986) Eating disorders in female adolescents with insulin dependent diabetes mellitus. *International Journal of Psychiatry in Medicine*, **16**, 49–57.

Rosen, J. C. and Leitenberg, H. (1985). Exposure plus response prevention treatment of bulimia. In: Garner, D. M. and Garfinkel, P. E. (Eds) *Handbook of Psychotherapy for Anorexia Nervosa and Bulimia*. New York: Guilford Press, pp. 193–209.

Russell, G. F. M. (1979). Bulimia nervosa: An ominous variant of anorexia nervosa. *Psychological Medicine*, **9**, 429–448.

Schwartz, R. C., Barrett, M. J. and Saba, G. (1985). Family therapy for bulimia. In: Garner, D. M. and Garfinkel, P. E. (Eds) *Handbook of Psychotherapy for Anorexia Nervosa and Bulimia*. New York: Guilford Press, pp. 280–307.

Shatford, L. A. and Evans, D. R. (1986). Bulimia as a manifestation of the stress process: A LISREL causal modeling analysis. *International Journal of Eating Disorders*, **5**, 451–473.

Steel, J. M., Young, R. J., Lloyd, G. G. and Clarke, B. F. (1987). Clinically apparent eating disorders in young diabetic women: Associations with painful neuropathy and other complications. *British Medical Journal*, **294**, 860–863.

Strober, M. J. (1984). Stressful life events associated with bulimia in anorexia nervosa: Empirical findings and theoretical speculations. *International Journal of Eating Disorders*, **3**, 3–16.

Stunkard, A. J. (1959). Eating patterns and obesity. *Psychiatric Quarterly*, **33**, 284–292.

Wardle, J. and Beinart, H. (1981) Binge eating: A theoretical review. *British Journal of Clinical Psychology*, **20**, 97–109.

Weeda-Mannak, W. L. and Drop, M. J. (1985). The discriminative value of psychological characteristics in anorexia nervosa. Clinical and psychometric comparison between anorexia nervosa patients, ballet dancers and controls. *Journal of Psychiatric Research*, **19**, 285–290.

Weeda-Mannak, W. L., Drop, M. J., Smits, F., Strybosch, L. W. and Bremer, J. J. (1983). Toward an early recognition of anorexia nervosa. *International Journal of Eating Disorders*, **2**, 27–35.

Wilson, G. T. and Smith, D. (1987). Cognitive-behavioral treatment of bulimia nervosa. *Annals of Behavioral Medicine*, **9**, 12–17.

CHAPTER 14

Gastrointestinal Disorders

H. M. van der Ploeg[1]

Leiden University, Leiden

ABSTRACT

The behavioural treatment of four gastrointestinal disorders—psychogenic vomiting, irritable bowel syndrome, stomach ulcers and colitis ulcerosa—is described. After some epidemiological data have been presented, attention is focused on the role of psychological factors in the development and maintenance of the complaints. The assessment of these factors by means of functional behavioural analysis is detailed.

The importance of a cooperative relationship between patient and therapist during behavioural treatment is emphasized. The behavioural methods of reinforcement, aversion, relaxation, desensitization, assertive training, cognitive approaches, rational emotive therapy, hypnotherapy, and biofeedback, are described as applied to the disorders discussed.

It is concluded that, in addition to medical and pharmacological treatment, behavioural methods are of substantial value in the assessment and treatment of gastrointestinal disorders.

INTRODUCTION

This chapter describes the behavioural treatment of some gastrointestinal disorders in which psychological factors play a role in their course and/or treatment: psychogenic vomiting, the irritable bowel syndrome, and stomach ulcers and colitis ulcerosa. For treatment descriptions of other disorders of the gastrointestinal system, such as faecal incontinence, see Whitehead and Schuster (1985).

Behavioural Medicine
Edited by A. A. Kaptein, H. M. van der Ploeg, B. Garssen, P. J. G. Schreurs and R. Beunderman
© 1990 John Wiley & Sons Ltd.

Vomiting is a common disorder. Vomiting in babies and small children is quite normal and seldom requires medical treatment. The incidence in general practice is about 35 per 1000 for 0–4-year-old children and 10 per 1000 for other age groups over a two-year registration period (Lamberts, 1984). Chronic (psychogenic) vomiting, however, is a potentially dangerous disorder.

The *irritable bowel syndrome (IBS)*, characterized by abdominal pain and change in bowel habit, is a common disorder, too. The incidence in general practice in The Netherlands is about 15 per 1000 per annum and the prevalence is about 20 per 1000 (Lamberts, 1984). In a recent survey of the American Gastroenterological Association, 40% of patients seen by gastroenterologists had functional gastrointestinal disorders and 70% of these had IBS (Mitchell and Drossmann, 1987a). The IBS probably accounts for most of the digestive complaints in general practice and for a large proportion of referrals to medical specialists.

Stomach ulcers and colitis ulcerosa are less common, although the extensive descriptions of the disorders in the classical psychosomatic literature may suggest otherwise (Groen, 1982).

In fact, there are no objective figures available on the incidence and prevalence of gastrointestinal disorders because of hidden morbidity (van de Lisdonk, 1985). But the above figures are reasonable indications of the number of cases presented.

The GP and/or medical specialist will often be able to help the patient effectively with the usual medical treatment, with prescription of certain regimens, modifications in lifestyles and dietary modifications, but in some cases the absence of results will lead to a more detailed psychological approach. Behavioural treatment is then one of the possibilities.

Gastrointestinal disorders cannot be fully understood, and therefore not adequately treated, if they are regarded solely as somatic digestive diseases. Therefore the following section will first briefly discuss the disorders from a psychological point of view. Then the behavioural treatment of the disorders is described.

PSYCHOLOGICAL BACKGROUND

The importance of psychological or psychosocial factors in relation to gastrointestinal disorders has often been indicated in the literature (Katz and Zlutnick, 1975; Walen, Hauserman and Lavin, 1977; Koopman, 1982; Latimer, 1983). Strains and emotions, especially anxiety and anger, can contribute to the development, maintenance or worsening of the complaints. Psychological problems, may, of course, also develop as a consequence of somatic disorders.

In many cases a number of accompanying symptoms other than gastrointestinal can be observed in patients with gastrointestinal complaints, and those other symptoms (such as expressions of strain, stress reactions and psychological problems) often cannot be explained by gastrointestinal physiological abnormalities (Weinstock and Clouse, 1987). Neither can gastrointestinal complaints simply be regarded as an expression of psychiatric illness, as most of the patients do not meet the criteria for such a diagnosis. Therefore, a psychophysiological model to explain the gastrointestinal complaints is more appropriate. Such a model comprises constitutional factors, somatic vulnerability, personality structure, social factors and the repeated occurrence of emotionally stressful periods. In addition, patients with these complaints often acquire an undesired or maladaptive behaviour pattern.

This maladaptive behaviour may consist of:

1. Verbal behaviour (the patient complains of abdominal pain, nausea, changes in bowel habit);
2. Motoric behaviour (the patient takes medications, laxatives, frequently visits the toilet, changes in food and drink);
3. Physiological behaviour (change in motility of the gut). Furthermore, the patient's social behaviour may change as a result of this (social contacts, participation in social activities, behaviour at work, at home).

The diagnosis should be made from this point of view (see also Latimer, 1983; Mitchell and Drossmann, 1987b) and proper diagnostic procedures are a necessary condition in the behavioural treatment. In addition to the somatic diagnosis, a detailed biographical history taking should be performed and a functional analysis of the behaviour and of the gastrointestinal complaints should be made. In doing this, the therapist should try to distinguish between cause and effect as much as possible. This may also result in the patient gaining insight into the factors that maintain or worsen (or reduce) the complaints.

Detailed problem identification and behavioural analysis can result in an improvement of the treatment results. The main complaint must be assessed as well as the accompanying complaints and limitations experienced by the patient. In order to do so, as many quantitative data as possible should be collected from, for example, diary notes, self-monitoring and registration of selected variables. It is of great importance that the patient has the opportunity to talk about how (s)he experiences these complaints and limitations. This will contribute to the therapist–patient relationship and gives the therapist the opportunity to identify details that may be important in the treatment of the patient.

In addition to a description of the complaints and the situations in which these occur, a more dynamic description will be necessary: the functional behavioural analysis. This analysis relates complaints, relevant conditions or stimuli on the one hand to effects and reinforcing reactions on the other hand, which helps in acquiring insight into the antecedents of the complaints and the factors that worsen and maintain them. Some questions during behavioural analysis are:

- In which situations does the complaint occur?
- How does the patient react?
- What is the frequency and intensity of the complaints?
- How does the partner/social environment of the patient react to the complaints?

- What factors worsen the complaints?
- What factors reduce the complaints?

THE TREATMENT

The first requisite is to perform a diagnostic examination in order to detect possible organic abnormalities. Before considering psychological treatment, the physician/therapist will usually implement somatic therapy, pharmacological treatment, modifications in lifestyle and dietary modifications, or even an operation.

Of course, psychological treatment will start only after history-taking and behavioural analysis have been performed. It is important that the patient (with all his/her complaints) is accepted unconditionally by the therapist. This means that the therapist does not put the patient off with remarks such as 'It's psychological' (meaning it is make-believe), but takes the patient seriously, and that the therapist tries to determine to what extent stresses influence the complaint. A relationship of trust and understanding is necessary to be able to complete psychological treatment successfully. Furthermore, adequate explanation and information about the complaints is of great importance, as is explanation and information about possible interactions with psychological factors (emotions) and the development of a conditioning process, which teaches the patient to pay attention to certain aspects of the complaint. This information or patient education may sometimes enable patients to change their behaviour by themselves and may also reduce the complaints.

VOMITING

Vomiting is potentially dangerous to the health. Furthermore, it often has consequences, especially of an interpersonal nature. The social environment will react by paying attention to and taking care of the patient, and by offering practical help (cleaning up, etc.). Psychogenic vomiting may sometimes give a person the opportunity to escape from unpleasant or difficult situations, or to avoid these. If the behavioural analysis gives reason to suspect that such reinforcers are operative, a relatively simple extinction therapy seems appropriate. This therapy concentrates on avoidance behaviour and other 'advantages' of the complaint. The implementation of extinction procedures implies that the social environment no longer pays (extra) attention, does not offer practical help, and refrains from or reduces social contact immediately after the vomiting so that there is no reinforcement of the tendency to avoid or escape from difficult situations.

In addition, it is advisable to reinforce desired behaviour and behaviour that is incompatible with or contrary to the vomiting reactions (such as swallowing, sucking sweets).

The problem of retching, for example, can occur in specific situations and under specific conditions. One can imagine a student who starts retching the morning before a test, then starts vomiting, does not go to school and need not do his test. When trying to modify this maladaptive behaviour, one may try to change the sequence of reactions itself or reward the student explicitly if (s)he does take the test. As a result of this positive reinforcement, the vomiting reactions may decrease without treatment of the actual vomiting. Modifying the social consequences of vomiting can thus influence this behaviour. A description has been given of the psychological treatment of a baby who was held extra tenderly if the (psychogenic) vomiting stayed away and was put back to bed if it threatened to vomit. If the baby stopped vomiting it was taken out again (Murray and Keele, 1976). The direct social environment, that is, the parents and educators, can be instructed about their interaction with the patient. Changing the influence of the social network can result in a reduction of the complaints, as is shown in the following example. In this treatment procedure with a 14-year-old girl, social reinforcement was provided by means of attention, giving the opportunity to play games and have contact with visitors if the vomiting stayed away. If the girl started vomiting, all reinforcers were removed for 15 minutes. This soon reduced the vomiting (Ingersoll and Curry, 1977).

A completely different approach to psychogenic vomiting is the application of aversion techniques. It should be stressed that the aversion technique should only be applied when all other methods have failed. Even then, it is only (ethically) permissible after a careful evaluation of the advantages and disadvantages. The aversion technique must not be unnecessarily prolonged in the hope of gaining results especially since its results are generally limited. In the literature, aversion therapy is used especially with severely retarded adults and very young children, probably because other and more suitable methods are less well applicable to these groups. In aversion therapy, harmless but painful electric shocks, lemon juice and Tabasco sauce can be used.

Aversion therapy directly suppresses the vomiting reaction, and can be followed by an attempt to teach the patient more desired behaviour by means of other behavioural procedures, such as positive reinforcement, shaping, retraining, and assertiveness training.

A description has been given of a therapy with a seven-and-a-half-month-old child which frequently vomited. Several kinds of treatments had been unsuccessfully applied, after which aversion therapy was tried. Immediately upon vomiting, the child was given a mild electric shock of half a second. The vomiting then soon stopped and in the days following the child gained weight (Toister et al., 1975). Other reports described comparable results with slight modifications in procedure. In addition to or instead of electric shocks, lemon juice (and Tabasco sauce) can be used as aversive stimuli. When the patient starts vomiting, drops of lemon juice are put on the tongue.

Psychogenic vomiting of retarded persons may partly be the result of stomach overloading. A single case study showed that vomiting decreased during spaced food intake and a slower eating pattern in a male retarded subject. Vomiting resumed during normal intake and decreased again during the reinstated spaced intake (Azrin, Jamner and Besalel, 1986).

A case of psychogenic vomiting in the context of social phobia was treated by a combination of exposure *in vivo*, social skills training, and cognitive restructuring. The intervention was not directly aimed at the vomiting, but at aspects of the patient's behaviour hypothesized to be instrumental in maintaining it. Change was assessed on the basis of the patient's records of daily frequency of vomiting, performance and anxiety. Change occurred only with the introduction of treatment. Clinically the vomiting was virtually eliminated after seven weeks. General improvements of performance and a decrease in anxieties have also occurred (Stravynski, 1983).

Finally, a recent development is reported briefly. Retching and vomiting appear to be conditioned, and systematic desensitization and relaxation may be beneficial. A 33-year-old patient stated that her fear of flying expressed itself by nausea, cold sweat and shivering, followed by vomiting. This continued until about 10 minutes after takeoff and then returned every 20 minutes. The therapy consisted of relaxation exercises and a form of desensitization of the frightening airplane experiences. After a couple of sessions and regular home exercises of relaxation and desensitization, the complaints had disappeared. Rebman (1983) reports that the procedures, especially the relaxation exercises, could also be useful in the treatment of conditioned nausea and vomiting caused by chemotherapy in cancer patients. Research confirms that nausea in cancer patients may be reduced by training them in deep muscle relaxation. Control groups consisting of cancer patients without relaxation training support the finding that the nausea and vomiting reactions can decrease significantly after relaxation training.

IRRITABLE BOWEL SYNDROME

As a first step here, a detailed somatic diagnosis is essential in order to exclude food allergies. Next, pharmacological treatment, dietary modifications and changes in lifestyle seem relevant. If these prove unsuccessful, behavioural techniques can be useful. However, relatively few behavioural therapies have been described for the irritable bowel syndrome.

In one case, the complaints of a 22-year-old woman with chronic diarrhoea had increased to such an extent that she constantly remained close to a toilet. It was found that the diarrhoea was particularly related to her fear of people. Muscle relaxation and systematic desensitization of the fear-inducing situations resulted in a completely successful treatment of 12 sessions. Follow-up after two years indicated that the favourable results had been maintained (Hedberg, 1973).

Other diarrhoea patients gained control over their bowel activity by means of biofeedback procedures. The bowel sounds were electronically amplified *via* a stethoscope and verbal positive reinforcement was given, which together appeared to be an effective treatment of the complaints. The favourable results appear to have been achieved mainly by correction of undesirable, learned or conditioned behaviour (Furman, 1973; see also Bleijenberg and Cluysenaer, 1983).

It is essential that behavioural analysis of patients with IBS is performed before an appropriate therapy may be considered. At a physiological level, methods checking the spasms could be considered. At a behavioural level, self-monitoring, self-registration and self-observation of pains, and stress-management techniques could be used. Indeed, registration and observation methods have proved to be therapeutically effective by themselves. At a social level, the consequences of the complaint could be targeted, involving the help of close relatives, partner, children, parents, and significant others.

In general, psychotherapy (insight and cognitive psychotherapy) *versus* routine medical treatment only seemed somewhat superior in the short term (Svedlund *et al.*, 1983). Comparisons between the two treatment groups of IBS patients after one year showed that the complaints of the medically treated group had remained the same or grown worse. Psychological intervention may improve the patient's ability to cope with everyday stresses that contribute to IBS symptoms (Svedlund *et al.*, 1983).

Hypnotherapy compared with psychotherapy in IBS patients showed that both treatment groups improved, but the hypnotherapy group also reported significant improvement in bowel habit. In the hypnotherapy group no relapses were recorded during the three-month follow-up period, and no substitution symptoms were observed (Whorwell, Prior and Faragher, 1984; Mitchell and Drossmann, 1987b).

A long-term follow-up with a mean duration of 18 months of hypnotherapy in patients with severe IBS also demonstrated the successful effect. Patients of over 50 responded very poorly, whereas those under 50 with classical IBS (as contrasted with atypical cases and cases exhibiting significant psychopathology) exhibited a 100% response rate (Whorwell, Prior and Colgan, 1987).

Sixteen clients with IBS were treated with progressive muscle relaxation, thermal biofeedback, cognitive therapy, and IBS education. Comparisons of pretreatment indices with one-year follow-up ratings showed significant reductions in ratings of abdominal pain and tenderness, diarrhoea, and flatulence. Nine patients met the criterion for clinical improvement of at least a 50% reduction in major symptom scores, and all but one of the 16 patients rated themselves as subjectively improved (Schwarz, Blanchard and Neff, 1986).

To compare the effects of conventional medical treatment with a combination of medical treatment and psychotherapy, 101 outpatients with IBS and 103 with peptic ulcer disease were randomly allocated to two treatment groups. Psychotherapy included dynamically oriented individual treatment in 10 one-hour sessions spread over three months. There was a greater improvement in the psychotherapy groups for patients with IBS after three months and for both the IBS and the peptic ulcer disease patients at follow-up after 15 months. The patients given psychotherapy showed further improvement, and the patients who had received medical treatment showed some deterioration at 15 months' follow-up. The combination of medical treatment with psychotherapy improved the outcome for both groups of patients (Svedlund and Sjoedin, 1985).

A more detailed case history is the following. The patient is a 32-year-old manager suffering from chronic diarrhoea. The treatment procedure first involved a number of sessions about his life situation, his family, his work and the consequences of his complaints. Medical examination by the GP and a specialist on earlier occasions had indicated that there were no somatic disorders and consequently medical treatment had yielded unsatisfactory results. In the course of these introductory conversations, a regularity in the urge to visit the toilet was discovered. Certain social situations and forms of interpersonal behaviour appeared to precede the complaints quite frequently. It was also found that the patient was able to suppress the urge for some time and that in a single case a delay of several hours was not too great a problem. The following therapeutic sessions mainly focused on the patient's social behaviour. Although subassertiveness was in fact hardly the problem, there were nevertheless certain stressful social situations which could almost invariably evoke the complaints. By means of role-play, assertiveness training and rational emotive training, these situations were practised. Furthermore, the patient was advised to actually suppress the urge to go to the toilet for several minutes in certain situations. Muscle relaxation exercises proved to be very useful here. It also appeared that a formerly prescribed diet had never been followed properly; with the help of behavioural instructions the patient was now able to do this. In relation to this, the diarrhoea frequency decreased stepwise from about 10 times per day to about three to five times. Further reduction of this number could only be achieved after the patient was willing to give more information about particular stressful situations at work and at home. These sources of stress had remained 'hidden' during the first phases of the therapy. It was not until the patient had observed an improvement of his complaints that he was willing to work on these too. It was found that the complaints could largely be made to disappear by means of stress management, a continuation of the relaxation exercises, rational emotive training, and the development of a more adjusted and more relaxed lifestyle and professional career. At follow-up some years later, the diarrhoea was reported to be unusually absent, although the complaints returned temporarily under extremely stressful circumstances. The occurrence of these situations was a sufficient indication for the patient to repeat certain parts of the therapy (relaxation and rational emotive training), after which the complaints usually soon disappeared.

In conclusion, the treatment of abdominal pain in children is briefly discussed. Using reward and punishment, operant conditioning may result in the ability to control the pain (especially if the consequences possibly influence the complaint). Pain is effectively 'punished' and no pain 'rewarded'. Especially in children, operant conditioning, for example *via* the parents or the children themselves, seems to yield good results. However, before these procedures are put into practice, it should be clear that the complaints have been present for quite some time and the contribution of psychological factors should have been established.

STOMACH ULCERS AND COLITIS ULCEROSA

In the behavioural literature it is described how by using relaxation exercises and especially relaxation of the abdominal muscles, colitis ulcerosa symptoms disappeared after some months (Susen, 1978).

Another treatment of a patient with colitis started with functional analysis of the complaints and with self-observation and registration of stress episodes preceding the attacks (which occurred usually three times a week). Next, the patient was taught how to relax so that he would be able to resist stress reactions. Finally, he was taught how to bring about changes in his environment and in his reactions to intrusive and troublesome thoughts about work-related activities. After the relaxation exercises the number of attacks diminished, while there was an obvious and further improvement after the last therapy phase. During a long follow-up period only a few attacks had recurred (Mitchell, 1978).

In a controlled study, relaxation training was also found to be highly successful in reducing pain in individuals with ulcerative colitis. Six weekly training sessions of 75 minutes' duration in the technique of progressive relaxation were given to 20 patients. Another 20 subjects with the same illness condition constituted an attention control group. Before treatment both groups were alike. Immediately after treatment and at follow-up experimental subjects were superior on a number of variables such as pain description, pain ratings, pain frequency, distress and amount of medications used, thereby showing the important contribution of relaxation training (Shaw and Ehrlich, 1987). Colgan, Faragher and Whorwell (1988) described a controlled trial of hypnotherapy in patients with duodenal ulcers in order to prevent relapses. After a successful drug treatment one half, the randomly selected treatment group, received hypnotherapy, the others received no hypnotherapy. Follow-up continued for 12 months and it was found that in the hypnotherapy group eight out of 15 patients had relapsed and in the control group all (15) patients had relapsed. These results suggest that hypnotherapy may be a useful adjunct for some patients with chronic recurrent duodenal ulceration.

The history of a hyperactive boy with colitis ulcerosa indicated that his hyperactivity especially seemed to influence the complaints. His treatment consisted of mediation therapy, which meant that the therapy was carried out by his parents. They were instructed to ignore his hyperactive behaviour and to reward his attention verbally. After some weeks the hyperactive behaviour had diminished considerably and the intestinal problems had become less severe, as could be confirmed at follow-up (Daniels, 1973).

Finally, a treatment programme for duodenal ulcers will be described (Brooks and Richardson, 1980). This programme consists of emotional skills training with components combating anxiety (relaxation, desensitization, cognitive restructuring) and assertiveness training. All patients received a booklet about the treatment in which among other things the relationship between anxiety, emotional inhibition and the complaints as well as the relationship between worry and anxiety was explained. Furthermore, irrational thoughts which can cause fear, as well as negative and positive self-reinforcement, and coping and assertiveness were discussed. By means of exercises in recognizing irrational thoughts and exercises in self-observation and self-registration of undesired behaviour and pain, the patients were trained in their newly acquired emotional skills. The control group only received descriptions of the relationship between anxiety, emotional inhibition and the complaints, and the opportunity to monitor daily ulcer pain. The treatment programme consisted of eight sessions of approximately one and a half hours of which the first four sessions dealt with anxiety management and the other four with assertiveness training. At follow-up, judging from the subjective report of the complaints, the treatment group appeared to have improved considerably, having experienced less pain and having used less medication. At follow-up three and a half years later, it was demonstrated that the treatment with relaxation, desensitization, identifying irrational thoughts, assertiveness training and cognitive restructuring had resulted in a significantly faster improvement with less relapse in periods of anxiety and stress than in the comparable control group.

CONCLUSION

In this chapter, some behavioural treatments of patients with gastrointestinal disorders—psychogenic vomiting, irritable bowel syndrome, and stomach ulcers and colitis ulcerosa—have been described. As may be clear from the discussions, there is no single treatment procedure which is preferred or which is the most effective in all cases. A careful diagnosis and behavioural analysis of the patient's complaints should precede every treatment. This is necessary because a large number of environmental as well as internal (physiological) factors can maintain the symptoms.

The physician/therapist will usually start with medical and pharmacological treatment, thus trying to reduce the complaints. This approach will often be successful, but in a number of patients the complaints will not be reduced. Furthermore, there will be patients in whom the gastrointestinal disorders are obviously related to stress or more generally to psychological factors. The behavioural methods described in this chapter seem appropriate here.

Part of these behavioural techniques can be applied by the physician him/herself. Some of the possibilities for him/her would be, for example, relaxation training, presenting the theory of and experiences with relaxation, and providing appropriate guidelines. The more laborious techniques, such as systematic desensitization, assertiveness training and cognitive methods, should be left to the behavioural therapist. This means that the physician, after an unsuccessful attempt to intervene medically, or after some conversations, will most probably decide to refer the patient. Depending on his/her knowledge and experience, and the individual possibilities, this referral will take place sooner or later in the treatment of the patient. Together with a behavioural therapist, the most appropriate and promising therapeutic strategy can then be decided upon. It will be clear that a patient with gastrointestinal disorders is best served by an extensive and multifaceted approach to his/her complaints.

NOTES

Address for correspondence: H. M. van der Ploeg, Division of Medical Psychology, Leiden University, PO Box 1251, 2340 BG Oegstgeest, The Netherlands.

REFERENCES

Azrin, N. H., Jamner, J. P. and Besalel, V. A. (1986). Vomiting reduction by slower food intake. *Applied Research in Mental Retardation*, **7**, 409–413.

Bleijenberg, G. and Cluysenaer, O. J. (1983). Behavioural treatment of the speaking stomach syndrome. *Journal of Behavioral Medicine*, **6**, 115–122.

Brooks, G. R. and Richardson, F. C. (1980). Emotional skills training: A treatment program for duodenal ulcer. *Behavior Therapy*, **11**, 198–207.

Colgan, S. M., Faragher, E. B. and Whorwell, P. J. (1988). Controlled trial of hypnotherapy in relapse prevention of duodenal ulceration. *Lancet*, **6**, 1299–1300.

Daniels, L. K. (1973). Parental treatment of hyperactivity in a child with ulcerative colitis. *Journal of Behavior Therapy and Experimental Psychiatry*, **4**, 183–185.

Furman, S. (1973). Intestinal biofeedback in functional diarrhea by systematic desensitization: A preliminary report. *Journal of Behavior Therapy and Experimental Psychiatry*, **4**, 317–321.

Groen, J. J. (1982). *Clinical Research in Psychosomatic Medicine*. Assen: Van Gorcum.

Hedberg, A. G. (1973). The treatment of chronic diarrhea by systematic desensitization: A case report. *Journal of Behavior Therapy and Experimental Psychiatry*, **4**, 67–68.

Ingersoll, B. and Curry, F. (1977). Rapid treatment of persistent vomiting in a fourteen-year-old female by shaping and time-out. *Journal of Behavior Therapy and Experimental Psychiatry*, **8**, 305–307.

Katz, R. C. and Zlutnick, S. (Eds) (1975). *Behavior Therapy and Health Care: Principals and Applications*. New York: Pergamon.

Koopman, H. M. (1982). Maag-darmklachten. In: Orlemans, J. W. G. *et al.* (Eds) *Handboek voor Gedragstherapie*. Deventer: Van Loghum Slaterus, p. C.5.9.

Lamberts, H. (1984). *Morbidity in General Practice*. Utrecht: Huisartsenpers.

Latimer, P. R. (1983). *Functional Gastrointestinal Disorders: A Behavioral Medicine Approach*. New York: Springer.

Lisdonk, E. H. van de (1985). Ervaren en aangeboden morbiditeit in de huisartspraktijk. Dissertation, Katholieke Universiteit, Nijmegen.

Mitchell, C. M. and Drossmann, D. A. (1987a). Survey of the AGA membership relating to patients with functional GI disorders. *Gastroenterology*, **92**, 1282–1284.

Mitchell, C. M. and Drossmann, D. A. (1987b). The irritable bowel syndrome: Understanding and treating a biopsychosocial illness disorder. *Annals of Behavioral Medicine*, **9**, 13–18.

Mitchell, K. R. (1978). Self-management of spastic colitis. *Journal of Behavior Therapy and Experimental Psychiatry*, **9**, 269–272.

Murray, M. E. and Keele, D. K. (1976). Behavioral treatment of rumination. *Clinical Pediatrics*, **15**, 591–596.

Rebman, V. L. (1983). Self-control desensitization with cue-controlled relaxation for treatment of a conditioned vomiting response to air travel. *Journal of Behavior Therapy and Experimental Psychiatry*, **14**, 161–164.

Schwarz, S. P., Blanchard, E. B. and Neff, D. F. (1986). Behavioral treatment of irritable bowel syndrome: A 1-year follow-up study. *Biofeedback and Self-Regulation*, **11**, 189–198.

Shaw, L. and Ehrlich, A. (1987). Relaxation training as a treatment for chronic pain caused by ulcerative colitis. *Pain*, **29**, 287–293.

Stravynski, A. (1983). Behavioral treatment of psychogenic vomiting in the context of social phobia. *Journal of Nervous and Mental Disease*, **171**, 448–451.

Susen, G. R. (1978). Conditioned relaxation in a case of ulcerative colitis. *Journal of Behavior Therapy and Experimental Psychiatry*, **9**, 283.

Svedlund, J. and Sjoedin, I. (1985). A psychosomatic approach to treatment in the irritable bowel syndrome and peptic ulcer disease with aspects of the design of clinical trials. *Scandinavian Journal of Gastroenterology*, **109**, 147–151.

Svedlund, J., Sjoedin, I., Ottoson, J. O. and Dotevall, G. (1983). Controlled study of psychotherapy in irritable bowel syndrome. *Lancet*, **2**, 589–592.

Toister, R. P., Condron, C. J., Worley, L. and Authur, D. (1975). Faradic therapy of chronic vomiting in infancy: A case study. *Journal of Behavior Therapy and Experimental Psychiatry*, **6**, 55–59.

Walen, S., Hauserman, N. M. and Lavin, P. J. (Eds) (1977). *Clinical Guide to Behavior Therapy*. Baltimore: Williams and Wilkins.

Weinstock, L. B. and Clouse, R. E. (1987). Area review: Gastrointestinal disorders. A focused overview of gastrointestinal physiology. *Annals of Behavioral Medicine*, **9**, 3–6.

Whitehead, W. E. and Schuster, M. M. (1985). *Gastrointestinal Disorders: Behavioral and Physiological Basis for Treatment*. Orlando, FL: Academic Press.

Whorwell, P. J., Prior, A. and Colgan, S. M. (1987). Hypnotherapy in severe irritable bowel syndrome: Further experience. *Gut*, **28**, 423–425.

Whorwell, P. J., Prior, A. and Faragher, E. B. (1984). Controlled trial of hypnotherapy in the treatment of severe refractory irritable bowel syndrome. *Lancet*, **2**, 1232–1234.

CHAPTER 15

Skin Disorders

A. A. Kaptein[1]

Leiden University, Leiden

ABSTRACT

Skin disorders quite often have substantial negative impact on the psychological and social functioning of the afflicted patients. In this chapter, behavioural aspects in the assessment, treatment and social consequences of acne, psoriasis and atopic dermatitis (eczema) are described. Epidemiological data on skin disorders are presented, and differences between dermatologists and psychologists with regard to the classification of dermatological disorders are pointed out.

In acne, psychological factors impact on the development, maintenance and treatment of the disorder. Studies on behavioural interventions in patients with acne are scarce, but results indicate that biofeedback, relaxation and guided cognitive imagery can improve the lesions. In psoriasis, the role of psychological factors in the course of the illness, psychological and social problems, and psychological intervention methods are described. Self-management training appears to be the most promising approach here. Atopic dermatitis is a condition which has been studied in some detail by psychologists. Research indicates that techniques such as habit reversal, hypnosis, and the combination of biofeedback, relaxation and guided imagery, do show promise for patients with this disorder.

It is emphasized that dermatological disorders deserve more adequate research from a behavioural medicine point of view and, also, that health care providers (e.g. general practitioners, dermatologists) and society at large, should be objects of research and intervention by psychologists.

Behavioural Medicine
Edited by A. A. Kaptein, H. M. van der Ploeg, B. Garssen, P. J. G. Schreurs and R. Beunderman
© 1990 John Wiley & Sons Ltd.

INTRODUCTION

'What is beautiful is good . . . physical beauty is the sign of an interior beauty, a spiritual and moral beauty (Dion, Berscheid and Walster, 1972, p. 285). In girls and boys, in women and men, physical appearance plays an important role in initiating and maintaining social interactions. Disorders of the skin quite often influence a persons physical appearance negatively. People suffering from acne, eczema, urticaria or psoriasis report that dating, employment, sexual behaviour, self-confidence and overall well-being are hindered because of not having an unblemished skin. Itching and scratching are behaviours which are painful for the sufferer of skin disorders, and may be embarrassing or annoying to the non-sufferer. Skin disorders, therefore, are a field of interest not only for dermatologists but for psychologists as well.

In the book *Touching—the Human Significance of the Skin*, Montagu (1986) elaborates on the intricate associations of the skin with, for instance, caressing, scratching, sexuality, immunology, somatic illness and love. The book is about the largest organ of the human body, the skin. In this chapter we will discuss the epidemiology and classification of skin disorders, the psychological and social consequences, and behavioural treatment of three disorders of the skin: acne, psoriasis and atopic dermatitis (eczema).

EPIDEMIOLOGY AND CLASSIFICATION OF SKIN DISORDERS

Data on the incidence and prevalence of skin disorders are hard to come by since most epidemiological studies do not focus specifically on distinct skin disorders. In general, acne affects some 20–30% of especially younger persons (Marks, 1985), psoriasis has a prevalence of about 2% (Zachariae, 1986), and atopic dermatitis of about 2% (Faulstich and Williamson, 1985). Dermatological complaints make up a substantial part of the workload of general practitioners; approximately 1% of the hospital population is admitted because of dermatological disorders (Office of Population Censuses and Surveys, 1974).

Dermatologists, psychiatrists and psychologists discuss and argue about how to classify dermatological complaints and disorders. Generally, a distinction is made between psychiatric syndromes with dermatological expression and skin diseases in which the course of the disease is also influenced by the behaviour of the patient (Cossidente and Sarti, 1984). Trichotillomania (the pulling out of hairs mainly from the scalp, but also from eyebrows, eyelashes or the pubic hairs), dermatitis artefacta (self-inflicted lesions of the skin), and parasitaphobia (a persistent and strong conviction that the skin is infested with parasites) are usually regarded as dermatological disorders which are the expression of psychiatric syndromes (Gupta, Gupta and Haberman, 1987a). Most patients with these disorders will deny any psychiatric illness and will, therefore, seek the help of a dermatologist. This usually leads to consultation of a liaison psychiatrist, which makes behavioural treatment by a hospital psychologist often unlikely. We will therefore not discuss the psychiatric syndromes with dermatological expression (see Friman, Finney and Christophersen, 1984, for an overview of the behavioural treatment of trichotillomania).

In almost any physical illness, behavioural factors affect the course of the affliction—this is also the case in skin disorders. In the remainder of this chapter, we will expand on these behavioural factors and examine the effects of psychological interventions in three specific skin disorders: acne, psoriasis and atopic dermatitis. They were chosen because of their high prevalence and associated psychological and social impact, and the availability of empirical studies in which psychological treatment has been applied. In addition, the impressive personal and social consequences of these dermatological disorders will be illustrated. For a review of the psychological reactions to and behavioural treatment of vitiligo, urticaria, hyperhidrosis, and warts, the reader is referred to Pinkerton, Hughes and Wenrich (1982), Porter *et al.* (1986) and Spanos, Stenstrom and Johnston (1988).

ACNE (ACNE VULGARIS)

Acne is an inflammatory disorder of the pilosebaceous follicles; the defining lesion of acne is the comedo. 'Acne can kill the personality, though not the person' (Medansky, 1980, p. 199): all papers on acne which are relevant for psychologists emphasize the negative impact of this skin disorder on the patient. Also, most authors stress the need to emotionally support the patient with acne. Empathy and acknowledgement that medical intervention in most cases is not omnipotent is more beneficial than any cream, ointment, skincleansing procedure or diet. Clinical observation and research show that emotional stress can exacerbate the flaring up of the lesions in the skin (Albers, 1985). The lesions themselves cause psychological tension in the patient, giving rise potentially to a vicious circle where the skin affliction and the psychological response to it reinforce each other.

Both Shuster *et al.* (1978) and Garrie and Garrie (1978) demonstrated that patients with acne scored significantly higher than persons without diagnosed dermatological disorders on the state and trait anxiety scales of the STAI. In addition, significant negative effects were observed, especially in women, on self-image and perceived social acceptance. The effects of acne on the occupational, social and emotional functioning of the patients are impressive. Jowett and Ryan (1985a) studied a group of outpatients with acne, aged 16–79. The patients were interviewed in their homes, using a non-structured interview schedule. Pain and itching were prominent symptoms: the actual appearance of their skin and the subsequent lack of self-confidence were the worst aspects of the affliction, according to the patients. Other people not realizing the physical and emotional suffering caused by acne was one of the reported social consequences of acne. Regarding employment, 66% of the patients reported interpersonal difficulties and limited job opportunities (e.g. not being accepted as an employee in a fashion store). Shame, embarrassment, anxiety, lack of confidence, depression, and concern about scarring were other outstanding psychological consequences of acne.

Marks (1985) writes about the myths surrounding causes and treatment of acne. Dietary manipulations (e.g. avoiding eating chocolate) and 'too much or too little sex' as factors causing acne are discarded as folk tales. He reports substantial negative effects on the employment status of 625 outpatients with acne: compared to matched controls, the acne patients in his study experienced about double the rate of unemployment.

An exhaustive literature search resulted in two papers in which psychologists report on the effects of behavioural interventions in patients with acne. In the first, 30 female students with acne of at least two-year duration were assigned to one of three treatment conditions (Hughes *et al.*, 1983). The first treatment condition consisted of biofeedback and relaxation with guided cognitive imagery training. The second experimental condition consisted of group sessions with rational behaviour therapy (considered as attention placebo), the third was the regular medical care condition. Acne gradings by means of photographs and self-evaluations of acne severity, and level of relaxation were the dependent variables which were assessed before and after the interventions and at follow-up at four weeks. Two major findings were observed. Patients in the first treatment condition experienced statistically significant and clinically relevant reductions in acne gradings, self-evaluations of acne severity, and higher levels of relaxation, compared with patients in the other two conditions. Also, those patients in the relaxation with guided cognitive imagery condition who reported continuing the therapeutic procedures after the treatment session had been concluded fared much better at follow-up than the patients who discontinued their therapy. Statements by two successful participants illustrate the contents of the imagery they applied: '. . . farmers shovelling out dirt from my pores and using a water bucket to nurture each pore with medication . . .', and '. . . imagining facial pores opening wider as relaxation deepened, allowing bacteria and oil to escape . . .' (pp. 189–190).

The second study (Flanders and McNamara, 1985) focused on an indirect method to improve acne, namely, improving compliance with the application to the afflicted skin of a medication which is supposed to be effective against acne. Forty-two undergraduate students were assigned randomly to four groups: a waiting-list control group, a self-monitoring group, a non-contingent contract group, and a contingent contract group. Compliance with the medication was increasingly supervised and reinforced in the three treatment conditions. The dependent measures in the study were compliance, acne severity and number of acne lesions, and satisfaction with the treatment. No significant differences were found between the groups on all dependent measures before or after the interventions: all patients noted some improvement in the number of acne lesions. Further, compliance with the acne medication increased in comparison with the usual, very low (12%) compliance of patients with acne.

Summarizing, it can be concluded that acne does have rather negative effects on psychological, social and employment issues. Psychologists have not yet explored the possibilities of various behavioural interventions in this category of patients. The study by Hughes *et al.* (1983) is the first one in this field. Apart from patients with acne, perhaps equally important for psychologists are two other potential target groups where behavioural interventions may benefit the patient with acne indirectly, namely, the public at large and dermatologists. Marks (1985) expresses his surprise over the relative sophistication of the general public about illnesses such as haemophilia or multiple sclerosis and their relative ignorance about a common affliction such as acne. He surmises that patients with acne might benefit from more enlightened attitudes of the public towards patients with this disorder of the skin. Second, most acne sufferers do not need extensive psychological treatment—they need a good dermatologist (Jowett and Ryan, 1985b). Psychologists might want to use their expertise in training dermatologists to become more empathetic in their encounters with patients with acne.

PSORIASIS

'On a full double-decker bus, at least two people will actually have psoriasis and another five a predisposition to it' (Henley, 1981, p. 1852). The prevalence of psoriasis in western Europe and North America is approximately 2%. The age of onset of psoriasis varies from the first to the final years of life; the ratio of male to female patients is about unity (Zachariae, 1986).

Psoriasis is a non-contagious skin condition that is associated with an increased rate of proliferation of the epidermal cells. The characteristic lesions are deep red, thickly scaling plaques that may affect any region of the skin, although plaques are classically found on the extensor aspects of the limbs, the lumbosacral region, and the scalp. As psoriasis becomes more severe, the skin grows dry and pruitic, and builds into heavy layers that may crack, bleed, and become painful. Itching can be a particular problem when the lesions are located in body flexures.

We will discuss three topics which are relevant for the psychologist working with these patients in a hospital or outpatient setting:

1. The role of psychological factors in the course of psoriasis;
2. The psychological and social problems associated with adaptation to a chronic and cosmetically disfiguring disease; and
3. Psychological intervention methods and their results in patients with psoriasis.

Psychological Factors and the Course of Psoriasis

Based on clinical observation, some authors describe patients with no previous skin disorders at all in whom the onset of psoriasis appeared to be caused by psychological factors. Duller and Van Veen-Viëtor (1986) portray a man in whom psoriasis begins and deteriorates after an unsuccessful change in employment. In another patient, mounting family problems were associated with the onset of psoriasis. It should be stressed, however, that these cases do not prove that psychological turmoil can lead to the onset of psoriasis, since the association may be based on coincidence. In a comprehensive review, Gupta, Gupta and Haberman (1987b) conclude that there is no evidence for the onset of psoriasis being caused by 'stress' or psychological factors. In addition, attempts to delineate a psychological profile of patients with psoriasis have failed to produce clear-cut conclusions.

Psoriasis does, however, seem to be affected in its course by psychological factors. Two studies deserve mention in this respect. Seville (1977) studied 132 inpatients with psoriasis and asked them what upset or illness there was just before the onset of the psoriatic rash. Major interpersonal upsets within the family, deaths or hospitalization of close relatives, examinations, accidents and sexual assaults were reported by 39% of the patients with psoriasis. In a control group of patients with infectious diseases, only 10% of the patients reported major emotional turmoil before the onset or exacerbation of the diseases. Although this study does have some methodological weaknesses, the data indicate that in patients with psoriasis, major disruptions of a psychological or social nature tend to be associated with exacerbation of psoriasis. Similar results were observed in a sample of 252 hospitalized patients with psoriasis: Baughman and Sobel (1971) found a significant but modest correlation between 'stress' (as measured by the Social Readjustment Rating Scale) and psoriasis severity.

Living with Psoriasis: Consequences in Daily Life

'Each morning, I vacuum my bed. My torture is skin deep: there is no pain, not even itching; we lepers (psoriatics) live a long time, and are ironically healthy in other respects. Lusty, though we are loathsome to love. Keen-sighted, though we hate to look upon ourselves. The name of the disease, spiritually speaking, is Humiliation' (Updike, 1976, p. 28).

Being a patient with psoriasis implies that virtually every aspect of daily life is influenced by the disease: working, social activities, sexual life, family interactions. Having psoriasis means, for instance, having to change the bed linen once (or more) every day, applying ointments to the lesions, which can be a messy, greasy and smelly undertaking, being rejected sexually by a partner or others, and being frowned upon in social places. One patient reports, when having dinner at a restaurant, overhearing from a nearby table '. . . you'd think they'd know better than to come to a public place where they can ruin our appetites' (Dungey and Buselmeier, 1982, p. 144).

A few studies have presented empirical data on the impact of psoriasis on the sufferer. Roenigk and Roenigk (1978) studied 84 outpatients and found male patients to be bothered by the illness when they were participating in outdoor activities, while female patients reported 'worry and stress' as the most significant effect of the illness on their daily functioning. In female patients, sex life, social life, sports activities and relations with the same sex were disrupted more severely than in male patients. In another study, the worst feature about having psoriasis was assessed in 94 outpatients (Stankler, 1981): avoidance of short sleeves and dark clothes (to avoid the 'dandruff effect') was reported by more than half of the patients; swimming, sunbathing and going to the hairdresser's were the activities that were most often avoided or disliked. Coen-Buckwalter (1982) stresses the negative effects of psoriasis on the sexual life of patients and their partners. In her study, 60% of the respondents admitted psoriatic lesions in the genital area and chest/breast region. Most patients felt embarrassed and restricted their sexual activities: '. . . psoriasis is not good for your social or sex life. I'm very withdrawn until I get drunk. The girls I've lived with would go along with it for a while until they saw it wasn't going to get any better' (Coen-Buckwalter, 1982, p. 104). Weinstein (1984) found that sexual functioning was negatively affected in 72% of the patients; comparable results were found by Ramsay and O'Reagan (1988).

The items which make up the Psoriasis Disability Index, drawn up by Finlay and Kelly (1987), mirror the previous studies. Interference because of psoriasis with carrying out work around the house or garden, types or colours of clothes worn, changing or washing clothes, problems at the hairdresser's, taking more baths than usual, career prospects, sports activities, problems with communal bathing, increased smoking and drinking more alcohol, and a messy or untidy home, make up the items of this index. Itching (in 87%) and pain (in 21%) were the most prominent symptoms in the patients with psoriasis studied by Jowett and Ryan (1985a). Encountering ignorance and misunderstanding, and limited job opportunities and functional difficulties figured prominently as problems in this patient group. Eighty-nine per cent experienced shame and embarrassment, while anxiety, lack of confidence and depression were reported by about 50% of the patients. There are some indications that patients with psoriasis drink more alcohol than the average population (Morse, Perry and Hurst, 1985; Parish and Fine, 1985), which may be explained as a response to perceived unattractiveness and depressive feelings.

Psychological Interventions in Psoriasis

It is rather disappointing to note the paucity of studies on the effects of psychological treatment in patients with psoriasis. An exhaustive literature search produced only two reports on this subject (Benoit and Harrell, 1980; Bremer-Schulte et al., 1985).

In the study by Benoit and Harrell, biofeedback on skin temperature was applied in three patients with psoriasis. The theoretical rationale for skin temperature biofeedback is based on the observation that in psoriasis, reduced heat production in the skin may, via vasoconstriction, decrease the metabolic activity of psoriatic tissue and affect cell proliferation. Temperature biofeedback on a psoriatic plaque was given and the subjects were instructed to reduce skin temperature. Biopsies from the lesions were taken before and after training to measure cell proliferation. Results indicated that after six sessions, skin temperature was reduced by about one degree Celsius in all subjects compared to pretraining level ($P < 0.02$). Cell proliferation was reduced (exact data are not given) and in two subjects all plaques showed clinical improvements. In the other patient, slight improvements were observed. In a follow-up conducted four months after training, the improvements were still evident but the lesions were beginning to show a return to their original condition. The authors quite rightly point to the small number of patients in the study, and suggest that replication with a larger sample is indicated. In addition, they speculate that the biofeedback procedure may have indirect effects *via* increased control of the patients over their illness, which in general has beneficial effects on coping with most illnesses (Bandura, 1982).

This last observation leads to the second study by Bremer-Schulte *et al.*, where the psychological intervention is not aimed at improving psoriatic symptoms as such but at strengthening self-care and coping skills, mutual aid, increasing the expertise of the patient about his illness, and encouraging the patient to become more assertive towards physicians. In a disease which has been described in the earliest written sources, and where medical treatment does not lead to complete cure of the illness, it is, in our opinion, not realistic to pretend that psychological treatment can lead to complete cure. The contribution of psychologists to the well-being of patients with psoriasis should rather be aimed at teaching patients what skills, cognitions and attitudes may help them experience as little discomfort as possible because of the illness.

Essentially, the study by Bremer-Schulte *et al.* illustrates a patient education format where somatic and emotional aspects of the disease are discussed in a group of patients with psoriasis. The unique feature of this particular study is that the group sessions are led by a physician and a 'fellow-sufferer', both of whom have been trained together to run a patient group, the so-called 'duo formula group treatment'. In 10 weekly sessions of two hours each, 28 patients in the experimental group discussed somatic issues (information on ointments, radiation, climatotherapy, diets) and emotional issues (worries about relapses, shame and shyness, sexual relationships, lack of understanding, etc.). In addition, relaxation and respiratory exercises aimed at relaxation were part of the treatment. The effects of the intervention were assessed by means of an interview and a questionnaire before and after the training, and at a follow-up three months after the end of the training. Fourteen patients served as a waiting-list control group. The results of the assessment showed significant reductions of medical consumption, shame and shyness, and significant improvements in interpersonal skills, identification with the skin and overall well-being. The authors emphasize the importance of training dermatologists at internship level to acquire the skills necessary to run comparable groups.

ATOPIC DERMATITIS

Atopic dermatitis is a skin disorder where the skin is chronically inflamed; it is characterized by a dry, irritable and itchy skin associated with and exacerbated by excessive scratching. The skin lesions are commonly seen on the flexures of the arms and legs, and on the nape of the neck, which are areas easily accessible to scratching. Multiple causative and maintenance factors have been postulated in atopic dermatitis: immunological and constitutional factors, autonomic imbalance, the itch–scratch cycle and psychological–emotional factors (Haynes *et al.*, 1979). Atopic dermatitis, neurodermatitis, and atopic eczema are considered here to be synonymous. Atopic dermatitis is frequently seen in patients with a personal or family history of atopic (allergic) manifestations, such as asthma, allergic rhinitis or hay fever. It is estimated that about 2% of the population suffer from atopic dermatitis (Faulstich and Williamson, 1985).

Research by psychologists on patients with atopic dermatitis tends to confirm clinical observations by dermatologists and patients: psychological factors exacerbate episodes of atopic dermatitis. Faulstich *et al.* (1985) compared patients with atopic dermatitis with active symptomatology and control subjects on reactions to a psychophysiological 'stress test' (intelligence test items, cold pressor test). The patients exhibited greater forearm electromyogram activity, higher heart rates and higher scores on some SCL-90 scales (anxiety, somatization, obsessive-compulsiveness and depression) than the control subjects. Garrie and Garrie (1978) found patients with atopic dermatitis to have significantly higher state and trait anxiety scores than healthy controls or other patient groups with dermatological disorders. Recently, Gil *et al.* (1987) demonstrated in a carefully designed study that measures of stress and quality of family interaction were important predictors of symptom severity, also after controlling for demographic and medical status variables such as age and serum IgE levels. In line with these findings, the work by McSkimming, Gleeson and Sinclair (1984)—although only a pilot study—on support groups for parents of children with atopic dermatitis should be mentioned. They found high levels of social and psychological problems in these parents because of negative community attitudes towards the children and their parents, and anger and hopelessness in dealing with the child and the child's reactions to the affliction.

In addition to medical care, different psychological treatment methods have been applied: (a) habit reversal, (b) hypnosis, and (c) a combination of biofeedback, relaxation and guided imagery.

Habit Reversal

Atopic dermatitis is almost always associated with itching ('pruritis'). As scratching provides immediate relief of the itching sensation, scratching is reinforced. Some patients continue this scratching, especially when they are in emotionally stressful situations. The already mentioned vicious circle of itching–scratching may give rise to a worsening of the skin disorder. It is apparent, then, that breaking this vicious circle may lead to improvements in the affected skin.

Rosenbaum and Ayllon (1981), Melin *et al.* (1986) and Cole, Roth and Sachs (1988) applied the behavioural method of habit reversal in patients with atopic dermatitis. In the first study, four cases were treated with this technique. In the second study, 17 patients were randomly assigned to two groups, one of which received a combination of habit reversal and hydrocortisone cream and the other the regular ointment treatment. Habit reversal consisted of various steps:

- 'Response description', the patient describes and demonstrates his scratching;
- 'Early warning', the patient is taught to recognize when he brings his hands towards the area which he scratches;
- 'Situation awareness', the patient describes those situations in which he usually scratches or does so more actively;
- 'Habit control motivation', unpleasant aspects of scratching are discussed; and
- 'Competing response practice', the patient is taught to develop behaviours incompatible with scratching (e.g. clenching his fist; see Melin *et al.*, 1986, for further details).

Finally, Cole, Roth and Sachs (1988) report the results of a pilot study on the effects of a behavioural treatment package (relaxation training, identification of behavioural triggers of scratching, habit reversal) on symptoms of eczema. After 12 weekly meetings, the 10 patients and medical raters reported significant improvement on all eczema symptoms (e.g. dryness of the skin, itching). This result was maintained at a one-month follow-up assessment. Also, the number of grammes of topical steroids supplied decreased during the active study period.

In all studies, skin status and frequency of scratching were significantly improved at the end of the treatment. In addition, in the studies where a follow-up was applied, the improvements continued to exist.

On the basis of the available studies, it may be concluded that behavioural treatment, particularly habit reversal, of patients with atopic neurodermatitis, in combination with medical care, has beneficial effects.

Hypnosis

Lehman (1978) describes a patient with atopic dermatitis where he used brief hypnotherapy. The therapist uncovered two major problems of the patient (a high need for achievement and a lack of assertiveness). He gave her hypnotic suggestions concerning clearing of the skin which were imagined by the patient. The author reports that after eight sessions 'the rash was gone and only a slight reddening of the skin attested to it ever having existed' (p. 50). At four-year follow-up, the skin condition had not reappeared. The literature on hypnosis and skin disorders, however, is not very convincing, due to the small numbers of patients in various studies (case reports are frequently described) and inadequate methodology.

Biofeedback, Relaxation and Guided Imagery

Another behavioural treatment method in patients with atopic dermatitis is biofeedback, supported by relaxation and guided imagery. Manuso (1977) describes a case-study where in 13 weekly sessions of 15 minutes' duration each, biofeedback-assisted hand-warming training and relaxation were applied to a woman with chronic eczematous dermatitis of the hands. In the course of the therapeutic sessions, the patient learned to raise her hand temperature. At the end of treatment, there were no lesions present, scaling had ceased, and dryness and discoloration were minimal. A medical examination concluded that the dermatitis had completely remitted. At six months' follow-up, the patient's previous dermatitis had been absent since the termination of the treatment, and she maintained her ability to increase hand temperature.

Gray and Lawlis (1982) used a combination of frontalis electromyogram (EMG) biofeedback, relaxation training, stress management and guided imagery in a similar case. The therapy entailed 10 sessions over a four-month period. During the guided imagery the patient visualized her skin cells as '. . . little, round persons basking on a beautiful warm, peaceful beach and imagining her skin cells as totally serene and completely relaxed in a state of utter contentment' (p. 630). EMG readings over the 10 sessions were not reduced, but ratings of rash and pruritis were reduced considerably. At one-year follow-up, the patient reported she had experienced only three brief exacerbations of her skin disorder.

The most elaborate study on biofeedback treatment of patients with atopic dermatitis has been performed by Haynes et al. (1979). Eight subjects were exposed to an intervention package involving three phases: no treatment, placebo treatment, and a treatment combination of frontal EMG feedback and relaxation instructions. Photographic analysis of involved skin areas, frontal EMG activity, and ratings of itching levels were the dependent measures. The results indicated reductions in affected skin areas and decreases in itching ratings during each session but not across sessions.

Controlled studies with fairly large numbers of patients in the various treatment modalities have not yet been done in patients with atopic dermatitis. The case-studies presented here warrant some optimism about the effectiveness of biofeedback in atopic dermatitis.

Atopic dermatitis is not a spectacular disease. The study of Jowett and Ryan (1985a), however, demonstrated that this skin disease does have negative psychological and social consequences. In their research, patients with atopic dermatitis said the irritation, constant itching, and the actual marks on one's skin were the worst aspects of having atopic dermatitis. Shame and embarrassment were reported by 78%, anxiety by 63% and depression by 38% of the patients. Clearly, more and better research on how psychologists can help these patients is needed.

CONCLUDING REMARKS

Widely held notions in society regarding health, beauty, cleanliness, and general physical appearance complicate an individual's psychological and social adjustment to skin disorders. Patients with skin disorders do suffer—not only somatic complaints, but the visibility of the disorders has many negative consequences for the patient in his relationships with partners, colleagues and the social environment as well. Psychological help seems in order for quite a number of patients.

The studies on psychological treatment of skin disorders that have been published suffer methodological weaknesses. True experimental designs, careful patient selection, subjective and objective assessment methods, adequate control groups and adequate follow-up should be applied in future research. The studies that have been done, however, indicate that some optimism is justified. There is a drastic need for replication and extension of the initial work. Various behavioural methods (relaxation, hypnosis, biofeedback) and, especially, training in adequate coping skills appear to have promising effects, not only in a somatic sense but, almost more important, also in improving the skills with which patients can manage the psychological and social consequences of the disorder. Dermatologists increasingly recognise the importance of encouraging patients to manage their skin disorder themselves (Logan, 1988).

Patients with dermatological diseases complain about the lack of empathy by dermatologists for the psychological and social impact of the skin problems (Weinstein, 1984). Patients report embarrassment over appearance as the most serious factor, while dermatologists rank this factor lowest (Duller and van Veen-Viëtor, 1986). As has been pointed out earlier in this chapter, not only the patient with a skin disorder can be the focus of psychological interventions— providers of medical care for this group of patients, such as nurses, general practitioners and dermatologists, and also society at large can be objects of psychological intervention and research.

NOTES

[1]Address for correspondence: A. A. Kaptein, Department of General Practice, Leiden University, PO Box 2088, 2301 CB Leiden, The Netherlands.

REFERENCES

Albers, H. J. (1985). Psychological dilemma and management of the acne patient. In: Cullen, S. I. (Ed.) *Focus on Acne Vulgaris*. London: Royal Society of Medicine Services, pp. 27–34.

Bandura, A. (1982). Self-efficacy mechanism in human agency. *American Psychologist*, **37**, 122–147.

Baughman, R. and Sobel, R. (1971). Psoriasis, stress, and strain. *Archives of Dermatology*, **103**, 599–605.

Benoit, L. J. and Harrell, E. H. (1980). Biofeedback and control of skin cell proliferation in psoriasis. *Psychological Reports*, **46**, 831–839.

Bremer-Schulte, M., Cormane, R. H., Dijk, E. van and Wuite, J. (1985). Group therapy of psoriasis. Duo formula group treatment (DFGT) as an example. *Journal of the American Academy of Dermatology*, **12**, 61–66.

Coen-Buckwalter, K. (1982). The influence of skin disorders on sexual expression. *Sexuality and Disability*, **5**, 98–106.

Cole, W. C., Roth, H. L. and Sachs, L. B. (1988). Group psychotherapy as an aid in the medical treatment of eczema. *Journal of the American Academy of Dermatology*, **18**, 286–291.

Cossidente, A. and Sarti, M. G. (1984). Psychiatric syndromes with dermatologic expression. *Clinic in Dermatology*, **2**, 201–220.

Dion, K., Berscheid, E. and Walster, E. (1972). What is beautiful is good. *Journal of Personality and Social Psychology*, **24**, 285–290.

Duller, P. and Veen-Viëtor, M. van (1986). Psychosocial aspects. In Mier, P. D. and van de Kerkhof, P. C. M. (Eds) *Textbook of Psoriasis*. Edinburgh: Churchill Livingstone, pp. 84–95.

Dungey, R. K. and Buselmeier, T. J. (1982). Medical and psychosocial aspects of psoriasis. *Health and Social Work*, **7**, 140–147.

Faulstich, M. E. and Williamson, D. A. (1985). An overview of atopic dermatitis: Toward a bio-behavioural integration. *Journal of Psychosomatic Research*, **29**, 647–654.

Faulstich, M. E., Williamson, D. A., Duchmann, E. G., Conerly, S. L. and Brantley, P. J. (1985). Psychophysiological analysis of atopic dermatitis. *Journal of Psychosomatic Research*, **29**, 415–417.

Finlay, A. Y. and Kelly, S. E. (1987). Psoriasis—an index of disability. *Clinical and Experimental Dermatology*, **12**, 8–11.

Flanders, P. A. and McNamara, J. R. (1985). Enhancing acne medication compliance: A comparison of strategies. *Behavior Research and Therapy*, **23**, 225–227.

Friman, P. C., Finney, J. W. and Christophersen, E. R. (1984). Behavioral treatment of trichotillomania: An evaluative review. *Behavior Therapy*, **15**, 249–265.

Garrie, S. A. and Garrie, E. V. (1978). Anxiety and skin diseases. *Cutis*, **22**, 205–208.

Gil, K. M., Keefe, F. J., Sampson, H. A., McCaskill, C. C., Rodin, J. and Crisson, J. E. (1987). The relation of stress and family environment to atopic dermatitis symptoms in children. *Journal of Psychosomatic Research*, **31**, 673–684.

Gray, S. G. and Lawlis, G. F. (1982). A case study of pruritic eczema treated by relaxation and imagery. *Psychological Reports*, **51**, 627–633.

Gupta, M. A., Gupta, A. K. and Haberman, H. F. (1987a). The self-inflicted dermatoses: A critical review. *General Hospital Psychiatry*, **9**, 45–52.

Gupta, M. A., Gupta, A. K. and Haberman, H. F. (1987b). Psoriasis and psychiatry: An update. *General Hospital Psychiatry*, **9**, 157–166.

Haynes, S. N., Wilson, C.C., Jaffe, P. G. and Britton, B. T. (1979). Biofeedback treatment of atopic dermatitis. Controlled case studies of eight cases. *Biofeedback and Self-Regulation*, **4**, 195–209.

Henley, L. A. (1981). Psoriasis. *British Medical Journal*, **282**, 1851–1852.

Hughes, H., Brown, B. W., Lawlis, G. F. and Fulton, J. E. (1983). Treatment of acne vulgaris by biofeedback—relaxation and cognitive imagery. *Journal of Psychosomatic Research*, **27**, 185–191.

Jowett, S. and Ryan, T. (1985a). Skin disease and handicap: An analysis of the impact of skin conditions. *Social Science and Medicine*, **20**, 425–429.

Jowett, S. and Ryan, T. (1985b). Dermatology patients and their doctors. *Clinical and Experimental Dermatology*, **10**, 246–254.

Lehman, R. E. (1978). Brief hypnotherapy of neurodermatitis: A case with four-year follow-up. *The American Journal of Clinical Hypnosis*, **21**, 48–51.

Logan, R. A. (1988). Self help groups for patients with chronic skin diseases. *British Journal of Dermatology*, **118**, 505–508.

Manuso, J. S. J. (1977). The use of biofeedback-assisted hand warming training on the treatment of chronic eczematous dermatitis of the hands: A case study. *Journal of Behavior Therapy and Experimental Psychiatry*, **8**, 445–446.

Marks, R. (1985). Acne—social impact and health education. *Journal of the Royal Society of Medicine*, **78** (Suppl. 10), 21–24.

McSkimming, J., Gleeson, L. and Sinclair, M. (1984). A pilot study of a support group for parents of children with eczema. *Australian Journal of Dermatology*, **25**, 8–11.

Medansky, R. (1980). Dermatopsychosomatics: An overview. *Psychosomatics*, **21**, 195–200.

Melin, L., Frederiksen, T., Noren, P. and Swebilius, B. G. (1986). Behavioural treatment of scratching in patients with atopic dermatitis. *British Journal of Dermatology*, **115**, 467–474.

Montagu, A. (1986). *Touching—the Human Significance of the Skin*, 3rd edn. New York: Harper and Row.

Morse, R. M., Perry, H. O. and Hurt, R. D. (1985). Alcoholism and psoriasis. *Alcoholism: Clinical and Experimental Research*, **9**, 396–399.

Office of Population Censuses and Surveys (1974). *Morbidity Statistics from General Practice. Second National Study 1970–1971*. London: Office of Population Censuses and Surveys.

Parish, L. C. and Fine, E. (1985). Alcoholism and skin disease. *International Journal of Dermatology*, **24**, 300–301.

Pinkerton, S. S., Hughes, H. and Wenrich, W. W. (1982). Skin disorders. In: Pinkerton, S. S., Hughes, H. and Wenrich, W. W. (Eds) *Behavioral Medicine—Clinical Applications*. New York: Wiley, pp. 248–260.

Porter, J. R., Beuf, A. H., Lerner, A. and Nordlund, J. (1986). Psychosocial effect of vitiligo: A comparison of vitiligo patients with 'normal' control subjects, with psoriasis patients, and with patients with other pigmentary disorders. *Journal of the American Academy of Dermatology*, **15**, 220–224.

Ramsay, B. and O'Reagan, M. (1988). A survey of the social and psychological effects of psoriasis. *British Journal of Dermatology*, **118**, 195–201.

Roenigk, R. K. and Roenigk, H. H. (1978). Sex differences in the psychological effects of psoriasis. *Cutis*, **21**, 529–533.

Rosenbaum, M. S. and Ayllon, T. (1981). The behavioral treatment of neurodermatitis through habit-reversal. *Behaviour Research and Therapy*, **19**, 313–318.

Seville, R. H. (1977). Psoriasis and stress. *British Journal of Dermatology*, **97**, 297–302.

Shuster, S., Fisher, G. H., Harris, E. and Binnell, D. (1978). The effect of skin disease on self image. *British Journal of Dermatology*, **99**, 18–19.

Spanos, N. P., Stenstrom, R. J. and Johnston, J. C. (1988). Hypnosis, placebo, and suggestion in the treatment of warts. *Psychosomatic Medicine*, **50**, 245–260.

Stankler, L. (1981). The effect of psoriasis on the sufferer. *Clinical and Experimental Dermatology*, **6**, 303–306.

Updike, J. (1976). From the journal of a leper. *The New Yorker*, July 19, 28–33.

Weinstein, M. Z. (1984). Psychosocial perspective on psoriasis. *Dermatologic Clinics*, **2**, 507–515.

Zachariae, H. (1986). Epidemiology and genetics. In: Mier, P. D. and van de Kerkhof, P. C. M. (Eds) *Textbook of Psoriasis*. Edinburgh: Churchill Livingstone, pp. 4–12.

CHAPTER 16

Cancer

A. L. Couzijn,[1,2] W. J. G. Ros and J. A. M. Winnubst

Utrecht University, Utrecht

ABSTRACT

The psychological and social problems which cancer patients and their families encounter are considered under four headings: the diagnostic period, the treatment phase, the terminal phase, and the period of surviving cancer. Some epidemiological data on the incidence and prevalence of various types of cancer are presented.

In the section concerning the process of diagnosing cancer, the authors describe psychological reactions, psychological and social morbidity in patients and their families, and the importance of information and social support. In the second phase, treatment, psychological reactions are described and behavioural interventions—supportive group therapy, patient education, coping skills training—are elaborated upon. Results of research on this topic are provided. Special emphasis is given to pain and the burden for the family during the treatment phase. In the terminal phase, the process of anticipatory grieving, quality of life issues, and terminal care are described. Finally, patients who survive cancer present an increasingly important category in which the value of behavioural assessment and treatment should be explored further by psychologists. Some intervention studies on this subject are presented.

The authors conclude that more psychological research is needed to gain insight into the problems of cancer patients and their families, in order to develop adequate intervention methods in the various stages of illness and medical treatment.

Behavioural Medicine
Edited by A. A. Kaptein, H. M. van der Ploeg, B. Garssen, P. J. G. Schreurs and R. Beunderman
© 1990 John Wiley & Sons Ltd.

INTRODUCTION

The word 'cancer' stands for various diseases which differ widely in cause, course, prognosis, complaints and treatment modalities. Research has shown that the general public is inclined to underestimate the incidence of cancer and the effectiveness of treatment (Weisman, 1981). Generally cancer is associated with serious pain and continuous invalidism.

A quarter of all deaths in western countries are due to neoplastic disease (Parkin, Stjernsward and Muir, 1984). Since breast cancer for women and lung cancer for men are the most frequent types, we will give some figures on these. The yearly incidence of breast cancer is 87 per 100,000 in North America and 84 per 100,000 in western Europe (Parkin, Stjernsward and Muir, 1984). The prognosis is strongly dependent on how far the cancer has advanced. Approximately 40–50% of patients with breast cancer have the cancer spread to axillary nodes. For these patients five-year relapse-free survival is about 40%. For patients with negative nodes five-year relapse-free survival is approximately 75% (Hellman *et al.*, 1982). For men, the yearly incidence of lung cancer is 68 per 100,000 in North America and 87 per 100,000 in western Europe (Parkin, Stjernsward and Muir, 1984). Five-year survival of lung cancer is 8% for men; many patients die within one year. In 17% lung cancer is diagnosed as local. Five-year survival is then estimated at 28% for men (Minna, Higgins and Glatstein, 1982).

These figures give an indication of the magnitude and variety of care to be provided for cancer patients. Since many patients cannot be cured, they must be cared for.

The course of cancer is difficult to predict, due to differences in prognosis, treatment, effect of treatment, rapidity of deterioration, symptoms (as a result of both illness and treatment) and physical invalidism. The physician cannot be very specific about the prospects of an individual patient because of the unpredictable character of the disease and the treatment. Therefore, cancer patients have in common great uncertainty about the course of the illness and the possible prospect of a period of suffering and often eventually death.

In addition to the severe problems that may be caused by the often very serious physical aspects of cancer, the patient is confronted with consequences of a social and financial nature.

For people in the direct proximity of the patient, cancer also has many consequences. First and foremost there are the family members of the patient. They need time to adjust emotionally to the changed situation. Besides that, they are especially heavily burdened if the patient needs a lot of care and cannot perform certain daily chores within the family.

In this chapter we will consider the psychological and social problems a cancer patient and his family encounter. First we will deal with the period associated with the diagnosis and describe which reactions are considered normal and which are pathological and thus require treatment. Then we will consider the phase which centres around treatment, which comprises the period after the initial diagnosis up until either the disease is clearly terminal and death is imminent or survival has become probable. Problems and interventions will be discussed. Third, the terminal phase will be described. Anticipatory grieving and terminal care and quality of life will be discussed. Finally, we will deal with the problems of survivors of cancer. Throughout the chapter attention will be given not only to the patient but also to the family.

THE DIAGNOSIS 'CANCER'

Psychological Reactions

For most patients the diagnosis 'cancer' will be followed by what Weisman (1979) refers to as an acute 'existential crisis' because of the association of cancer with death. This crisis is marked by shock, uncertainty, confusion, anxiety, sorrow and depression (Weisman, 1979; Northouse, 1984). The family members of a patient experience a similar crisis (Thomas, 1978). Individual differences in coping with the diagnosis will show in the degree of denial, anger, aggression and bargaining. This crisis may last from a few days up to several months. Often grief reactions are noticed in patients soon after the diagnosis of cancer is made. This grief may find expression in either an angry or a fearful depression. It is the length of time over which such a depression occurs that distinguishes between a grief-related depression and a longer-term depression for which a cancer patient should be referred to a psychologist or psychiatrist (Kriesel, 1987).

Furthermore, Kriesel points to the fact that a patient's coping mechanisms in dealing with the diagnosis 'cancer' are the same as used in other situations (Kriesel, 1987). Likewise, certain aspects of personality make a person more vulnerable to stress. Worden and Sobel (1978) showed that people who suffer from reduced self-esteem are also more susceptible to stress caused by a chronic or life-threatening disease. Health care professionals should take this individual variance into account in their dealings with the patient and his/her family.

Information

Information is important in coping with a diagnosis of cancer, because lack of knowledge about the disease, the course of the illness, the treatment and the medical system seem to add to stress and problems for the patient (Krumm, Vanatta and Sanders, 1979).

It is difficult to find out what a cancer patient really wants to know about the disease. Research on supplying information gives no unequivocal answer to the question whether or not everything should be told. Patients with a relatively good prognosis seem to be better off (that is to say they experience less anxiety and tension) with information than do patients with a bad prognosis (Gordon *et al.*, 1980; Jacobs *et al.*, 1983).

A study with 79 cancer patients shows that patients want information about their disease and treatment from their physicians (Dunkel-Schetter, 1984). Patients stated that too much information was never a reason for a negative judgement about the doctor or the hospital: on the contrary, too little information was. The complaint was often that medical care was given without emotional support. Patients described their doctors as too cold, too clinical and insensitive to the emotions of the patient. In conclusion, whatever information is given, the way in which it is presented is of major importance.

Also, it is important for information to be given in different ways and repeatedly, because not all information can be absorbed at once. Information in writing is effective because people can reread the information at home. A study in Canada demonstrated that patients who received an information booklet prior to their first visit to an outpatient clinic of a cancer centre felt less overwhelmed and better informed than patients who were given the same booklet during their first visit (Hutchcroft *et al.*, 1984).

In addition, a patient may be limited because he cannot cope (at that moment) with the meaning of the information. At such a time denial is a healthy defence mechanism. It enables the patient to cope with the information gradually. It is important to stress that such reactions may (re)appear at different moments in various degrees. Thus the situation may occur that a physician has had an open and clear talk with the patient about his illness, yet at the next visit the patient appears completely ignorant. This is also true for family members. A check at the beginning of a visit as to the state of knowledge of the patient, and of the family members, can prevent misunderstandings and unpleasant situations. It is definitely advisable to have several consultations with the family members as well.

Kriesel (1987) stresses that sharing the diagnosis is much more than simply the delivery of information. A genuine dialogue may help the patient in coping with the diagnosis and in his attitude towards treatment. The point is stressed that the ordinary mode of conversation is not adequate for doctor–patient communication. Rather, it is suggested that, after each piece of information the physician presents, the patient is asked what he or she has heard and, if needed, the information is clarified.

Communication between doctors is indispensable in order to avoid the risk that the patient is given contradictory information (Sangster, Gerace and Hoddinott, 1987).

Family

The consequences of a life-threatening disease are not only limited to the patient. Those involved with the patient also bear the consequences. One of the main problems for the family members is the feeling of being excluded from care (Northouse, 1984). Family members also have a need for information from physicians (Kriesel, 1987), but this need is certainly not always met (Bond, 1982; Speedling, 1980). Krant and Johnston point to the fact that communication between the doctor and the family members during the time the diagnosis is made is indicative of the amount of contact between the doctor and the family in later phases of the illness and of the amount of support felt to be given by the doctor (Krant and Johnston, 1977–78).

Social Support

Research in the field of health and stress indicates more and more strongly that social support is of major importance in coping with serious events (Taylor et al., 1986). Coping with cancer starts the moment the diagnosis is made and continues even when the patient is considered cured. A patient may receive social support from various people. Important sources are the direct environment of the patient, such as the spouse and the family, but also friends, neighbours, colleagues, acquaintances and, especially for cancer patients, (para)medical personnel (Wortman, 1984).

A distinction is made between emotional support, with the accent on understanding, instrumental support, which deals with acquiring help, and informational support, which is concerned with adequate information. The effectiveness of each type of support seems in part dependent on the source. In a study on cancer patients it has been reported that information pertaining to illness and treatment has a more positive effect when given by the medical network rather than by the family network. Emotional support was perceived as helpful regardless of whether it came from family, friends or medical personnel (Dunkel-Schetter, 1984).

An alternative to dealing with cancer through family, friends and medical caregivers is provided by social support groups. A study which evaluated six structured group counselling sessions for 30 newly diagnosed adult patients with advanced cancer showed that shortly after counselling the patients had a significantly more positive self-concept, better hospital adjustment and more knowledge of the disease as compared to 30 matched control subjects (Ferlic, Goldman and Kennedy, 1979). Another study compared the long-term (i.e. one year) benefits of a thematic counselling model used as a structure for group support and for individual counselling. The patients were women newly diagnosed with gynaecological cancer and were assessed within one month of diagnosis (i.e. before counselling), immediately after counselling, and again six months later (i.e. about one year after diagnosis). Both counselling groups showed significantly more improvement than the controls on the three focal areas of counselling, namely, information about illness, resumption of participation in sexual relationships and return to participation in leisure activities. Group and individual counselling were found to be equally effective (Cain et al., 1986).

Psychological Morbidity

In a study of newly diagnosed cancer patients aiming at preventive intervention for patients at risk of developing psychosocial problems, 33% of the patients were shown to have high emotional distress (Worden and Weisman, 1984). It is remarkable that in the literature on survivors of cancer a similar percentage of psychological morbidity is mentioned (Bos-Branolte et al., 1988). Another recent study (Houts et al., 1986) presents the finding that for 25% of patients with cancer the most frequently mentioned unmet need is 'help in dealing with emotional problems'. This would seem to indicate that about a quarter to one third of the cancer population has so much trouble in coping with the disease that intervention is called for.

It should be noted that in several studies on psychiatric disorders in cancer patients, much higher percentages are found. As Stam, Bultz and Pittman (1986) point out, this seems due to two factors. One is the fact that such studies use the DSM-III classification of psychiatric disorders, which does not take into account the specific somatic aspects of a chronically ill population and thus will give a higher incidence of mental disorders. The other factor is that in these studies frequently the assessment is made within three months of diagnosis; this period is generally considered to be the most distressing (De Haes and Van Knippenberg, 1985; Cassileth et al., 1984). Assessment during that period, will cause inflation of the percentage of mental disorders. Therefore the percentage of 20–33% seems to be a realistic indication of psychological morbidity in the diagnostic phase of cancer. As Weisman and Worden (1984) state, there are generally three approaches to psychological intervention for cancer patients. One is to provide services to everyone, the other is to wait and see and refer a patient once he/she has serious psychological problems and the third is aimed at preventive mental health. Generally, the second option is used.

In view of what has been stated above, it seems not only worthwhile but plainly imperative that a screening instrument is devised to identify patients that are at risk of psychological morbidity. Taylor et al. (1986) give another reason for doing so. They point to the finding that support group attenders, while bothered more by cancer-related and general concerns than non-attenders, show less psychological distress than non-attenders. They give two possible explanations of this curious finding. One is that support group attenders show less distress because the support group is helping them solve cancer-related and other concerns. The other is that perhaps the use of a social support group causes a person to make mountains out of molehills. This would seem to indicate that help should be offered and used selectively only by those in real need of it, since for some people negative effects may occur.

Worden and Weisman (1984) developed a screening instrument for assessing high *versus* low emotional distress in newly diagnosed cancer patients and designed two interventions for the high-distress group. The screening took place within 10 days of the initial diagnosis; intervention followed shortly thereafter and follow-up was at two, four, six and 12 months. The interventions were based on the findings in previous descriptive research (Weisman and Worden, 1976), in which the authors identified specific coping deficits in the group of highly distressed newly diagnosed patients. The patients did not have significantly *more* problems than the low distress group, but lacked the ability to generate strategies to cope adequately with them, thus leading to more distress. One of the interventions was based on a psychotherapeutic model. The focus was on specific problems the patient was currently facing and on ways to handle such problems. The other intervention was more didactic, based on cognitive skills training programmes and behaviour therapy. The focus was on common problems that cancer patients encounter in the course of the illness. For the intervention groups, emotional distress at the end of the intervention was found to be significantly lower and problem-solving capacities significantly higher. No significant difference was found between the two interventions in their effectiveness in reducing distress.

PERIOD OF TREATMENT

This phase is characterized by further medical diagnostic procedures and treatment that may be either curative or palliative. In this chapter we consider this phase to comprise the whole period of treatment as long as the disease is not clearly terminal and death imminent, nor has survival become probable.

Psychological Reactions

Psychologically the transition between the first period of coping with the diagnosis and the period of—in the words of Weisman (1979)—accommodation and mitigation is a gradual one. At first, frequent visits to physicians and hospitals for in- and/or outpatient treatment severely disrupt daily life and form a psychological burden in addition to the physical consequences of illness and treatment. Then, gradually, most patients will get back into (part of) their daily routine. Especially if a period of remission follows, some patients will feel relatively tranquil and less preoccupied with the disease and will be able to lead their life more or less in the same way as before their illness; others will have to make more adjustments due to changes in physical status (e.g. after surgery).

When it becomes evident that the disease is progressive and treatment is no longer effective, the unavoidable expectation of death causes another period of great anxiety in which reactions such as fear, aggression and denial, as in the phase of existential crisis, are not uncommon.

Psychological Interventions

Intervention strategies can be divided into three types: supportive group therapy, patient education and training in coping skills (Telch and Telch, 1985).

The majority of psychological interventions focus on the effect of *supportive group therapy* (Taylor *et al.*, 1986). The underlying idea is that group support and the possibility of sharing fear, needs and worries with other patients has a positive effect. A research project has been described involving a group of women with advanced breast cancer (Spiegel, Bloom and Yalom, 1981). This group met once a week over a year to talk about their problems and experiences with cancer. It was found after a year that these women were less tense, less depressed, less tired and less anxious than a control group which had not partaken in such a group.

Methodologically, the informal and unstructured character of support groups gives rise to measurement problems in assessing effects of treatment. It is difficult to determine what causes the effects that are found. Yet, there are indications that the positive effect of supportive groups for patients lies in becoming aware of the fact that other people too experience similar problems and that one is not unique in feelings of fear and insecurity. Results of recent Dutch research with groups of cancer patients confirm the favourable effect that the sharing and learning of each other's experiences has (Van den Borne, Pruyn and Van den Heuvel, 1987).

Despite the potential benefits of social support groups, such groups are utilized only by a distinct minority of cancer patients, namely, one that is disproportionally white and female, with high socioeconomic status: the same individuals that also use traditional mental health services (Taylor *et al.*, 1986).

Intervention by means of *patient education* assumes that psychological stress which accompanies physical illness is in part due to a lack of knowledge about the disease, the course of the illness, the treatment and the medical system (Krumm, Vanatta and Sanders, 1979). Therefore fear and other symptoms of stress will diminish as knowledge and information increase. Intervention may consist of written material, films, audiotapes and educational groups, with subjects such as the hospital system, medical terminology, description of the illness, treatment and side-effects, aetiology and the doctor–patient relationship. A study in which patients with Hodgkin's disease were prepared by sending them a 27-page information booklet to their home address showed that they were less anxious, had fewer problems concerning the treatment, were less depressed, experienced less disruption in their lives, and finally that their knowledge of the disease was greater as compared to patients who did not receive such a booklet (Jacobs *et al.*, 1983).

Training in coping skills aims at teaching specific behavioural and cognitive skills. This approach presumes that stress is caused partly by a too limited or ineffective set of skills for coping with stress. Cancer patients are taught mainly relaxation techniques and self-instruction procedures.

A number of researchers have been studying a very troublesome phenomenon, namely, nausea and vomiting due to and in anticipation of chemotherapy. Pharmacologically caused nausea and vomiting usually begins one or two hours following chemotherapy and lasts from six to 12 hours up to several days. Conditioned nausea and vomiting is thought to develop through a classical conditioning process in which anxiety plays a critical potentiating role (Burish and Carey, 1986). It can occur before, during and after chemotherapy. Approximately 18% (Nicholas, 1982) to 57% (Jacobsen, Redd and Holland, 1985) of the patients who receive chemotherapy are bothered by anticipatory nausea and vomiting (Morrow and Morrell, 1982; Redd, Andresen and Minagawa, 1982).

Both the effect of progressive muscle relaxation (Lyles *et al.*, 1982) and of muscle relaxation in combination with hypnotic relaxation (Redd, Andresen and Minagawa, 1982) was positive. Not only did anticipatory nausea and vomiting decrease, but nausea and vomiting after treatment were less severe and frequent as well. Cognitive/attentional distraction in the form of playing video games resulted in significantly less nausea in paediatric cancer patients receiving chemotherapy (Redd *et al.*, 1987).

That relaxation techniques can be quite effective in improving mood and in reducing anxiety and depression is well illustrated by a study on relaxation and relaxation plus imagery in early breast cancer patients (Bridge *et al.*, 1988).

Other frequently used behavioural interventions are hypnosis and systematic desensitisation. Data suggest that behavioural interventions can be highly effective for reducing and even preventing much of the distress accompanying cancer chemotherapy, including conditioned nausea and vomiting (Burish and Carey, 1986). It is beyond the scope of this chapter to review behavioural interventions in more detail. For excellent review articles see Burish and Carey (1984) and Burish, Redd and Carey (1985).

Pain

A special problem in patients with cancer is the management of pain. It is indicated that moderate to severe disease-related pain is experienced by 40% of adult patients in the intermediate stages of cancer and by 60–80% of those in the advanced stages (Bonica, 1980). In a Dutch study it was found that 45% of a group of cancer patients (unselected for cancer type, stage or source of pain) reported having pain (Dorrepaal *et al.*, 1986). The intensity of pain was not markedly different in the hospital from at home. In 65% of the cases it was found that the patient's mood was influenced by pain. In 25% of the cases sleeping problems were aggravated by pain. Further, 50% of the patients indicated that they used little or no analgesics, fearing, often irrationally, side-effects and addiction. Another reason was the fear that later on 'when it would really be necessary' the painkillers would no longer be effective. In 54% of the cases in that same study, medical pain management was judged to be inadequate. Therefore it seems that more attention should be paid to adequate (medical) pain management in the various kinds of medical training for doctors. It is of major importance to inform the patient, particularly when he is at home, about (side-) effects of analgesics and to remove unjustified fears about this.

Jay, Elliott and Varni (1986) point to the paucity of controlled investigations on psychological interventions for cancer-related pain, although interventions such as hypnosis, cognitive restructuring and biofeedback seem promising.

The Family During the Treatment Phase

Adapting to the changed situation is one of the major tasks for family members. Often changes in roles and lifestyle within the family take place, because the patient may not be able to perform certain tasks, needs care, and so forth (Meyerowitz, Watkins and Sparks, 1983; Silberfarb, Maurer and Grouthamel, 1980). For the sake of their own health, family members must continue life, including enjoying things and having fun. Frequently this proves to be rather complicated. If the patient exclusively gets all the attention, resentment and anger towards the patient may occur (Thomas, 1978; Wortman and Dunkel-Schetter, 1979). If family members do take time for themselves, feelings of guilt towards the patient are not merely hypothetical.

Open communication about the illness within the family seems desirable both for the patient and for the family members. A 'conspiracy of silence' may have long-lasting negative effects for the family members (Kriesel, 1987). Patients who receive little support are anxious more frequently and experience more problems than patients who can speak openly about their uncertainties and who feel they receive emotional support from their family (Lichtman, Wood and Taylor, 1982). However, this may not be within everyone's reach. It is reported by several investigators that up to 50–55% of patients indicate the desire to speak more openly with their family members or spouse about the cancer (Taylor et al., 1986; Bos-Branolte, 1987).

TERMINAL PHASE

There is no one definition of when cancer is terminal. We shall here adopt the meaning which seems most commonly used, namely, when the disease can no longer be treated—except palliatively—and death has become inevitable. In the literature on terminal cancer patients, definitions are not given explicitly but can be inferred. For example, of the sample of terminal cancer patients in the National Hospice Study (Mor, 1987), 89% died within six months, with a median survival of 39 days. We will discuss the following topics: anticipatory grieving, terminal care, and quality of life. Also the impact on the family will be considered.

Anticipatory Grieving

Hermann (1985) defines anticipatory grieving as the process by which patients and families begin to mourn in advance of the actual death. It begins when death is perceived as inevitable and that may be as early as the initial diagnosis. Behavioural clues that this process has started are, for example, expressions of sadness and crying, acceleration of life review processes and a compressed sense of time (Kriesel, 1987). Although anticipatory grieving is a process which has been described regarding the family in the first place, several authors point to the fact that patients also experience this (Kriesel, 1987; Paterson, 1987). Patients grieve not only over the final loss of their life, but also over the partial losses they undergo in the course of the illness, such as loss of bodily parts and physical capability but also of autonomy.

Quality of Life and Terminal Care

In the National Hospice Study (NHS) a vast amount of data on psychological issues has been gathered concerning cancer patients, including terminal cancer patients. Of the many reports using these data, we will select a number of findings which are particularly relevant for this chapter (Greer et al., 1986; Mor, 1987; Morris and Sherwood, 1987; Morris et al., 1986). Except for pain and symptom control, which may be better in the inpatient hospice setting, patients' quality of life was found to be similar in the hospice to that in conventional care systems. Hospice care is less costly and more likely to keep patients in their home environments than conventional care (Greer *et al.*, 1986). However, since two-thirds of the terminal sample of cancer patients reported at least some pain, of whom 25% reported severe or worse pain (Mor, 1987), inpatient hospice care would seem required for a considerable percentage of cancer patients as well.

In a study of the quality of life of terminal cancer patients, using three samples of terminal cancer patients (one of the NHS, one of patients in nursing homes and one of patients in the community), it was reported that changes (i.e. deterioration of life quality) among cancer patients in nursing homes were observed about four weeks earlier than in terminal cancer patients in the community (Morris and Sherwood, 1987). Since this could have major implications in deciding the management strategies for terminally ill patients, further research must be done, both to corroborate this finding as well as to gain more insight into the specific process of deterioration of life quality. The findings of several researchers suggest that cancer patients, whether in the community, the hospital or in a nursing home, share a common trajectory of decreased quality of life in most areas during the last few weeks of life (Morris and Sherwood, 1987; Gotay, 1985). Although there are some indications of a decline in quality of life prior to the last few months of life, more research is needed to specify this process.

Family

This phase may constitute a heavy burden for the family as well. Insomnia and fear that the patient will die are mentioned (Vachon *et al.*, 1977). For partners, keeping the house, managing the children and at the same time preparing for the impending loss of the spouse is by no means a light task.

During the process of anticipatory grieving, changes in the intensity of patient–family bond (closer or more distant) are mentioned, as well as the fact that it may create more open communication between family members which enables them to support each other after the patient's death (Kriesel, 1987).

Since lack of forewarning of death is considered a precursor of complicated or pathological grief, it is important to inform the patient and the family that a fatal outcome is likely as soon as this is recognized (Paterson, 1987; Parkes and Weiss, 1983).

SURVIVORS OF CANCER

The problems that a cured cancer patient may encounter are many: impaired psychological and social adjustment, difficulties at work, lack of energy, depression, perceived diminished physical and/or sexual attractiveness, impaired sexual functioning, infertility, medical and life insurance discrimination, work discrimination (Fobair *et al.*, 1986; Cella, 1987).

Psychological Morbidity

In reviewing the literature on the incidence of psychological morbidity after successful treatment of cancer, a similar phenomenon is encountered as in determining the incidence of psychological morbidity when the diagnosis of cancer is first made and during treatment. Some authors claim little or no psychological morbidity (Cella and Tross, 1986), others find percentages of 20–40 (Fobair et al., 1986; Greer and Moorey, 1987; Bos-Branolte et al., 1988). This difference may be due to the use of different measurement instruments (Cella and Tross, 1986). More specifically, when conventional psychiatric instruments are used, few or no differences are found compared to a healthy population. When psychological instruments are used which are especially devised for cancer patients and their specific problems, clear indications are obtained that the experience of cancer may leave scars even many years after cure (Greer and Moorey, 1987; Bos-Branolte, 1987). In their follow-up study on survivors of Hodgkin's disease, Fobair et al. (1986) report that 42% had difficulties at work, 37% complained of persistent lack of energy, 26% considered their physical attractiveness diminished by the illness, sexual function was impaired in 20% and 18% suffered from depression.

Another important issue in many studies on the sequelae of cancer cure is the lack of specificity. That is to say, often the patient sample is not controlled for such important intervening variables as age, site of cancer, prognosis, treatment or time since treatment (see also Cella and Tross, 1986; Cella, 1987).

Interventions

Only some studies on interventions with cured cancer patients use well-specified samples, for example a study on the results of professional psychotherapy for patients who had been in remission for at least six months or were cured of gynaecological cancer (Bos-Branolte, 1987). The author reports that 30% of the patients accepted the offer of psychotherapy. The patients were offered a choice between group psychotherapy, which consisted of eight 90-minute sessions during the course of 10 weeks, and individual psychotherapy, with no fixed number of sessions; individual therapy was started on a weekly basis, the frequency being reduced gradually. Individual therapy was more insight-oriented than group therapy. In both types of psychotherapy the emphasis was on the following items: anxiety, depression, body image, self-esteem, partner/proximity relation, and well-being. The patients that accepted psychotherapy suffered significantly more frequently from severe anxiety and depression than patients who refused such treatment. The author concludes that most of the cured gynaecological cancer patients 'knew' themselves whether they needed psychotherapy. Therefore, the author recommends that screening for patients 'at risk' be done in the form of a diagnostic interview, which should be offered to cancer patients who are cured or in remission approximately 1–2 years after the end of medical treatment. The effects of psychotherapy were evaluated six months after the last session in terms of numbers of patients reporting moderate or severe problems with respect to six variables, namely, anxiety, depression, body image, self-esteem, partner/proximity relation, and well-being. Overall, about two-thirds of the psychotherapy patients had improved, whereas about two-thirds of the untreated patients with severe problems remained unchanged. Individual therapy was found to be more effective than group therapy, especially with respect to anxiety and depression.

Especially in the field of psychosocial care of the cured cancer patient only a beginning has been made. Many careful, well-designed studies are necessary in order to obtain more insight into the problems of these people and their families and to develop appropriate kinds of interventions for the various problems.

CONCLUDING REMARKS

Research on psychological and social problems of cancer patients and their families has shown that the majority of people manage to adapt quite well to cancer. However, a substantial minority of approximately 20–30% continue to have serious psychological problems. Thus the value of a valid and reliable instrument to identify patients and their family at risk of developing psychological morbidity cannot be exaggerated.

In trying to understand the process of coping with cancer it is useful to distinguish various phases of treatment. Psychological reactions of both patient and family at the time the diagnosis has just been made will be different from the reactions during treatment, during the terminal phase and after survival of cancer.

As reactions differ according to what the patient is facing, psychological interventions should be tailored to the various specific problems. For instance, during the period of diagnosis adequate information is extremely important. The majority of interventions during the period of treatment focus on the effect of supportive group therapy. Behavioural interventions seem quite effective in managing anticipatory vomiting and nausea associated with cancer chemotherapy. During the terminal phase anticipatory grieving is important both for the patient and for the family. The field of psychosocial care for survivors of cancer is relatively new.

Psychosocial research is needed to gain more insight into the problems of cancer patients and their families in order to develop adequate intervention methods in the various stages of illness and/or treatment.

NOTES

[1]Addresses for correspondence: A. L. Couzijn, W. J. G. Ros and J. A. M. Winnubst, Department of Clinical and Health Psychology, Utrecht University, Heidelberglaan 1, 3584 CS Utrecht, The Netherlands.
[2]Supported by a grant from 'Koningin Wilhelmina Fonds', No. NUKC 85–30.

REFERENCES

Bond, S. (1982). Communication with families of cancer patients. I.: The relatives and doctors. *Nursing Times*, **78**, 962–965.

Bonica, J. J. (1980). Cancer pain. In: Bonica, J. J. (Ed.) *Pain*. New York: Review Press, pp. 335–362.

Borne, H. W. Van den, Pruyn, J. F. A. and Heuvel, W. J. A. Van den (1987). Effects of contacts between cancer patients on their psychosocial problems. *Patient Education and Counseling*, **9**, 33–51.

Bos-Branolte, G. (1987). Psychological problems in survivors of gynaecological cancer—a psychotherapeutic approach. Doctoral dissertation, De Kempenaer, Oegstgeest. The Netherlands.

Bos-Branolte, G., Rijshouwer, Y. M., Zielstra, E. M. and Duivenvoorden, H. J. (1988). Psychologic morbidity in survivors of gynaecologic cancers. *European Journal of Gynaecologic Oncology*, **9**, 168–177.

Bridge, L. R., Benson, P., Pietroni, P. C. and Priest, R. G. (1988). Relaxation and imagery in the treatment of breast cancer. *British Medical Journal*, **297**, 1169–1173.

Burish, T. G. and Carey, M. P. (1984). Conditioned responses to cancer chemotherapy: Etiology and treatment. In: Fox, B. H. and Newberry, B. H. (Eds) *Impact of Psychoendocrine Systems in Cancer and Immunity*. Toronto, Ontario: Hogrefe, pp. 147–178.

Burish, T. G. and Carey, M. P. (1986). Conditioned aversive responses in cancer chemotherapy patients: Theoretical and developmental analysis. *Journal of Consulting and Clinical Psychology*, **54**, 593–600.

Burish, T. G., Redd, W. H. and Carey, M. P. (1985). Conditioned nausea and vomiting in cancer chemotherapy: Treatment approaches. In: Burish, T. G., Levy, S. M. and Meyerowitz, B. E. (Eds) *Cancer, Nutrition and Eating Behavior: A Biobehavioral Perspective*. Hillsdale, NJ: Erlbaum, pp. 205–224.

Cain, E. N., Kohorn, E. I., Quinlan, D. M., Latimer, K. and Schwartz, P. E. (1986). Psychosocial benefits of a cancer support group. *Cancer*, **57**, 183–189.

Cassileth, B. R., Lusk, E. J., Strouse, T. B., Miller, D. S., Brown, L. L., Cross, P. A. and Tenaglia, A. N. (1984). Psychosocial status in chronic illness: A comparative analysis of six diagnostic groups. *New England Journal of Medicine*, **311**, 506–511.

Cella, D. F. (1987). Cancer survival: Psychosocial and public issues. *Cancer Investigation*, **5**, 59–67.

Cella, D. F. and Tross, S. (1986). Psychological adjustment to survival from Hodgkin's disease. *Journal of Consulting and Clinical Psychology*, **54**, 616–622.

Dorrepaal, K. L., Dam, F. S. A. M. Van, Hanewald, G. J. F. P. and Overweg-van Kints, J. (1986). Pijn bij kanker. *Nederlands Tijdschrift voor Geneeskunde*, **130**, 634–638.

Dunkel-Schetter, C. (1984). Social support and cancer: Findings based on patient interviews and their implications. *Journal of Social Issues*, **40**, 77–98.

Ferlic, M., Goldman, A. and Kennedy, B. J. (1979). Group counseling in adult patients with advanced cancer. *Cancer*, **43**, 760–766.

Fobair, P., Hoppe, R. T., Bloom, J., Cox, R., Varghese, A. and Spiegel, D. (1986). Psychosocial problems among survivors of Hodgkin's disease. *Journal of Clinical Oncology*, **4**, 805–814.

Gordon, W. A., Freidenbergs, I., Diller, L., Hibbard, M., Wolf, C., Levine, L., Lipkins, R., Ezrachi, O. and Lucido, D. (1980). Efficacy of psychosocial intervention with cancer patients. *Journal of Consulting and Clinical Psychology*, **48**, 743–759.

Gotay, C. C. (1985). Why me? Attributions and adjustment by cancer patients and their mates at two stages in the disease process. *Social Science and Medicine*, **20**, 825–831.

Greer, S. and Moorey, S. (1987). Adjuvant psychological therapy for patients with cancer. *European Journal of Surgical Oncology*, **13**, 511–516.

Greer, D. S., Mor, V., Morris, J. N., Sherwood, S., Kidder, D. and Birnbaum, H. (1986). An alternative in terminal care: Results of the national hospice study. *Journal of Chronic Diseases*, **39**, 9–26.

Haes, J. C. J. M. De and Knippenberg, F. C. E. Van (1985). The quality of life of cancer patients: A review of the literature. *Social Science and Medicine*, **20**, 809–817.

Hellman, S., Harris, J. R., Canellos, G. P. and Fisher, B. (1982). Cancer of the breast. In: De Vita, V. T., Hellman, S. and Rosenberg, S. A. (Eds) *Cancer Principles and Practice of Oncology*. Philadelphia, Pennsylvania: J. B. Lippincott, pp. 914–970.

Hermann, J. F. (1985). Psychosocial support: Interventions for the physician. *Seminars in Oncology*, **12**, 467–469.

Houts, P. S., Yasko, J. M., Kahn, B., Schelzel, G. W. and Marconi, K. M. (1986). Unmet psychological, social and economic needs of persons with cancer in Pennsylvania. *Cancer*, **58**, 2355–2361.

Hutchcroft, S., Snodgras, T., Troyan, S. and Wares, C. (1984). Testing the effectiveness of an information booklet for cancer patients. *Journal of Psychosocial Oncology*, **2**, 73–84.

Jacobs, C., Ross, R. D., Walker, I. M. and Stockdale, F. A. (1983). Behavior of cancer patients: A randomized study of the effects of education and peer support groups. *Journal of Clinical Oncology*, **6**, 347–350.

Jacobsen, P. B., Redd, W. H. and Holland, J. C. (1985). Parameters of chemotherapy-induced anticipatory nausea in cancer patients. Paper presented at the meeting of the Society of Behavioural Medicine. New Orleans, LA (March).

Jay, S. M., Elliott, C. and Varni, J. W. (1986). Acute and chronic pain in adults and children with cancer. *Journal of Consulting and Clinical Psychology*, **54**, 601–607.

Krant, M. J. and Johnston, L. (1977–1978). Family members' perception of communication in late stage cancer. *International Journal of Psychiatry in Medicine*, **8**, 203–216.

Kriesel, H. T. (1987). The psychosocial aspects of malignancy. *Primary Care*, **14**, 271–281.

Krumm, S., Vanatta, P. and Sanders, J. (1979). A group for teaching chemotherapy. *American Journal of Nursing*, **16**, 916.

Lichtman, R. R., Wood, J. V. and Taylor, S. E. (1982). Close relationships after breast cancer. Paper presented at the American Psychological Association, Washington DC.

Lyles, J. N., Burish, T. G., Krozley, M. M. G. and Oldham, R. K. (1982). Efficacy of relaxation training and guided imagery in reducing the aversiveness of cancer chemotherapy. *Journal of Consulting and Clinical Psychology*, **50**, 509–524.

Meyerowitz, B., Watkins, I. K. and Sparks, F. C. (1983). Quality of life for breast cancer patients receiving adjuvant chemotherapy. *American Journal of Nursing*, **83**, 232–235.

Minna, J. D., Higgins, G. A. and Glatstein, E. J. (1982). Cancer of the lung. In: De Vita, V. T., Hellman, S. and Rosenberg, S. A. (Eds) *Cancer Principles and Practice of Oncology*. Philadelphia, Pennsylvania: J. B. Lippincott, pp. 396–474.

Mor, V. (1987). Cancer patients' quality of life over the disease course: Lessons from the real world. *Journal of Chronic Diseases*, **40**, 535–544.

Morris, J. N. and Sherwood, S. (1987). Quality of life of cancer patients at different stages in the disease trajectory. *Journal of Chronic Diseases*, **40**, 545–554.

Morris, J. N., Suissa, S., Sherwood, S., Wright, S. M. and Greer, D. (1986). Last days: A study of the quality of life of terminally ill cancer patients. *Journal of Chronic Diseases*, **39**, 9–26.

Morrow, G. R. and Morrell, L. (1982). Behavior treatment for anticipatory nausea and vomiting induced by cancer chemotherapy. *New England Journal of Medicine*, **307**, 1476–1480.

Nicholas, D. R. (1982). Prevalence of anticipatory nausea and emesis in cancer chemotherapy patients. *Journal of Behavioral Medicine*, **5**, 461–463.

Northouse, L. (1984). The impact of cancer on the family: An overview. *International Journal of Psychiatry in Medicine*, **14**, 215–242.

Parkes, C. M. and Weiss, R. S. (1983). *Recovery from Bereavement*. New York: Basic Books.

Parkin, D. M., Stjernsward, J. and Muir, C. S. (1984). Estimates of world wide frequency of twelve major cancers. *Bulletin of the World Health Organisation*, **62**, 163–182.

Paterson, G. W. (1987). Managing grief and bereavement. *Primary Care*, **14**, 403–416.

Redd, W. H., Andresen, G. V. and Minagawa, R. Y. (1982). Hypnotic control of anticipatory emesis in patients receiving cancer chemotherapy. *Journal of Consulting and Clinical Psychology*, **50**, 14–19.

Redd, W. H., Jacobson, P. B., Die Trill, M., Dermatis, H., McEvoy, M. and Holland, J. C. (1987). *Proceedings of the 4th European Conference on Clinical Oncology and Cancer Nursing, Madrid, 1–4 November.*

Sangster, J. F., Gerace, T. M. and Hoddinott, S. N. (1987). Family physicians' perspective of patient care at the London Regional Cancer Clinic. *Canadian Family Physician*, **33**, 71–74.

Silberfarb, P. M., Maurer, L. H. and Crouthamel, C. S. (1980). Psychosocial aspects of neoplastic disease: I. Functional status of breast cancer patients during different treatment regimens. *American Journal of Psychiatry*, **137**, 450–455.

Speedling, E. J. (1980). Social structure and social behavior in an intensive care unit: Patient–family perspectives. *Social Work in Health Care*, **6**, 1–15.

Spiegel, D., Bloom, J. R. and Yalom, I. D. (1981). Group support for patients with metastatic cancer. *Archives of General Psychiatry*, **38**, 527–533.

Stam, H. J., Bultz, B. D. and Pittman, C. A. (1986). Psychosocial problems and interventions in a referred sample of cancer patients. *Psychosomatic Medicine*, **48**, 539–549.

Taylor, S. E., Falke, R. L., Shoptaw, S. J. and Lichtman, R. R. (1986). Social support, support groups and the cancer patient. *Journal of Consulting and Clinical Psychology*, **54**, 608–615.

Telch, C. F. and Telch, M. J. (1985). Psychological approaches for enhancing coping among cancer patients: A review. *Clinical Psychology Review*, **5**, 325–344.

Thomas, S. (1978). Breast cancer: The psychological issues. *Cancer Nursing*, **1**, 53–60.

Vachon, M. L., Freedman, K., Formo, A., Rogers, J., Lyall, W. W. and Freeman, S. (1977). The final illness in cancer: The widow's perspective. *Canadian Medical Association Journal*, **117**, 1151–1153.

Weisman, A. D. (1979). A model of psychosocial phasing in cancer. *General Hospital Psychiatry*, **1**, 187–195.

Weisman, A. D. (1981). Understanding the cancer patient: The syndrome of the caregiver's plight. *Psychiatry*, **44**, 161–168.

Weisman, A. D. and Worden, J. W. (1976). The existential plight in cancer: Significance of the first 100 days. *International Journal of Psychiatry in Medicine*, **7**, 1–15.

Worden, J. W. and Sobel, H. J. (1978). Ego strength and psychosocial adaptation to cancer. *Psychomatic Medicine*, **40**, 585–591.

Worden, J. W. and Weisman, A. D. (1984). Preventive psychosocial intervention with newly diagnosed cancer patients. *General Hospital Psychiatry*, **6**, 243–249.

Wortman, C. B. (1984). Social support and the cancer patient: Conceptual and methodological issues. *Cancer*, **53**, (Suppl.), 2339–2360.

Wortman, C. B. and Dunkel-Schetter, C. (1979). Interpersonal relationships and cancer: A theoretical analysis. *Journal of Social Issues*, **35**, 120–156.

CHAPTER 17

Diabetes Mellitus

L. J. M. Pennings-van der Eerden[1]

Utrecht University, Utrecht

and

A. Ph. Visser

Limburg University, Maastricht

ABSTRACT

This chapter focuses on both major types of diabetes mellitus: insulin-dependent and non-insulin-dependent diabetes mellitus. Psychosocial factors are discussed such as anxiety, depression, stress, locus of control and health beliefs. Attention is given to psychological interventions in managing diabetes: behaviour therapy, patient education, family intervention, group therapy and self-help groups.

INTRODUCTION

Recent developments in the care of patients with diabetes, such as the opportunity of self-monitoring of blood glucose and the attention to diabetes education, have important consequences for psychologists who help patients suffering from this chronic disease. This chapter is intended to introduce the reader to the psychological aspects of these and other issues. The central theme is the patient with diabetes and the patient's management of the illness. The chapter has three main sections: one reports on the disease and its management, another deals with the impact of psychological factors on diabetes and its management, and the last section discusses interventions such as behaviour therapy, patient education, family intervention and the significance of self-help groups.

Behavioural Medicine
Edited by A. A. Kaptein, H. M. van der Ploeg, B. Garssen, P. J. G. Schreurs and R. Beunderman
© 1990 John Wiley & Sons Ltd.

WHAT IS DIABETES MELLITUS?

In 1985 the World Health Organization (WHO) Study Group on Diabetes Mellitus published the revised classification of diabetes mellitus. Two major types of diabetes were distinguished: insulin-dependent (or type I) diabetes mellitus (IDDM), formerly juvenile onset diabetes, and non-insulin-dependent (or type II) diabetes mellitus (NIDDM), formerly adult onset diabetes. NIDDM can be further subclassified into obese and non-obese types, primarily for the reason that 60–80% of NIDDM patients in western countries are obese (Bajaj, 1987). An additional category in the classification of the WHO Study Group is malnutrition-related diabetes mellitus (MRDM), which has been found in a substantial proportion of young people in developing countries in the tropics (WHO, 1985).

Diabetes mellitus is characterized by chronic elevation of the concentration of glucose in the blood, called hyperglycaemia. Although it may occur at any age, insulin-dependent diabetes usually begins before 40 years of age, most often in childhood and adolescence. The disease usually has an abrupt onset, and expresses itself in symptoms such as increased thirst and appetite, excessive urination, and weight loss. The insulin deficiency is absolute, which is why ketoacidosis (i.e. elevated concentrations of fatty acids, glycerol, and ketones in the blood, because glucose cannot be used effectively as a metabolic fuel in the absence of insulin) is a characteristic feature of IDDM. If left untreated, the disease will be fatal. Life can be maintained only with supplemental insulin from external sources.

Non-insulin-dependent diabetes mellitus usually begins after 40 years of age, although it may occur at a younger age. The onset is usually insidious; not infrequently, the diagnosis of diabetes is made in a completely asymptomatic person. Patients with NIDDM are not dependent on insulin, and are not prone to ketoacidosis.

Aetiology

For some IDDM patients, and more often those with NIDDM, there is evidence that the aetiology has a genetic basis (Pyke, 1979). Frequently, environmental factors play a role. There is evidence that infections in IDDM patients, either viral or bacterial, and pancreatic disturbances caused by toxic substances may be responsible (WHO, 1985). In NIDDM patients, environmental factors inherent in the western lifestyle are probably involved, such as an increased life expectancy, food both of poor quality and in large amounts, increased prevalence of obesity, decreased physical activity, and increased stress (Zimmet and Dowse, 1987).

Epidemiology

Epidemiological data of Jarrett (1986) yielded IDDM prevalence rates of approximately 0.2–2.4 per 1000 in the countries of western Europe and the USA, and lower rates of approximately 0.02–0.09 per 1000 in China and Japan. Studies of several populations in western Europe showed incidence rates to be highest in the Scandinavian countries (0.14–0.19/1000) and intermediate in central Europe.

There are no reliable figures on the incidence of NIDDM in western countries, but the data of Zimmet (1982) revealed rates of approximately 1.0/1000. According to the National Commission on Diabetes (1975) of the United States, NIDDM accounts for about 90% of the diabetic population in western countries.

Medical Treatment

The goal of medical treatment of diabetes is to normalize the concentration of glucose in the blood within the following limits: 3.3–5.6 mmol/l under fasting conditions, and not exceeding 10.0 mmol/l after meals (WHO, 1985). Patients with diabetes have a long-term risk of developing progressive damage to the retina, kidney, and the peripheral nerves, and of aggravated atherosclerotic disease of the heart, legs, and brain. Medical research strongly suggests that maintenance of nearly normal levels of blood glucose concentration reduces complications (e.g. Keen and Rifkin, 1987).

Self-monitoring of blood glucose (SMBG) is a relatively new development in diabetes management. Colour changes of reagent strips for blood glucose determination, to be interpreted by the patient, yield a direct measure of the blood glucose concentration. Patients can change blood glucose concentration themselves in order to actively normalize blood glucose levels (i.e. self-regulation). Three main components of diabetes management help normalize blood glucose levels: meal planning, physical exercise, and medication.

Meal planning is the primary element of treatment for all diabetic patients. For the IDDM patient, the timing of meals and snacks needs to be attuned to the insulin injections. The carbohydrate distribution of the food, spread out over the various meals in a day, needs to be adjusted to blood glucose levels and insulin dosage. For the NIDDM patient, timing is less important than the quantity and the composition of the diet. In case of overweight the first objective is to reduce body weight, for which caloric intake needs to be restricted.

The second element, physical exercise, benefits diabetic patients in two ways. It improves the body's absorption of insulin and it benefits the cardiovascular system. For many NIDDM patients, diet adherence combined with exercise can affect blood glucose levels effectively without any medication.

The medication is the third component in diabetes management. The medication of the IDDM patient consists of multiple injections of insulin which are needed on a daily basis to mimic the normal insulin release of the non-diabetic person. During the last decade, progress has been made in perfecting insulin delivery methods such as insulin infusion pumps, pen technique, and needle-less injecting. The continuous subcutaneous insulin infusion (CSII) pump is an alternative insulin injection method that may provide greater lifestyle flexibility, particularly with regard to meal schedules and travel (Chanteleau et al., 1982). Investigations suggest that CSII is demanding for some individuals (Ballegooie et *al.*, 1983), but it also enhances the feeling of well-being (Rudolf *et al.*, 1982) and yields less depression, less anxiety and greater family cohesion (Shapiro *et al.*, 1984). Intensified treatment has recently become possible with the pen technique, leading to better health outcomes and improved psychosocial functioning (Berger *et al.*, 1985). The technique of needleless injection also seems to have benefits as it reduces insulin requirements (Malone *et al.*, 1986). This technique seemed not to be very helpful to the patient, however. Evaluations of this injector for patients with and without needle phobia revealed poor acceptance of the device (Houtzagers *et al.*, 1988).

Most NIDDM patients need either an oral hypoglycaemic agent or insulin. The oral hypoglycaemic agent is needed when the NIDDM patient cannot regulate diabetes without medication. Insulin is needed when an oral agent alone cannot regulate blood glucose levels. NIDDM is often associated with additional physical disorders such as hypertension and cardiac failure. Gries and Alberti (1987) found that medical treatment of these symptoms may be more important for the prevention of complications than blood glucose regulation. In a study by Jenny (1986), NIDDM patients frequently experienced hypertension as a problem, whereas IDDM patients frequently reported they were in poor control.

To summarize, the substances of the medical treatment of IDDM and NIDDM may well differ from each other. However, both treatments require patients to play an active role in regulating the disease: a diabetic patient, especially an IDDM patient, largely has the control of the illness in his own hands.

PSYCHOLOGICAL REACTIONS TO DIABETES AND ITS MANAGEMENT

Diabetes: The Patient's Response

Immediate reactions to the discovery of having IDDM diabetes may encompass grief and mourning, feelings of helplessness and fear of death (e.g. Kovacs and Feinberg, 1982). Anxiety and depression are common reactions, even in long-term diabetic patients (Sullivan, 1978). The sources of anxiety and depression are most often related to fears of the future, and to worries about severe hypoglycaemia with symptoms such as weakness, sweating, irritability, unconsciousness, and convulsions. The possibility of early death and incapacitating complications haunts some patients, and the continuing regime of insulin injections, regular meals and the need for constant vigilance weigh heavily upon the patient and his family (Sanders *et al.*, 1975).

The types of immediate and long-term reactions to having diabetes that occur in IDDM patients have not been found in NIDDM patients. The latter tend to minimize the consequences of having diabetes, perhaps, as Podolsky (1983) suggested, as a consequence of the misconception among health care professionals that NIDDM diabetes is not life-threatening. In the study by Jenny (1986) NIDDM patients compared with IDDM patients showed a tendency to think that self-care behaviour had no positive consequences, and they were less compliant with the prescription regimen. However, both groups were equally motivated to improve health.

An important issue in diabetes mellitus is that exposure to stressful life situations can lead to fluctuations in blood glucose level in IDDM (Kemmer *et al.*, 1986) and NIDDM patients (Naliboff, Cohen and Sowers, 1985). Furthermore, it has appeared that IDDM patients who showed high levels of anxiety and depression (Hauser and Pollets, 1979) and who had poor quality of life scores (Mazze, Lucido and Shamoon, 1984) also had poorer health outcomes compared to IDDM patients with low levels of anxiety and depression. It should be noted that different emotions cause different fluctuations in blood glucose: fear or anger is generally associated with higher blood glucose levels, depression or frustration mostly with lower blood glucose levels, while feelings of happiness also usually result in a fall in blood glucose levels (Cox *et al.*, 1984). The relationship between stress and blood glucose levels is not unidirectional. The reverse pattern also occurs: hyperglycaemia may increase nervous system activity (insulin-regulating stress hormones). Lustman, Carney and Amado (1981) found that hyperglycaemia itself might result in increased feelings of anxiety, depression and a greater susceptibility to environmental stress. In a review of the literature, Czyzewski (1988) argued that an interaction of factors is the most likely explanation of the relationship. According to this author, most of the evidence tends in the direction that psychological stressors 'negatively affect diabetic control when the person is already experiencing metabolic decompensation' (p. 278).

Diabetes is probably perceived as more serious by IDDM subjects than by NIDDM subjects, as it has more negative effects on daily life. These and other stressors can influence metabolic control, and *vice versa*. Health care professionals might facilitate optimal self-management by helping the patient to cope with stress.

Diabetic Self-care and Psychological Predictions

Self-care behaviour includes taking medication (different options for subjects injecting insulin and those taking oral hypoglycaemic agents), diet, physical activity, foot care, testing urine and blood glucose, preventing hypo-/hyperglycaemia and carrying out self-regulative actions (adjustments by the patient in the quantity of food, the amount of insulin or the degree of exercise to normalize blood glucose level). Interindividual differences have been found in self-care behaviour. Pennings-van der Eerden and Schrijvers (1985) found that monitoring of urine glucose and blood glucose in IDDM patients was generally done by the physician alone (49% for urine glucose and 49% for blood glucose). If monitoring was performed by the patients it was often in cooperation with the physician (20% and 29% respectively). Forty-six per cent followed dietary prescriptions. Hypoglycaemia and hyperglycaemia were often treated by diabetic patients themselves (75% and 55% respectively). Ninety-two per cent of the patients performed their insulin administration on time. Seventeen per cent of the patients had never inspected their feet. If it is performed, regulatory action in the event of infection or illness is done by the physician (35%). In the case of stress and physical exercise, diabetic patients take action themselves (52% and 72% respectively). These and other findings among IDDM patients (Holstein, Jorgensen and Sestoft, 1986; Wysocki et al., 1978) as well as NIDDM patients (Ary et al., 1986) indicate some similarity in the occurrence of the components of self-care. Diabetic subjects reported the lowest levels of self-care behaviour in testing urine for glucose, diet and prevention of hyperglycaemia; they reported the highest levels of self-care behaviour in taking medication and preventing hypoglycaemia. Concurrently, Jenny (1986) found that diabetic patients experienced a great many obstacles in adhering to dietary prescription and physical exercise. In a comparative study by Pennings-van der Eerden and Post (1985), 35 elderly IDDM and 40 elderly NIDDM subjects reported equal levels of self-care behaviour. The self-regulative actions of these groups of patients have so far scarcely been studied.

For patients poor self-care behaviour may have a quite rational basis, for example they may not be willing to participate in self-monitoring of blood glucose (SMBG) because they will endure pain, they have poor expectations of its efficacy and like the continued dependency on doctors (Krosnick, 1980). What are predictors of diabetic self-care, when several components of self-care are taken together to measure one concept? Several predictors have been established for an understanding of individual differences in diabetic self-care. It appears that self-care is negatively related to the traditional patient–provider relationship, in which medical workers are active experts while patients remain uninformed and passive (Stone, 1979; Anderson, 1985). An important fact is that knowledge has been found not to be directly related to self-care (e.g. Graber et al., 1977) but is moderated by the conception of the patient–provider relationship. Only if a patient tends to perceive his or her diabetes management as independent of medical practitioners does knowledge predict self-care (Pennings-Van der Eerden, 1988). Locus of control as measured by Rotter's locus of control scale is related to knowledge of diabetes in a special way. Internally controlled patients had more knowledge of diabetes, although this superiority diminished with the duration of the disease. Contrary to prediction, internally controlled diabetic patients seemed to develop more problems with the disease than externally controlled as the disease progressed (Lowery and Ducette, 1976). Edelstein and Linn (1987) found that externally controlled individuals were more receptive to instructions than internally controlled patients, who tended to be more autonomous in learning. In neither of the locus of control studies did it become clear if knowledge and locus of control were related to levels of self-care. Finally, in a questionnaire with an open response format, Jenny (1986) found that barriers to self-care behaviour were generated by discomfort, low self-efficacy and lack of planning in self-care activities.

Next we shall discuss variables brought together into theoretical models, the health belief model (HBM) and the behavioural intention model (BIM). The health belief model as applied to diabetic patients emphasizes that they will not perform self-care behaviour unless they have at least a minimal level of motivation and knowledge, see themselves as vulnerable to complications and the illness as threatening (Bloom-Cerkoney and Hart, 1979; Alogna, 1980), are convinced of health behaviour's efficacy and perceive few barriers to action (Harris and Linn, 1985). Harris and Linn (1985) also found health beliefs to be significantly associated with physiological measures. A second model, the behavioural intention model of Fishbein and Ajzen (1975), predicts behaviour by a person's intention to perform or not perform the behaviour, which is a function of two basic determinants: the attitude towards the behaviour (behavioural beliefs) and the person's perception of social pressure to perform or not to perform the behaviour (normative beliefs). This model was partly tested in the case of diabetes mellitus (McCaul, Glasgow and Schafer, 1987; Wilson *et al.*, 1986). Health beliefs specific to the performance of diabetes self-care behaviours (e.g. 'Do you think that testing blood glucose can be helpful in controlling your diabetes?') and social support also specific to the performance of diabetes self-care behaviours proved to be the most important factors in predicting self-care.

PSYCHOLOGICAL INTERVENTIONS

Several psychological interventions are available for diabetic patients, such as behaviour therapy, patient education, family intervention and self-help groups.

Behaviour Therapy

Systematic desensitization is a much applied method of behaviour therapy through which anxiety may be reduced. Leenaars and Rombouts (1986) reported a case study of a 19-year-old male student. This case study provides an example of the use of systematic desensitization of anxiety about being out of diabetic control. The anxiety had arisen after several hypoglycaemic reactions. In an eight-week period, the compulsive self-monitoring of blood glucose (up to four times an hour) of the student was counteracted. Using information gathered from the patient, a set of anxiety-producing stimuli was identified, such as visits to friends at the weekend, eating a snack in the morning, etc. These stimuli were arranged in hierarchical order from most disturbing to least disturbing. The patient was asked to relax, first imaginally and later on actually, when visiting someone. He learned to separate rational thoughts ('I did everything to maintain normal blood glucose, so why should I bother?') from irrational thoughts ('My blood glucose level isn't normal'). During the eight-week training he exercised step by step, resulting in a decrease of self-monitoring activities. After training, the patient no longer felt compulsive in his monitoring behaviour. He generally felt more relaxed; and at a follow-up a year and a half later, the positive results were still present.

This case study offers a clear illustration of the risks of SMBG. The daily performance of SMBG may become a stressor in itself for the patient (Turk and Speers, 1983). Diabetic patients seem to have to balance between fear of metabolic destabilization and rigid self-management behaviour. In patient education, psychologists should be alert to situations in which high levels of self-care turn into unpleasant compulsive behaviour.

There are other major categories of behaviour therapy: biofeedback, physical relaxation, imaginal relaxation and hypnosis. We will discuss two procedures: the most frequently applied intervention in diabetes, EMG biofeedback, and meditation as a form of imaginal relaxation.

Fowler, Budzinsky and VandenBergh (1976) utilized EMG biofeedback and taped relaxation training in a single case study with an IDDM patient for one college semester in an endeavour to lower insulin requirements. During the training period the patient learned to relax her frontalis muscle with a portable EMG feedback unit which produced a click feedback. A cassette tape series was used along with the portable EMG. The patient was encouraged to practise twice each day and to attempt to maintain a relaxed state even when not in the practice situation. The daily use of the portable unit was terminated at the end of the semester. Results indicated a decrease in daily insulin from 85 units to 59 units during training. Follow-up six months later found insulin to be at 43 units per day. The patient herself reported that anxiety and tension levels had decreased. The authors concluded that this kind of training may be effective in patients who are continuously out of control.

Surwit and Feinglos (1983) reported that EMG biofeedback training significantly improved glucose tolerance in NIDDM patients. Twelve patients in poor control were hospitalized on a clinical research ward under identical conditions. Half of the patients were given five days of training with EMG feedback, after which all patients were retested. The training was found to improve glucose tolerance significantly without affecting insulin sensitivity.

Meditation may also improve diabetes control, due to the decline of anxiety and stress. In a non-controlled study, Maras et al. (1984) compared blood glucose tolerance in eight patients with IDDM before, during and after participating in a structured meditation programme which lasted four weeks. Participants received instructions in the use of progressive muscle relaxation techniques. They were given a cassette tape and were instructed to meditate 20 minutes twice daily, following the taped instructions. After learning to recognize the relaxation response, patients were encouraged to develop their own type of meditation to include a personally chosen mantra. The analysis revealed no statistically significant differences in the dosages of insulin and metabolic control measures. But there was a significantly improved perception of well-being as a result of the meditation experience, and stressful situations could be more effectively handled. The authors hypothesized that the poor findings of physical health outcomes were the result of the relatively short training period.

Despite favourable findings in some studies, relaxation therapy as a stress-management procedure has been criticized. Progressive muscle relaxation might cause problems in well-controlled diabetic patients, such as frequent episodes of hypoglycaemia as a consequence of physiological stress-reducing effects (Seeburg and DeBoer, 1980). Czyzewski's review (1988) concluded that methodological problems (e.g. non-random samples, questionable experimental conditions) in several studies are the reason why relaxation therapy has not been proved to enhance the patient's quality of life. Moreover, Czyzewski argued, adding another behaviour to the complicated regimen can increase the probability that patients neglect parts of the regimen. So medical practitioners and other health professionals should be cautious, because a rapid decrease in insulin requirements in the treatment phase can cause not inconsequential problems.

Patient Education and Self-management

When compared to other chronic diseases, the diabetes treatment regimen is remarkable both for its complexity and for the amount of responsibility it places on the patient. Since 1920, when E. P. Joslin and R. D. Lawrence published the first studies on diabetes education, a variety of educational programmes have been developed to improve indirectly the physical condition of patients with diabetes. Recent survey studies show the need for the integration of education with medical treatment of diabetes (Assal et al., 1983; Alogna, 1985). Three examples of evaluation studies of education programmes will be reported here: (a) the first is an evaluation study of education programmes with NIDDM patients; (b) the second study is concerned with education of IDDM and NIDDM patients; and (c) the third study considers the education of physicians and NIDDM patients.

In the first study, Hartwell, Kaplan and Wallace (1986) compared the effects of diet, physical exercise, the combination of diet plus exercise, and non-training (control group) on NIDDM patients. Patients were randomly assigned to one of the four treatment conditions. The 10-week treatment interventions were developed by incorporating principles of both behaviour modification (e.g. contracts, self-monitoring) and cognitive modification strategies (e.g. goal-setting, planning, the use of reinforcements and contingencies, negative and positive self-talk). The findings of the study suggest that a dietary intervention is more efficacious in the management of NIDDM than a short-term physical conditioning programme or a combination of the two. The diet group experienced a decrease in blood glucose, an increase in high-density lipoprotein cholesterol concentration (HDL), and greater weight loss in comparison to the control group. The study did not reveal if normality in blood glucose level had been achieved.

Another set of studies is concerned with education of IDDM and NIDDM patients. Berger, Mühlhauser and Jörgens (1984) described a five-day inpatient IDDM diabetes education programme to normalize blood glucose and decrease hospital admissions. Patients were taught simultaneously in groups up to 10. A central theme in patient education of IDDM patients was the use of regular insulin whereby the patients should be able to adapt their insulin individually according to their daily requirements. The short-term results are mentioned first. The patients were motivated to take responsibility for their metabolic control. They decided the amount of daily insulin injections and learned to adapt their insulin dosage to a variable carbohydrate intake. The patients made continual notes in a diabetes log book and learned to judge the efficacy of using regular insulin dosages.

A one-year follow-up of three groups of consecutively admitted IDDM patients ($N = 205$; mean age 28 yr), without a control group, revealed that HbAlc levels were significantly reduced to a normal range and that hospital admissions and hospital days were significantly reduced, except for patients with late complications (Assal et al., 1985).

In another study, the basis for long-term guidance of NIDDM patients is a structured programme focusing on metabolic self-monitoring (urine glucose), diet and foot care (Mühlhauser et al., 1985). The programme is administered by the physician him/herself to groups of four to 10 of their NIDDM patients (and their partners). Before starting, the physician (and his/her assistant) took an in-service training of four sessions in educating their patients. The first results of the physicians' programme with the patients are encouraging. Significant weight reduction and optimal HDL profiles in patients have been reached, but not better metabolic control yet.

The third study is the 'Diabeds' (Diabetes Education Study), an experimental investigation. Mazzuca et al. (1986) recruited over 500 patients from the general medicine clinic of a university medical centre. Of these patients, 275 participated in the postintervention assessment; 95% of them had NIDDM. Most of them were elderly (m = 58.1 yr), female (79%) and had a medical treatment of 'diet plus insulin' (70%). The patients' physicians usually treated their diabetic patients at fixed time intervals in the clinic. In the study, of which two progress reports are available, researchers investigated to what extent physician education, patient education, or both affected: (a) physicians' and patients' knowledge, attitudes and skills, and (b) relevant physiological and metabolic patient health outcomes. There were four experimental conditions: condition 1 was a control group in which diabetic patients received only diabetes education that was routinely available in the clinic; in condition 2, diabetes patients received a systematic education programme; in condition 3, only physicians and not their patients received a special educational programme; and in condition 4, both physicians and their patients received training programmes.

In this study, patient education was focused on self-care behaviour, but also on patient's health beliefs and attitudes. According to the results of patients' educational diagnosis, they are enrolled in one or more appropriate modules of instruction (e.g. understanding diabetes mellitus, urine testing, diet composition). Each educational module contains three elements: (1) 'didactic instruction' (lecture, discussion, audiovisual presentation), (2) 'skills exercises' (via modelling and feedback), and (3) 'behavioural methods' (individually tailored goal-setting with signed contracts).

In the physician education training programme, clinical knowledge and skills, clinical support systems (e.g. retrospective practice audits of resident adherence to protocols), and attitudes and beliefs about diabetes were all emphasized.

The experimental results showed that patient education yielded positive differences in knowledge and self-care behaviour (patients did not take all modules offered). Unfortunately, beliefs and attitudes were not measured. After patient education only, there was a significant decrease in body weight and a moderate improvement in metabolic control compared with the control group.

When both patients and their physicians participated in education, patient outcomes were significantly improved for fasting plasma glucose, two-hour postprandial blood glucose, glycosylated haemoglobin, diastolic blood pressure and body weight (Vinicor *et al.*, 1987). However, the favourable results with measures of metabolic control should be questioned. After treatment, the means for all groups, despite previous drops, remained high (> 10.0 mmol/l).

There are two problems in judging the results of qualified evaluation studies. The first problem is that a great many programmes in the seventies (and sometimes still now) focus on urine glucose monitoring alone, a kind of direct feedback that is not very helpful to the self-regulation of blood sugar levels. So poor metabolic control in these studies may reflect the poor tools that patients are given (Fischer *et al.*, 1982), rather than unwillingness to comply (Watts, 1980). This might be the case in the studies with NIDDM patients mentioned above. Both groups of patients, IDDM and NIDDM, profit by the opportunity to SMBG (Scott, Beaven and Stafford, 1984).

Another problem in judging the research is that it hardly ever indicates if and how psychological principles were applied in the programmes, as in the three examples mentioned above. Wing *et al.* (1986) reviewed the literature about formative evaluation and concluded that behavioural strategies specifically comprised goal-setting, contingency contracting procedures and feedback. With respect to the summative evaluation, the majority of the behavioural research on self-care has been directed at urine and blood glucose monitoring for IDDM patients, and primarily at weight reduction for NIDDM patients. Other components of the treatment regimen, such as following dietary guidelines in IDDM patients and self-monitoring in NIDDM patients, and foot care and self-regulative behaviours to effect changes in blood glucose level in both groups of patients, have been disregarded (Wing *et al.*, 1986).

Brittle Diabetes and Family Intervention

Brittle diabetes has been defined by Tattersall (1977) as a condition in which the life of a person with diabetes is constantly disrupted by repeated episodes of hypoglycaemia or hyperglycaemia. These patients—less than 5% of those who are insulin-treated—are in good control in the hospital on simple regimens and develop hypoglycaemia or ketoacidosis on returning home (Santiago, 1986). Brittle diabetes mostly occurs in adolescents or young adults. The majority of these patients are dealing with family problems that interfere with treatment (Orr *et al.*, 1986).

Minuchin *et al.* (1975) reported on family therapy strategies with 13 cases of brittle diabetes. With young diabetic patients and their families, the therapist explained the cause of poor control in terms of the family system. Some of the diabetic children in the study grew up in a family that encouraged and maintained 'psychosomatic responses' by using the illness as a point of concentration, or as a method of diffusing system stresses, or both. In these cases it is the family, rather than the child, which develops 'attacks' that challenge medical management. To change the family organization, the family homeostasis is challenged by the therapist. The age of the patient influences the selection of treatment strategies. When working with families in which the identified patient is an adolescent, the therapist will challenge the parents to place themselves in the position of the child, so that they can support the child's right to explore the extrafamilial world. The results of the therapy with 13 diabetic patients yielded a few admissions in hospital after treatment as opposed to over 100 admissions before family therapy. A case of therapy with the family of a 20-year-old IDDM patient was extensively reported by Frey (1984). This author also formulated general phases of the therapy process on the basis of tasks for the therapist.

Some unique characteristics have been found in the families of adolescent brittle diabetic patients, such as involvement with family conflicts, overprotection and excessive care for each other's well-being (Minuchin et al., 1975). Family problems may lead to refusal to supply insulin and sustain dietary prescriptions but these problems in themselves may directly influence fluctuations in blood glucose levels. Treating the family problems can improve metabolic control.

Medical practitioners and other health professionals should be attentive to possible family problems when they encounter adolescents with brittle diabetes. Interventions that modify the life context of the diabetic adolescent seem to achieve a faster and more sustained remission of the problems than interventions that focus exclusively on the individual.

Self-help Groups

In self-help groups, diabetics with a shared problem learn from the example of others while having the gratifying experience of helping others with similar problems. Most groups have a leader who facilitates group interaction by interpretation, focusing the discussion and providing information. Self-help groups may be composed of several kinds of diabetic populations.

1. Diabetic adolescents. Marrero et al. (1982) conducted a controlled study with 23 diabetic adolescents who needed psychosocial support. During the group sessions they practised coping strategies by role-playing and experimentation. The effects consisted of a reduction of depression, an increase in self-esteem and an increase in the size of the social support networks in the experimental group. For some participants, the group sessions were the only place where they could share and explore their problems in the process of adaptation to their illness.
2. Parents of children with diabetes. In volunteer support groups for parents of children with diabetes (Baumgardner et al., 1984), the members meet parents' educational and emotional needs. The group offers the parents a chance for 'sharing, caring and understanding'.
3. Diabetic adults. Patients experience support in gathering knowledge about the disease during group discussions (Groen and Pelser, 1982). In an experimental study (Visser and Bloks, 1980), knowledge about the disease appeared to be significantly enhanced, while anxiety levels decreased. In another controlled study, Van der Boogaard and Boomsma (1983) after group

discussions found significantly decreased external locus of control, which seemed a prerequisite for gains in knowledge and metabolic control.

4. Blind diabetic patients. Oehler-Giarratana and Fitzgerald (1980) reported on group sessions with four adult diabetic patients (< 40 yr) who were going blind. The group intervention comprised seven consecutive weekly two-hour group sessions which helped participants to understand and accept their condition and to begin rehabilitation.

5. Participation in patient organizations. Another kind of interaction between diabetic patients takes place in their patient organizations. The members are supplied with information about coping with the disease in daily life. It has been demonstrated that IDDM and NIDDM patients who are members of the Dutch Diabetes Association get significantly more information about the illness compared with patients who are not members. This information actually resulted in significantly more knowledge about the illness and affected self-care behaviours positively for both IDDM and NIDDM patients. (Pennings-van der Eerden and Post, 1985).

Enrolment in self-help groups seems to play a vital role in coping with diabetes, which is why diabetic patients (and their families) should be encouraged to join self-help groups and to participate in patient organizations.

CONCLUSION

In this chapter we described both types of diabetes mellitus. This chronic illness forms a threatening feature in daily life for patients with insulin-dependent diabetes mellitus as well as for patients with non-insulin-dependent diabetes mellitus, a fact which has psychological implications. Diabetes has a great impact on the lives of the patients with regard to the acceptance of their illness, the organization of the diabetic regimen in daily life, and provisions for the future. Diabetic patients themselves perceive only IDDM as an illness with far-reaching consequences for daily life as compared with NIDDM.

There is a relationship between psychological, environmental and physiological stress and metabolic control: the chicken-and-the-egg problem. Stress may thwart the patients' attempts to normalize blood glucose levels. Relaxation therapy is not recommended as a stress-management procedure. The psychologist should try to teach the patient to cope with stress by the use of other cognitive and behavioural strategies, family intervention, self-help group attendance or patient education.

The patient is required to take responsibility for the management of the illness. Medical treatment alone will not achieve optimal control unless the diabetic patient, especially the IDDM patient, is an active participant. In the research literature we find relatively low levels of self-care behaviour such as diet adherence and physical exercise. Unfortunately, self-regulative actions, which could be presumed to be related to diabetic control, have hardly been studied. These considerations might be one reason for the modest correlations between self-care and physiological outcomes.

Enhancing self-care requires an optimal patient–provider relationship in which the patient is allowed to be (become) relatively independent in controlling the illness. Locus of control, health beliefs and social support are important personality characteristics determining the degree of advancement made.

The major focus of attention in the recent literature on diabetes mellitus is patient education as a part of diabetes care. The modest results in studies so far could possibly be enhanced if some educational principles were better taken into account. First, in constructing a curriculum it is necessary to establish goals explicitly, to analyse all different tasks to be mastered and to choose appropriate didactic methods. Second, there are some behavioural recommendations for the educator concerning the intervention which include: (a) the educator should actively model the desired activities, thereby making them explicit and concrete. (b) The educator should question and clarify beliefs and perceptions of patients in reaching a more appropriate attitude towards self-care behaviour. (c) The patients must have the opportunity to practise the modelled behaviour. (d) The educator should provide feedback tailored to patient's conprehension levels, encouraging them to progress gradually by practising towards full competence. (e) The educator should teach both groups of patients how to use feedback instruments. (f) The responsibility for the activity of the patients must be transferred to the patients. As patients master one level of involvement, the educator increases the demands so that they are gradually called upon to function at a more challenging level.

NOTES

[1]Addresses for correspondence: L. J. M. Pennings-van der Eerden, Department of General Health Care and Epidemiology, Utrecht University, Bijlhouwerstraat 6, 3511 ZC Utrecht, The Netherlands; A. Ph. Visser, Department of Health Economy, Section on Aging Studies, Limburg University, PO Box 616, 6200 MD Maastricht, The Netherlands.

REFERENCES

Alogna, M. (1980). Perception of severity of disease and health locus of control in compliant and noncompliant diabetic patients. *Diabetes Care*, **3**, 533–540.
Alogna, M. (1985). CDC diabetes control programs—overview of diabetes education. *Diabetes Educator*, **11**, 32–40.
Anderson, R. M. (1985). Is the problem of non-compliance all in our heads? *Diabetes Educator*, **11**, 31–36.
Ary, D., Toobert, D., Wilson, W. and Glasgow, R. E. (1986). Patient perspective on factors contributing to nonadherence in diabetes mellitus. *Diabetes Care*, **9**, 186–172.
Assal, J.-Ph., Berger, M., Gay, N. and Canivet, J. (1983). *Diabetes Education: How to Improve Patient Education*. Amsterdam: Excerpta Medica.
Assal, J. P., Mühlhauser, I., Pernet, A., Gfeller, R., Jörgens, V. and Berger, M. (1985). Patient education as the basis for diabetes care in clinical practice and research. *Diabetologia*, **28**, 602–613.

Bajaj, J. S. (1987). New WHO classifications and diagnostic criteria of diabetes mellitus. *IDF Bulletin*, **32**, 165–168.

Ballegooie, E. van, Leitsma, W. D., Sluiter, W. J. and Doornbos, H. (1983). De verbetering van diabetes mellitus bij patiënten die zichzelf controleren en reguleren onder poliklinisch toezicht (Enhancing diabetic care with outpatients who self-monitor blood glucose). *Nederlands Tijdschrift voor Geneeskunde*, **127**, 44–50.

Baumgardner, P. B., Berry, R. H., Rinaldi, F. W., Wheeler, F. C. *et al.* (1984). A volunteer support group for parents of children with diabetes. *Diabetes Educator*, **10**, 53–57.

Berger, A. S., Saarbrey, N., Kühl, C. and Villuorsen, I. (1985). Clinical experiences with a new device that will simplify insulin injections. *Diabetes Care*, **8**, 73–76.

Berger, M., Mühlhauser, I. and Jörgens, V. (1984). The role of patient education in the treatment of type I diabetes mellitus. *Front. Diabetes*, **4**, 193–199.

Bloom-Cerkoney, K. A. B. and Hart, L. K. (1979). The relationship between the health belief model and compliance of persons with diabetes mellitus. *Diabetes Care*, **2**, 594–598.

Boogaard, P. R. F. van den and Boomsma, A. Y. (1983) Machteloosheid en het effect van een gespreksgroep voor diabetespatiënten (Helplessness and the effect of a group discussion with diabetic patients). *Gezondheid en Samenleving*, **4**, 264–272.

Chanteleau, E., Sonnenberg, G. E., Stanitzek-Schmidt, I., Best, F., Altenähr, R. and Berger, M. (1982). Diet liberalization and metabolic control in type I diabetic outpatients treated by continuous subcutaneous insulin infusion. *Diabetes Care*, **5**, 612–616.

Cox, D. J., Taylor, A. G., Nowacek, G., Holley-Wilcox, P., Pohl, S. L. and Guthrow, E. (1984). The relationship between psychological stress and insulin-dependent diabetic blood glucose control: Preliminary investigations. *Health Psychology*, **3**, 63–75.

Czyzewski, D. (1988). Stress management in diabetes mellitus. In: Russell, M. (Ed.) *Stress Management for Chronic Diseases*. Oxford: Pergamon, pp. 270–289.

Edelstein, J. and Linn, M. W. (1987). Locus of control and the control of diabetes. *Diabetes Educator*, **13**, 51–54.

Fischer, E. B., Delamater, A. M., Bertelson, A. D. and Kirkley, B. G. (1982). Psychological factors in diabetes and its treatment. *Journal of Consulting and Clinical Psychology*, **50**, 993–1003.

Fishbein, M. and Ajzen, I. (1975). *Belief, Attitude, Intention and Behaviour: An Introduction to Theory and Research*. Reading, Mass: Addison-Wesley.

Frey, J. (1984). A family/system approach to illness-maintaining behaviors in chronically ill adolescents. *Family Process*, **23**, 251–260.

Fowler, J. E., Budzynski, T. H. and VandenBergh, R. L. (1976). Effect of an EMG biofeedback relaxation program on the control of diabetes. *Biofeedback and Self-Regulation*, **1**, 105–112.

Graber, A. L., Christman, B. G., Alogne, M. T. and Davidson, J. K. (1977). Evaluation of diabetes-education programs. *Diabetes*, **26**, 61–64.

Gries, F. A. and Alberti, K. G. (1987). Management of non-insulin-dependent diabetes mellitus in Europe: A consensus statement. *IDF Bulletin*, **32**, 169–173.

Groen, J. J. and Pelser, H. E. (1982). Newer concepts of teaching, learning and education and their application to the patient–doctor cooperation in the treatment of diabetes mellitus. *Pediatric Adolescent Endocrinology*, **10**, 186–177.

Harris, R. and Linn, M. W. (1985). Health beliefs, compliance, and control of diabetes mellitus. *South Medical Journal*, **78**, 162–166.

Hartwell, S. L., Kaplan, R. M. and Wallace, J. P. (1986). Comparison of behavioral interventions for control of type II diabetes mellitus. *Behavior Therapy*, **17**, 447–461.

Hauser, S. T. and Pollets, D. (1979). Psychological aspects of diabetes mellitus: A critical review. *Diabetes Care*, **2**, 227–232.

Holstein, B. E., Jorgensen, H. V. and Sestoft, L. (1986). Illness-behaviour, attitude and knowledge in newly diagnosed diabetics. *Danish Medical Bulletin*, **33**, 165–171.

Houtzagers, C. M. A. J., Visser, A. Ph., Berntzen, P. A., Heine, R. J. and Veen, E. A. van der (1988). The medi-jector II: Efficacy and acceptability in insulin-dependent diabetic patients, with and without needle phobia. *Diabetes Medicine*, **5**, 135–138.

Jarrett, R. J. (1986). *Diabetes Mellitus*. London: Croom Helm.

Jenny, J. L. (1986). Differences in adaptation to diabetes between insulin-dependent and non-insulin-dependent patients: Implications for patient education. *Patient Education and Counseling*, **8**, 39–50.

Keen, H. and Rifkin, H. (1987). Guest Editor's Introduction: Complications of diabetes: A solvable problem. IDF *Bulletin*, **32**, 121–122.

Kemmer, F. W., Bisping, R., Steingruber, H. J., Baar, H., Hardtmann, F., Schlaghecke, R. and Berger, M. (1986). Psychological stress and metabolic control in patients with type I diabetes mellitus. *New England Journal of Medicine*, **314**, 1028–1034.

Kovacs, M. and Feinberg, T. L. (1982). Coping with juvenile onset diabetes mellitus. In: Baum, A. *et al.* (Eds) *Handbook of Psychology and Health, Vol. II, Issues in Child Health and Adolescent Health*. New York: Columbia University Press, pp. 212–239.

Krosnick, A. (1980). Self-management, patient compliance and the physician. *Diabetes Care*, **3**, 1.

Leenaars, P. E. M. and Rombouts, R. (1986). Diabetes mellitus en ontspoorde zelfcontrole (Diabetes mellitus and deranged self-control). *Gedrag & Gezondheid*, **14**, 105–113.

Lowery, B. J. and Ducette, J. P. (1976). Disease related learning and disease control in diabetics as a function of locus of control. *Nursing Research*, **25**, 358–362.

Lustman, P., Carney, R. and Amado, H. (1981). Acute stress and metabolism in diabetes. *Diabetes Care*, **4**, 568–569.

Malone, J. I., Lowitt, S., Grove, N. P. and Shah, S. C. (1986). Comparison of insulin levels after injection by jet stream and disposable insulin syringe. *Diabetes Care*, **9**, 637–640.

Maras, M. L., Rinke, W. J., Stephens, C. R., Chaplain, M. A. J. and Boehm, T. M. (1984). Effect of meditation on insulin dependent diabetes mellitus. *Diabetes Educator*, **10**, 22–26.

Marrero, D. G., Myers, G. L., Golden, M. P., West, D., Kershnar, A. and Lau, N. (1982). Adjustment to misfortune: The use of a social support group for adolescent diabetics. *Pediatric Adolescent Endocrinology*, **10**, 213–218.

Mazze, R. S., Lucido, D. D. and Shamoon, H. (1984). Psychological and social correlates of glycemic control. *Diabetes Care*, **7**, 360–366.

Mazzuca, S. A., Moorman, N. H., Wheeler, M. L., Norton, J. A., Fineberg, N. S., Vinicor, F., Cohen, S. J. and Clark, C. M. (1986). The Diabetes Education Study: A controlled trial of the effects of diabetes patient education. *Diabetes Care*, **9**, 1–10.

McCaul, K. D., Glasgow, R. E. and Schafer, L. C. (1987). Diabetes regimen behaviours. *Medical Care*, **25**, 868–881.

Minuchin, S., Baker, L., Rosman, B. L., Liebman, R., Milman, L. and Todd, T. C. (1975). A conceptual model of psychosomatic illness in children, family organization and family therapy. *Archives of General Psychiatry*, **32**, 1031–1038.

Mühlhauser, I., Jörgens, V., Kronsbein, P., Scholz, V. and Berger, M. (1985). Behandlung von nicht insulinpflichtigen Typ 2 Diabetikern in der ärtzlichen Praxis (Medical care of non-insulin-dependent diabetes mellitus by physicians in primary care). *Allgemeinmedizin*, **14**, 39–43.

Naliboff, B. D., Cohen, M. J. and Sowers, J. D. (1985). Physiological and metabolic responses to brief stress in non-insulin dependent diabetic and control subjects. *Journal of Psychosomatic Research*, **29**, 367–374.

National Commission on Diabetes. (1975). *Report of the National Commission on Diabetes to the Congress of the United States*. Washington, DC: Department of Health, Education and Welfare.

Oehler-Giarratana, J. and Fitzgerald, R. G. (1980). Group therapy with blind diabetics. *Archives of General Psychiatry*, **37**, 463–467.

Orr, D. P., Eccles, T., Lawlor, R. and Golden, M. (1986). Surreptitious insulin administration in adolescents with insulin-dependent diabetes mellitus. *Journal of the American Medical Association*, **256**, 3227–3230.

Pennings-Van der Eerden, L. J. M. (1988). Testing a self-care model with IDDM diabetics via linear structural equations with latent variables. Poster presented at the Second Meeting of the European Health Psychology Society, Trier.

Pennings-Van der Eerden, L. J. M. and Post, M. (1985). Zelfzorg bij oudere diabetici (Self-care with elderly diabetic patients). Unpublished report, RUU/AGE, 85. 15, Utrecht.

Pennings-Van der Eerden, L. J. M. and Schrijvers, G. (1985). Self-care and motivation in diabetics in Holland. Paper presented at the Annual Meeting of the IDF, Madrid.

Podolsky, S. (1983). Special medical problems of the elderly diabetic. *Diabetes Educator*, **9**, Special issue.

Pyke, D. A. (1979). Diabetes: The genetic connections. *Diabetologia*, **17**, 333–343.

Rudolf, M. C. J., Ahern, J. A., Genel, M., Bates, S. E., Harding, P., Hochstadt, J., Quinlan, D. and Tamborlane, W. V. (1982). Optimal insulin delivery in adolescents with diabetes: Impact of intensive treatment on psychosocial adjustment. *Diabetes Care*, **5**, (Suppl. 1), 53–57.

Sanders, K., Mills, J., Martin, F. I. R. and DelHorne, D. J. (1975). Emotional attitudes in adult insulin-dependent diabetics. *Journal of Psychosomatic Research*, **19**, 241–246.

Santiago, J. V. (1986). Another facet of brittle diabetes. *Journal of the American Medical Association*, **256**, 3263–3264.

Scott, R. S., Beaven, D. W. and Stafford, J. M. (1984). The effectiveness of diabetes education for non-insulin dependent diabetic persons. *Diabetes Educator*, **10**, 36–39.

Seeburg, K. N. and DeBoer, K. F. (1980). Effects of EMG biofeedback on diabetes. *Biofeedback and Self-Regulation*, **5**, 289–293.

Shapiro, J., Wigg, D., Charles, M. A. and Perley, M. (1984). Personality and family profiles of chronic insulin-dependent diabetic patients using portable insulin infusion pump therapy: A preliminary investigation. *Diabetes Care*, **7**, 137–142.

Stone, G. C. (1979). Patient compliance and the role of the expert. *Journal of Social Issues*, **35**, 34–39.

Sullivan, B. J. (1978). Self-esteem and depression in adolescent diabetic girls. *Diabetes Care*, **1**, 18–22.

Surwit, R. S. and Feinglos, M. N. (1983). The effects of relaxation on glucose tolerance in non-insulin-dependent diabetes mellitus. *Diabetes Care*, **6**, 176–179.

Tattersall, R. B. (1977). Brittle diabetes. *Clinical Endocrinol. Metab.*, **6**, 403–419.

Turk, D. C. and Speers, M. A. (1983). Diabetes mellitus: A cognitive-functional analysis of stress. In: Bradley, L. A. and Burish, T. C. (Eds) *Coping with Chronic Disease*. New York; Academic Press, pp. 191–217.

Vinicor, F., Cohen, S. J., Mazzuca, S. A., Moorman, N., Wheeler, M., Kuebler, T., Swanson, S., Ours, P., Fineberg, S. E., Gordon, E. E., Duckworth, W., Norton, J. A., Fineberg, N. S. and Clark, C. M. (1987). Diabeds: A randomized trial of the effects of physician education and/or patient education on diabetes patient outcomes. *Journal of Chronic Disease*, **40**, 345–356.

Visser, A. Ph. and Bloks, H. (1980). De psycho-sociale begeleiding van diabetes. Een onderzoek naar het effect van een gespreksgroep (The psychosocial guidance of diabetes: A study of the effects of a discussion group). *Tijdschrift voor Sociale Genees-kunde*, **58**, 90–95.

Watts, F. N. (1980). Behavioural aspects of the management of diabetes mellitus: Education, self-care and metabolic control. *Behaviour Research and Therapy*, **18**, 171–180.

Wilson, W., Ary, D. V., Biglan, A., Glasgow, R. E., Toobert, D. J. and Campbell, D. R. (1986). Psychosocial predictors of self-care behaviors (compliance) and glycemic control in non-insulin-dependent diabetes mellitus. *Diabetes Care*, **9**, 614–622.

Wing, R., Epstein, L., Nowalk, M. and Lamparski, D. (1986). Behavioral self-regulation in the treatment of patients with diabetes mellitus. *Psychological Bulletin*, **99**, 78–89.

World Health Organization (1985). *Diabetes Mellitus*. Report of a WHO Study Group, Geneva, TRS 727.

Wysocki, M., Czyzyk, A., Slonska, Z., Krolewski, A. and Janeczko, D. (1978). Health behaviour and its determinants among insulin-dependent diabetics, results of the diabetes Warsaw study. *Diabete & Metabolisme*, **4**, 117–122.

Zimmet, P. (1982). Type 2 (non-insulin-dependent) diabetes—an epidemiological overview. *Diabetologia*, **22**, 399–411.

Zimmet, P. and Dowse, G. (1987). Epidemiology of diabetes mellitus. *IDF Bulletin*, **32**, 174–175.

CHAPTER 18

Nocturnal Enuresis

M. J. M. van Son[1]

Utrecht University, Utrecht

R. Beunderman

University of Amsterdam, Amsterdam

D. J. Duyvis

University of Amsterdam, Amsterdam

and

M. C. Rientsma

Regional Institute for Outpatient Mental Health Care, Hilversum

ABSTRACT

Nocturnal enuresis is a widespread phenomenon, occurring also in the adult population (1.5%); no single therapy is 100% effective in dealing with enuresis. The most promising therapies are derived from behaviour therapy: urine-alarm training, retention control training and dry-bed training. Research data indicate that dry-bed training may be effective for both children and adults. However, a thorough diagnosis in each case is necessary.

INTRODUCTION

In psychological practice much attention has been paid to the subject of enuresis nocturna or bedwetting, in particular to childhood enuresis.

At least 5000 papers on the subject have been published, only a minor part of which are focused on enuresis in adults. The problem of bedwetting has been observed in earlier times, and was described as early as in the Middle Ages. It was treated then by means of 'psychological' methods such as urinating in the

Behavioural Medicine
Edited by A. A. Kaptein, H. M. van der Ploeg, B. Garssen, P. J. G. Schreurs and R. Beunderman
© 1990 John Wiley & Sons Ltd.

grave of a dead person, going on pilgrimages, and loving care, as well as by more medical practices such as drinking extracts of shepherd's purse and safflower, or eating soot and pancakes of woodlice.

Under present health care, attention is given to somatic and psychological causes. In this chapter the focus will be on the aetiology and on treatment procedures, based upon behavioural theories, for both children and adults.

DESCRIPTION, SYMPTOMS AND DIAGNOSIS

Bedwetting or enuresis nocturna is the involuntary loss of urine during sleep. This symptom is generally considered pathologic in our culture after the age of six. In some other cultures the critical age seems to be higher (Beunderman et al., 1984).

There is no agreement about what frequency of bedwetting should be seen as pathological. In the DSM-III-R the criterion is specified as: 'at least two such events per month for children between the ages of five and six and at least once a month for older children' (APA, 1987, p. 84). An additional criterion may be the degree to which the bedwetting negatively affects the patient's quality of life.

In itself enuresis nocturna is easy to assess: it applies to people above the age specified above who (still) more or less regularly wet their beds. Enuresis nocturna may be primary—the anamnesis shows that there has been no proper dry period—or secondary. In the latter case, it is evident from the patient's history that the patient has been dry for a considerable time during any period of his life. The DSM-III-R stipulates '(a period) of urinary continence lasting at least one year' (p. 84). The diagnosis of enuresis nocturna, which leads to an indication of treatment, ought to be further differentiated on the basis of ideas about its causal factors or conditions.

Furthermore it should be stated that enuresis nocturna may be accompanied by other complaints such as high micturition frequency or frequent urgency and by different disorders which are possibly related to enuresis—an organic lesion, a retarded maturation of the nervous system, or a myoneurogenic disorder of the bladder. Enuresis nocturna may also be related to relational and emotional problems or disorders. Whether the relationship between these phenomena and enuresis is a causal one, and what phenomenon exactly brings about the other, must be examined individually. It is also possible that a third factor (e.g. being in a bad shape physically and psychologically) causes both the enuresis and the emotional disorder. In this chapter we will discuss *functional* enuresis nocturna, that is, enuresis in the aetiology of which organic factors have been excluded. The possible organic factors which should be excluded are:

- *Organic defects.* Disturbance in maturation, epilepsia nocturna, a too small capacity of the bladder, urinary infections, urinary obstructions, functional disturbances in the lower urinary tracts, pathology of the vertebral column, an allergic food disorder (e.g. for eggs, chocolate, carbonated drinks), polyuria (urinating too much) as a consequence of diabetes mellitus, and polyuria caused by too much drinking, by decreased kidney function or by diabetes insipidus.

- *Genetic predisposition.* A genetic predisposition is often mentioned: In 35% of enuretic patients one of the parents would also be enuretic. With monozygotic twins, if one of them is enuretic then the other is also enuretic in 68% of the cases (Timmreck, 1983; Sorotzkin, 1984).
- *Diet and medical treatment.* If the enuresis started only recently, it may be the consequence of a change in diet (e.g. drinking coffee) or of a medical treatment, like gynaecological surgery or catheterization. It is important to note that these medical procedures may affect the patient both somatically and psychologically, and both effects may contribute to the development and the continuation of enuresis nocturna. It may be assumed that these organic effects are accompanied by other related problems besides enuresis nocturna, such as micturition problems or enuresis diurna (Edelstein, Keaton-Brasted and Burg, 1984).

It appears from what was mentioned above that one must ascertain in cases of enuresis nocturna what exactly are the symptoms of the enuresis (what its frequency and regularity are, whether it also happens during the day, and what the frequency of micturition is during the day). Moreover, one must include possible correlated somatic phenomena in the process of diagnosis.

DEVELOPMENT OF URINATION HABITS

Generally it is assumed that functional enuresis is determined by more than one condition. Tanagho (1979) states that there are several hypotheses about the mechanism of micturition and continence, but that none of them sufficiently explains it. The mechanism that functions during infancy—involuntary urination occurs by means of the urination reflex—differs from the mechanism that functions in the next developmental phase. In this phase the child gains control over the urination: then it learns to interrupt urination, to hold the urine and to urinate at any moment. With this mechanism the synergic activity of diaphragmatic abdominal and pelvic-floor muscles is important. The synergic activity must affect the lowering of the bladder cervix, so that the muscle of the bladder contracts as a reflex and urination occurs. In the case of interruption or holding up, a raising of the bladder cervix must occur so that the bladder is impermeably closed (Resnick and King, 1976). This very precise synergic activity may be disturbed as a consequence of physical or psychological strain.

The transition from involuntary to voluntary urination encompasses four phases:

1. Becoming aware that the bladder is full. The neural maturity of the higher nervous centres is essential for this sensation.
2. Being able to hold the urine for a short while when the bladder is full. This implies some control of the levator ani and the pubococcygeus. Most children

of two years are able to exercise this control and by doing so the bladder's capacity is gradually enlarged.

3. At the age of four to five years, the child is generally capable of urinating voluntarily when the bladder is full, by making use of the diaphragmatic and pelvic muscles.

4. At the age of six to seven, the child has generally developed the capacity to urinate whenever there is some urine in the bladder, as a result of simultaneous contraction of the diaphragmatic and the pelvic muscles, and relaxation of the pubococcygeus.

In the course of the period during which the child gains control, the capacity of the bladder increases. It is assumed that a capacity of 400 ml is necessary to prevent involuntary urination at night.

EPIDEMIOLOGY

In the case of enuresis nocturna in children the ideas of the parents determine what is acceptable and proper: whether the bedwetting is considered a symptom, a transitional phenomenon, something that is normal, or an unavoidable annoying phenomenon. In the case of adult enuretics it is often the idea of the patient involved or the idea of the partner that determines how the bedwetting is experienced.

Therefore, it is difficult to establish how many children are enuretic. With adults this is even more difficult, as it seems that certainly not all of them apply for treatment. The prevalence of enuresis nocturna in a so-called 'open' population has been estimated by several authors. There are no recent data available, so we rely in this matter upon early research. Lovibond (1964) estimated the prevalence of enuresis in children and youngsters from data in Bransby, Bloomsfield and Douglas (1955). He concluded that ±40% of children of the age of two years wet their beds; this percentage is strongly declining: at four years only ±15% of them are regular bedwetters. After that the decline is gradually less till after the age of 14 the curve follows an asymptotic course (Bransby, Bloomsfield and Douglas, 1955). At six years ±11% are still enuretic, at 10 ±7%; at the age of 14 1.7% of youngsters still wet their beds, and this percentage remains unchanged with higher ages. However, it is unclear whether the same (14 years old) persons keep wetting their beds later on. It is quite possible that some of them learn to control their urination, while others take their place (Bransby, Bloomsfield and Douglas, 1955).

Data from medical examinations of American army recruits show that the percentage of enuretics (and so unfit for military service) is 1.6 throughout. An investigation by Cushing and Baller in a group of American (post)graduate students shows that 3.8% of the male students and 3.6% of the female students report that they more or less regularly wet their beds (Cushing and Baller, 1975). There was no particular advantage for these respondents in the nature of the answer they gave in this investigation. The numbers therefore seem to be closer to reality than those of the American recruits. It is noteworthy that the difference between men and women is not very large, while data on children show that there are twice as many bedwetting boys as there are girls.

Who seeks medical care for enuresis nocturna? Beunderman *et al.* tried to establish the number of patients seeking medical care for enuresis nocturna from their general practitioner. The authors asked 35 general practitioners how many of their patients—to their knowledge—were enuretic. The general practitioners reported only 143 cases: 138 children and five people above the age of 18 years (Beunderman, Duyvis and Rientsma, 1985). This number is quite small considering that the total number of all patients of these general practitioners is well above 70,000. Thus, the number of those who seek help for enuresis nocturna does not match assumed prevalence of enuresis nocturna.

The difference may be explained by the ideas of parents and patients—for example, enuresis nocturna is just a transitional phenomenon or an annoying but untreatable phenomenon, or shame on the part of parents and patients. Another explanation may be found in the attitude of the general practitioners involved, as the authors suggest. They base their suggestion upon the finding that female general practitioners reported more cases than their male colleagues, and suggest that female doctors were more inclined to ask explicitly about enuresis and were more focused upon enuresis in their medical examination. Moreover, Beunderman *et al.* suggest that the female doctors were less inclined to believe that a formerly reported enuresis had disappeared, so these doctors inquired after it on a later visit by the patient. Thus, characteristics of the doctor may influence the detection of cases.

AETIOLOGY AND ANALYSIS

It is improbable that only one common factor would cause the various symptoms of all enuretic patients. Nor is it probable that only one general condition would lead to continuation of the enuresis. In this chapter we discuss functional enuresis nocturna, though we do not exclude that for some patients organic factors may be involved. In the literature about bedwetting, three major groups of conditions for development and continuation of functional enuresis nocturna are mentioned.

- *Skill deficiencies.* The person—child or adult—has not learned to wake up when the bladder is full, or has not sufficiently learned to control the muscles of the pelvic floor. This may be a consequence of a too strict or a too permissive upbringing, but also of major events in the sensitive (learning) period between the age of two and four, like moving out, birth of sibling or divorce of the parents. Also, the practice of some parents in not awakening the child properly when they let it urinate at night might end in the child not learning to wake if its bladder is full.
- *Psychological strain.* The sources of strain may vary: school problems, problems

in relationships with parents, partner or colleagues, financial problems, job problems or demands and, of course, the consequences of bedwetting itself. It is unknown how exactly psychological strain affects the synergism of the muscles of diaphragm, abdomen, pelvic floor, bladder and cervix of the bladder. Neither do we know if, and in what way, strain influences the perception of a full bladder and the capacity to wake up if one does perceive that the bladder is full.

- *Secondary gain*. We do not wish to assert that the enuretic patient wets his bed on purpose, but certainly, in some cases, enuresis may fulfil a function in the patient's life. One consequence of enuresis may be attention from the parents. Another function may be diverting attention to the enuretic (child or adult) so that potential threatening situations, like quarrels between parents or quarrels with partners, do not occur. In some cases, the enuresis may eventually end in the child not being able to leave home, not going and living on his own, and in not being able to make friends and have close relationships outside the family. So the enuresis may prevent the patient from having to meet the uncertainties of adult life. Enuresis may also be a safe way to express aggression: others are saddled with the wet sheets, while the consequences of overt aggression are avoided.

The 'choice' of enuresis nocturna 'in order' to get the 'secondary gains' mentioned above may in part result from the habits of the child's family, such as being overconcerned or, on the other hand, being indifferent, fostering feelings of insufficiency, siblings claiming too much attention and communicating by way of complaints. A family with such habits may be the basis for isolation from the outside world, the basis for seeking security in the parental home and thus, sometimes, for the continuation of bedwetting, which in turn protects against appeals to become self-reliant ('because you wet your bed, you cannot live on your own!').

The assumption that enuretic patients would manifest neurotic symptoms, like social anxiety, thumb-sucking, nail-biting, dependency on others, shame, concentration disturbances, and so on, has not been verified (Baller, 1975). It is, however, plausible that, if these symptoms have been diagnosed in an enuretic patient, they may be the indirect consequence of bedwetting. The direct negative consequences may be accountable for these 'neurotic' symptoms. The direct negative consequences may involve: reduction of the patient's range of social actions—no staying with friends or family, no nights at hotels, no bedpartners—being badgered when bedwetting is discovered, disapproval by the next of kin and being treated like an infant. It needs no explaining that some of these consequences may lead to a negative self-image, which in turn may end in narrowing the scope of the patient. Moreover, they may eventually lead to secondary psychological problems, such as depression and social anxiety.

TREATMENT OF NOCTURNAL ENURESIS

It is obvious that with a phenomenon that is maintained by so many conditions, more than one particular therapy may be successful. The following approaches may be observed:

- *Simply waiting for the bedwetting to pass over.* This may be combined with encouragement to keep dry, encouragement to be patient and encouragement to accept the bedwetting. It may be put into practice by keeping a calender of successful nights and by rewarding them. With children of the age of two to six years, therapy is often confined to this simple approach.
- *Pharmacological treatment.* Contemporary pharmacological treatment consists, according to Blackwell and Currah (1973), of various types of drugs: cerebral stimulants, tricyclic antidepressants (imipramine and amitriptyline), diuretics, tranquillizers and anti-epileptic drugs. Of these, the tricyclic antidepressants administered for a few months before going to sleep in a 25–100 mg dose proved to be effective in 70% of the cases. After termination of the medication, there is a relapse of about 50% of the cases (Blackwell and Currah, 1973). Despite the development of all kinds of new drugs in other areas in recent years, and despite the fact that psychotherapists—especially behaviour therapists—have become more sensitive to the role of pharmacotherapy (Mountjoy, Ruben and Bradford, 1984), the conclusions of Blackwell and Currah still apply to recent practice, as Sorotzkin states in his overview (Sorotzkin, 1984).
- *Urological treatments.* The following procedures are mentioned in the literature: longlasting hydrostatic bladder distension, physical transsection of the bladder, sacral plexis blockade and selective sacral neurectomy. With respect to the transsection and the supratrigonal denervation, it has been reported that only a very few cases were successful and that the danger of consequent fibrotization with accompanying shrivelling of the bladder is far from imaginary. It will be clear that before deciding on such drastic and unpromising procedures other possibilities must be taken into consideration (van Son *et al.*, 1984; Mountjoy, Ruben and Bradford, 1984).
- *Psychological treatments.* See below.

PSYCHOLOGICAL TREATMENTS

According to van Londen (1986), parents employ various educational practices in order to try to overcome bedwetting in their children, such as: exercises in holding the urine as long as possible, rubbing the patient's nose in the urine, advice to sleep on the back, advice not to sleep on the back, advice to drink just before going to sleep, advice not to drink before going to sleep, making the patient ridiculous or praising the child for his qualities, etc. Such educative practices would be effective in 20–40% of the cases, possibly as a result of the attention itself on the part of the parents towards the child involved.

In medical and mental health care, one may observe a variety of therapeutic approaches to enuresis nocturna, including such treatments as: analytic psychotherapy, hypnotherapy, rational emotive therapy, family therapy, life-style instructions (e.g. not drinking, Edelstein, Keaton-Brasted and Burg, 1984), sleep interruptions, punishment and reward, and behaviour therapy (Beunderman, *et al.*, 1984).

As most outcome research has been reported with three behavioural methods, we discuss these in the following paragraphs. The bell-and-pad method, retention-control training and dry-bed training have been applied with both children and adults.

The Bell-and-pad Method or Urine-alarm Method

The name of this method refers to two important parts of the apparatus that is used during the treatment: the bell—the device that must awaken the patient if urine has touched the pad—and the pad, which is mostly a water-absorbent paper or cloth with wires woven into it on which the patient sleeps.

The bell-and-pad machine consists of a small box which contains a battery that is connected with the pad and the bell. When the patient urinates, the urine is absorbed by the cloth, which enables a small electrical current to run from the battery wire to the other wires in the cloth, thereby closing an electrical circuit that triggers a buzzer, a siren or a lamp (Mowrer and Mowrer, 1938; Mountjoy, Ruben and Bradford, 1984; Sorotzkin, 1984).

The treatment consists of informing the patient—the adult or the child and, in the latter case, the child's parents too—extensively about the method, practising some of the procedures in the consultation room and presenting written instructions for the use of the apparatus. Moreover it is agreed that as soon as the patient goes to bed, he or she puts on the pants (the pad) or puts down the pad in the bed and the buzzer is connected. It is also agreed that, as soon as the patient hears the buzzer, he gets out of his bed immediately and goes to the bathroom to urinate (further).

With children who sleep deeply and are difficult to arouse, an additional alarm may be put beside the parents' bed. When the parents hear the buzzer, they awaken the child and let him get up and visit the toilet. The designers of the method, Mowrer and Mowrer (1938), advise against awakening the child in between and putting him on the toilet. Their argument is that by doing so the connection would not be established between 'high tension of the bladder', 'awakening' and 'contracting the sphincter'. The procedure may be combined with giving a reward for each dry night or—later on—for each dry period.

Contraindications for this treatment are: organic disturbances, other severe neurotic disturbances or psychoticism and serious personality disorders, implying that the child is unable to cooperate.

The results are generally favourable, although not in 100% of the cases as achieved by Mowrer and Mowrer, and indicate that about 75% of the cases are successful. However, relapse in successful cases is considerable (30%), and frequently occurs as early as some weeks after termination (Doleys, 1977; Turner and Taylor, 1974; Sorotzkin, 1984). Relapse may be prevented by—intermittently—rewarding consistently the dry nights and by 'overlearning'. Overlearning means the continuation of treatment after the criterium has been reached, combined with drinking a lot before going to sleep (Doleys, 1977; Fielding, 1985).

In cases of relapse one may retrain with the same procedure; most of the subsequently retrained patients become dry (Fielding, 1985).

In general, only low dropout rates have been mentioned, but they may still be substantial—up to 30%. Moreover, there may be a significant number of referred patients who do not attend the therapist (about 12%). Most studies do not reveal this selection from the potential patient group (Fielding, 1985).

There are no well-documented data about the treatment of adult enuretics and only three studies about adolescent enuretics. These studies reveal contradictory results and do not confirm that the bell-and-pad method is as successful here as it is with younger children (Turner and Taylor, 1974; de Haan and Hoogduin, 1981; Sacks and DeLeon, 1983).

Retention-control Training (RCT)

This training aims at achieving voluntary control of urination, and at enlarging the bladder capacity. It consists of exercises asking the patient to start urinating and subsequently to interrupt it. Moreover the patient learns to inhibit urination for an increasingly longer time. These exercises are combined with drinking a lot and systematically rewarding the patient for both the drinking of fluids and the retention of urine. Contrary to the other two procedures described here, this procedure is carried out during the daytime.

Muellner (1960) and later on Kimmel and Kimmel (1970) developed this procedure, meant to enlarge the capacity of the bladder (Paschalis, Kimmel and Kimmel, 1972). The criterion for success of treatment is seven nights without bedwetting. The success rate first reported—100% by Kimmel and Kimmel (1970) and 48% by Paschalis, Kimmel and Kimmel (1972)—has not been found again by Harris and Purohit (1977). Fielding (1985) reported that RCT was inferior to the bell-and-pad procedure for enuresis nocturna.

It is known, however, that an increase in bladder capacity, or an increase in retentive capacity as such, does not directly result in dry nights (Harris and Purohit, 1977). Geffken, Johnson and Walker (1986) speculate that the therapeutic agent may be found in the attention which is paid to the urinating behaviour during the day and so to the proprioceptive cues, resulting in the awareness of control. (But it may also increase the urination frequency.) Like Fielding (1985), Geffken *et al.* stipulate that this control may be crucial in retention-control training.

No outcome studies involving adult enuretic patients have been published yet.

Dry-bed Training (DBT)

This extensively investigated and comprehensive procedure is a combination of the main features of the above-described methods, the bell-and-pad method and retention-control training. The emphasis lies on operant conditioning, in other words upon rewarding taking part in the training and especially staying dry. The operant conditioning implies also, on the part of the patient, taking the negative consequences of being wet: awakening when the bed gets wet, carrying out exercises during the night if one is wet, and changing the wet sheets and pyjamas (Azrin, Sneed and Foxx, 1973, 1974).

The procedure consists of two phases: the so-called 'intensive night' and the subsequent training during the following nights. Before the intensive night, the patient and his partner or his parents are instructed about what each is expected to do, and they are urgently requested to carry it through as it is a very demanding programme that lays great strain on all subjects involved. Before the patient goes to bed the first night he engages in extra drinking. Then the urine-alarm machine (bell-and-pad device) is switched on and the 'positive practice procedure' is performed. The lights are switched off, the patient lies in his bed and counts to 50. Next, the patient rises and goes to the toilet, tries to urinate and returns to bed. He repeats this procedure 20 times. After that the patient drinks as much as he can. In the case of a child, the parents might very well then explain one more time the procedure to be followed that night. The patient then goes to sleep. During the night the patient is awakened by the partner or a parent every hour to go to the toilet. At the toilet the patient is asked by the partner or parent whether he can inhibit urination for another hour. In the event of 'no', the patient is allowed to urinate and in the event of 'yes' the patient returns to bed. In both cases he is allowed to return to sleep, but only after he has felt that the sheets are still dry, has been praised for it and has had another drink.

If the patient wets his bed, the urine alarm, the bell, sounds. Then the partner or parent switches off the alarm, eventually awakens the patient, reprimands the patient and sends him to the toilet to finish urinating. The patient must wash himself and change his night clothes and bedding. This is the so-called 'cleanliness-training'. Next, the patient switches on the urine-alarm device and carries out the 'positive practice procedure' another 20 times, as described above. In the event of bedwetting during this night, the patient starts again the subsequent night—before going to sleep—performing the positive practice procedure 20 times. The patient is awakened by partner or parent the next night a few hours after his bedtime and sent to the toilet. During the following nights, the awakening for toileting is 30 minutes earlier each night, until the awakening is about one hour after the patient went to sleep. After each dry night the patient is explicitly praised and rewarded for his achievement. The criterion for terminating the treatment is seven consecutive dry nights.

This procedure can be performed at home with the patient and his parents but also—in the case of an adult enuretic patient—with a partner or friend. It is also possible to perform the procedure with a professional in an inpatient setting. All kinds of variations of this procedure have been reported since its introduction (Sorotzkin, 1984). A feature intrinsic to the procedure is the extensive praising and rewarding of the patient by partner or parents and other significant people.

The procedure applied to children and to adult retarded persons by Azrin, Sneed and Foxx (1973, 1974) proved to be very successful. These authors reported a 100% short-term success, but also a relapse rate of 30%. Other researchers were less successful, but the results were still more favourable than those of the bell-and-pad method or the retention-control therapy alone (Doleys, Ciminero and Tollison, 1977; Bollard and Nettelbeck, 1981; Bollard, Nettelbeck and Roxbee, 1982; Bennett et al., 1985).

In a recent study the success rate, relapse rate and duration of treatments appeared not so favourable as reported by other researchers. The authors suggest that this is due to the fact that the age of the patients in their study ranged from 5 to 12 years with a mean of 8.5 years (whereas other researchers included much younger children in their study—from as young as three years) (Bennett et al., 1985). So it is quite possible that there may be a difference between effectiveness in older children compared with younger ones.

On the other hand, Mulder et al. (1988) concluded from their outcome research with adult enuretics that DBT may be 100% successful in the short term (10 weeks), the relapse—between post-treatment assessment and follow-up assessment—being 22%. There were no dropouts during the therapy. A comparable result was obtained by de Haan and Hoogduin (1981).

Fincham and Spettell (1984) did not find support for the view that DBT is a more acceptable or more effective treatment for enuresis than the traditional bell-and-pad method. Moreover, they report that parents who had implemented the bell-and-pad method rated the treatment more favourably than those who carried out DBT. Both methods were considered to be more acceptable when offered by a clinic than when presented by self-help manuals. On the other hand, Bollard and Nettelbeck (1981) found that DBT administered by parents, with professional supervision, is as effective as administered by professionals. And in a later study (Bollard, Nettelbeck and Roxbee, 1982) the authors found that instructing parents in small groups does not reduce the effectiveness of DBT.

However, the procedure makes high demands on the persons concerned. In particular, the 'positive practice procedure' is experienced as tedious and overly demanding (Fincham and Spettell, 1984; Bennett et al., 1985). Thus the modification Azrin et al. introduced (Azrin et al., 1979; Besalel et al., 1980), letting parents administer the training using only a manual, does not seem likely to be an effective approach. Other modifications proposed by Azrin (Azrin and Thienes, 1978) were to shift the 'intensive training night' to an earlier time—during the afternoon and evening, from 4 pm to 12.00 pm—and to eliminate the urine-alarm device. Bollard and Nettelbeck (1981) and Keating et al. (1983) compared DBT with and without such an alarm device. They found only a slightly better outcome for the DBT involving the use of the urine-alarm device.

Which Therapy is the Treatment of Choice?

To summarize: none of the methods is 100% successful. Comparing DBT—including the use of the urine-alarm device—and retention-control training, we may conclude that retention-control is the least effective procedure. DBT without the urine alarm is less effective than DBT with the use of such a device. DBT alone seems not always more effective than the bell-and-pad procedure alone, and in the case of older children the bell-and-pad method may be the method to be preferred. However, a recent study also demonstrates the effectiveness of DBT for older children (Van Londen, 1989).

Whether DBT is to be administered by partners, friends, parents or professionals depends in the first place upon the availability of partners, etc. or parents but also upon their compliance.

There are only very few studies involving adult enuretics and, as far as one may draw conclusions from them, one may observe that the results are not very different from those obtained with younger people (Mulder et al., 1988). On the whole, one may conclude that for children and adults the available studies have their limitations, especially caused by methodological factors. Fielding (1985) points out that in most studies there is no mention of dropout rates, so that it is unknown with how many patients the therapy may be successful. Another aspect concerns the impossibility of finding the exact ages of the children involved in a number of studies and, if they are known, it is quite possible that, in respect of outcome, very young children may differ quite significantly from older children. This is especially the case when the studies involve children below the age of six years (Breit et al., 1984). It may also be possible that the method of obtaining subjects in the treatment studies may influence the success rate: patients applying for therapy as a response to an advertisement from the researchers in the local campus journal may respond quite unlike patients who apply for therapy as a result of the misery of the enuresis nocturna. Moreover, 'academic' patients may respond favourably to 'academic' therapies while patients from another cultural background do not. In addition, the criteria for success are not always available for the reader of the relevant studies, and if they are they are not always comparable.

Applying one of the three above-described behavioural procedures rests upon the premise that the patient is enuretic because of a skill deficiency: he did not learn the appropriate responses which are necessary for control of the urination. Perhaps he 'unlearned' already acquired skills (as may be the case in secondary noctural enuresis). Other premises involve psychological strain and secondary gain of nocturnal enuresis, as pointed out earlier.

The fact that other factors besides skill deficiency may play a role in the aetiology of nocturnal enuresis may well be responsible for the finding that the standard methods, as described above, seem not always equally effective for younger and older children. The possibility of other aetiological factors than skill deficiency may account for the finding in a small survey in two Dutch outpatient mental health care centres. The therapists in these centres treated the 17 adult enuretics who applied for therapy with a battery of various psychotherapeutic methods (Beunderman et al., 1984) such as: bell-and-pad procedures, muscle relaxation exercises, assertiveness training, training in how to cope with stress, learning how to recognize and to cope with emotions, etc. It is striking that only one of the five patients who gained complete remission had been treated by a therapy especially designed for bedwetting, that is, a combination of DBT, relaxation exercises and retention-control training. It is also notable that, in three out of the five successful cases, the therapy aimed at young adult patients separated from their parents. Moreover, all but one of the patients treated by 'classic' methods aimed directly at nocturnal enuresis showed no improvement. A plausible explanation for the low success rate in this group may be the assumption that adults are more resistant to therapy because of their longer history and because of the function that bedwetting might have provided.

For this reason we advise—tentatively—making a careful diagnosis or a functional analysis before treatment starts. In particular, we advise doing this in dealing with adults and older children with persistent enuretic problems. In such an analysis one has to take into account the antecedents as well as the consequence of the enuretic incidents, and the consequences of the fact that one is enuretic (positive as well as negative). Moreover, the therapist must consider facilitating and organic factors, the history of the complaints, the ideas of the patient and his family concerning bedwetting, lifestyle, earlier treatments, possible reinforcers for remission of the enuresis and the social circumstances (as possible beneficial or limiting factors). Baseline recording of frequency of enuretic incidents and quantity and urine involved, time of enuresis and number of times the patient awakes and goes to the toilet may also constitute part of the diagnosis.

On the basis of such an individual analysis the therapist may opt for a therapy comprising one or a combination of methods. On the other hand, recent evidence allows us to suggest that the dry-bed training is an option which may well be taken into consideration in this process (de Haan and Hoogduin, 1981; Mulder *et al.*, 1988).

HOW TREATMENT MAY WORK OUT—SOME CASE HISTORIES

Case A

A is a 10-year-old boy who came with his mother to the general practitioner's surgery because of bedwetting complaints. He is the eldest of three children. His two younger brothers (six and eight years old) keep their beds dry at night. With the exception of some short periods during the holidays, A has never been completely dry at night.

Previously, the parents of A attempted to control the enuresis by waking him at night and sending him to the toilet, and also by not allowing him to drink anything after supper. After taking the history, the general practitioner proposed the following programme to A and his parents:

1. During the following weeks A himself will keep a record of the nights he was dry.
2. If he wakes up at night after wetting his bed, A will wash himself, remove the wet bed sheets, and place these together with his wet pyjamas in the washing machine. Next, A will remake his bed and put on dry pyjamas.
3. The 'prohibition' on drinking after supper is removed.
4. The parents and A agree that if A keeps his bed dry for at least five nights a week, the family will pay a visit to a motor museum.

During the consultation the physician gives A and his mother information about bedwetting. They are also provided with a general booklet about bedwetting to read at home. The information particularly concerns knowledge of the importance of skill-learning in the process of acquiring control over urination and the facilitating factors for such learning. When A returns two weeks later with his mother, he has been dry for five nights during one week. To reward this achievement the family has gone to the motor museum. It is then agreed that the criterion for a reward will be raised from five nights dry in one week to six nights dry. If the procedure is successful, the criterion will again be raised by one dry night. On the basis of this programme, A has been dry after 10 weeks. After a small relapse, the programme is repeated by A and his parents, after which A no longer wets his bed.

The procedure as applied by this general physician is a simplified version of the dry-bed training, in which the child is rewarded for 'being dry' and in which he has to deal with the negative effects of wetting his bed.

Case B

B is an 11-year-old boy, the youngest of a family of five children. The history shows that B did not wet his bed from the age of three to six years. From then, he has wet his bed each night. As soon as he wakes up wet, he wakes up the whole family by his crying. His parents, in particular the father who suffers from insomnia, react strongly to his crying. More than once, B has been beaten black and blue by his father. Former treatments, as advised by the general practitioner, included first medication and next application of the urine-alarm device. No results were achieved. Upon inquiry the parents told the doctor that they thought the urine-alarm method as dreadful as the bedwetting ('father wakes up and cannot sleep any more'); after some nights the father had switched off the urine alarm.

Because of this, the physician decided to consult the behaviour therapist at the children's hospital in a nearby town. By mutual agreement, it is decided that B will take part in the children's hospital's dry-bed programme. Three weeks later B participates in this programme and is dry for two weeks after termination of the therapy. After a small relapse in the month following the termination, B is trained in the hospital once more for one night according to the DBT procedures. Since this retraining B has been dry at night.

Case C

Mrs C, a student in social work, 33 years old, divorced and mother of two children, seeks medical help because of bedwetting problems. She does not wet her bed every night but from time to time and, if so, for a few consecutive nights. The physician sees no reason to suppose an organic cause. Because he has observed that the periods of bedwetting often coincide with periods of strain and despondency, he refers the patient to a psychotherapist. The psychotherapist concludes, together with the patient, that the bedwetting strongly interferes with her social life, especially because she feels ashamed of her bed-wetting. When looking for detailed information it turns out that the bedwetting periods often coincide with the menstrual period. It also appears that Mrs C. urinates 15–20 times a day. What is more, the bedwetting periods coincide with stressful events. It turns out that the patient generally finds it difficult to express herself about matters that are important to her: she withdraws as soon as emotions come up for discussion. While talking with the therapist, she also rationalizes strongly and does not recognize her feelings (she often phrases her problems in global terms, such as: 'I believe that it is quite difficult'). It is assumed that the bedwetting is related to a low tolerance for bladder tension, in combination with stress that cannot be solved by discussing it or by expressing the emotions involved.

Therefore the therapy aims at reducing the frequency of urination during the day by means of retention-control training, which allows urination only nine times a day. After five weeks the frequency of urination is diminished to 7–9 times a day.

The diary she keeps shows that the bedwetting periods coincide especially with disappointments about how people treat her. Therapist and patient decide to train the patient during the therapy sessions to name her emotions and to learn to solve emotional problems by expressing them and talking them over with those involved, and, if necessary, to go into conflict. She is also taught to realize that some events are hurtful, disappointing and sad. The sessions involve detailed assignments to try out in normal life what has been discussed during the therapy sessions. The therapy is terminated when the patient thinks she has reasonable control over the urination: she can predict enuresis, and the frequency of bedwetting has dropped from an average of once in two weeks to once in seven weeks.

CONCLUSION

Despite the fact that there are about 5000 articles dealing with nocturnal enuresis, knowledge about enuresis and micturation is quite limited.

Only global knowledge is available about the mechanism of micturition; specific details about factors playing an important role in this mechanism and in the development of micturition and continence are in need of further research. This is also the case for data about the prevalence and incidence of nocturnal enuresis: most figures derive from relatively old studies and from not really representative samples. However, one may conclude that at least 15% of six-year-olds are enuretic and possibly about 1.5% of 15-year-olds and older persons.

Knowledge of the aetiology of nocturnal enuresis is far from complete because of the lack of proper research. The available data point to a different aetiology for different enuretic persons: organic disturbances, including dietary and drinking habits, pathology of the vertebral column, urinary infections, and so on; genetic predispositions, skill deficiences, as a result of not having been taught the proper control responses; psychological strain and secondary gain from the complaint.

As a consequence, the diagnosis and treatment in individual cases must involve attention to all possible factors influencing the control mechanism of urination.

On the other hand, a few behavioural therapy procedures in particular seem to result in a significant remission in enuresis: bell-and-pad or urine-alarm therapy, retention-control therapy and dry-bed training. The data from the relevant studies do not as yet indicate whether one of them is suitable for all enuretics—old and young—and what characteristics of the patients may result in more or less reduction in enuresis. There is a slight tendency for all of the three standard methods to help in some cases and for the DBT as the most promising therapy.

Considering the state of the art in this area, it is best to make an extremely thorough diagnosis in each particular patient before deciding which procedure or combination of procedures gives the best chance of remission of the nocturnal enuresis. This is especially true for older adolescents and adults as most studies do not involve these groups.

NOTES

[1]Addresses for correspondence: M. J. M. van Son, Department of Clinical and Health Psychology, Utrecht University, Heidelberglaan 1, 3584 CS Utrecht, The Netherlands; R. Beunderman, Department of Medical Psychology, University of Amsterdam, Meibergdreef 15, 1105 AZ Amsterdam, The Netherlands; D. J. Duyvis, Department of Gynaecology and Obstetrics, University of Amsterdam, Meibergdreef 15, 1105 AZ Amsterdam, The Netherlands; M. C. Rientsma, Regional Institute for Outpatient Mental Health Care, Hilversum, The Netherlands.

REFERENCES

American Psychiatric Association (1987). *Diagnostic and Statistical Manual of Mental Disorders*, 3rd edn, revised. Washington DC: APA.

Azrin, N. H., Sneed, F. J. and Foxx, R. M. (1973). Dry bed training: A rapid method of eliminating bedwetting (enuresis) in the retarded. *Behaviour Research & Therapy*, **11**, 427–434.

Azrin, N. H., Sneed, F. J. and Foxx, R. M. (1974). Dry bed training: rapid elimination of childhood enuresis. *Behaviour Research & Therapy*, **12**, 147–156.

Azrin, N. H. and Thienes-Hontos, P. M. (1978). Rapid elimination of enuresis by intensive learning without a conditioning apparatus. *Behavior Therapy*, **9**, 342–354.

Azrin, N. H., Thienes-Hontos, P. M. and Besalel-Azrin, V. (1979). Elimination of enuresis without a conditioning apparatus: An extension by office instruction of the child and parents. *Behavior Therapy*, **10**, 14–19.

Baldew, J. M. (1986). Medische aspecten van enuresis. In: van Londen, A. (Ed.) *Enuresis*. Lisse: Swets & Zeitlinger, pp. 59–62.

Baller, W. R. (1975). *Bedwetting: Origins and Treatment*. New York: Pergamon.

Besalel, V. A., Azrin, N. H., Thienes-Hontos, P. and McMorrow, M. (1980). Evaluation of a parents' manual for training enuretic children. *Behaviour Research & Therapy*, **18**, 353–360.

Bennett, G. A., Walkden, V. J., Curtis, R. H., Burns, L. E., Rees, J., Gosling, J. A. and McQuire, N. L. (1965). Pad-and-buzzer training, dry-bed training and stop-start training in the treatment of primary nocturnal enuresis. *Behavioural Psychotherapy*, **13**, 309–319.

Beunderman, R., Duyvis, D. J. and Rientsma, M. C. (1985). Enuresis nocturna: Een enquête onder huisartsen. *Medische Psychologie*, **5**, 68–76.

Beunderman, R., Son, M. J. M. van, Duyvis, D. J. and Rientsma, M. C. (1984). Nocturnal enuresis in adults. Paper presented at the European Association for Behaviour Therapy Congress, Brussels.

Blackwell, B. and Currah, J. (1973). The psychopharmacology of nocturnal enuresis. *Clinical Developmental Medicine*, **48/49**, 231.

Bollard, J. (1982). A two year follow-up of bedwetters treated by dry-bed training and standard conditioning. *Behaviour Research & Therapy*, **20**, 571–580.

Bollard, J. and Nettelbeck, T. (1981). A comparison of dry-bed training and standard urine-alarm conditioning treatment of childhood bedwetting. *Behaviour Research & Therapy*, **19**, 215–226.

Bollard, J., Nettelbeck, T. and Roxbee, L. (1982). Dry-bed training for childhood bedwetting: A comparison of group with individually administered parent instructions. *Behaviour Research & Therapy*, **20**, 209–217.

Bransby, E. R., Bloomsfield, J. M. and Douglas, J. (1955). The prevalence of bedwetting. *The Medical Officer*, **94**, 5–7.

Breit, M., Kaplan, S. L., Gauthier, B. and Weinhold, C. (1984). The dry bed method for the treatment of enuresis: A failure to duplicate previous reports. *Child & Family Behaviour Therapy*, **6**, 17–23.

Cushing, F. C. and Baller, W. R. (1975). The problem of nocturnal enuresis in adults: Special reference to managers and managerial aspirants. *Journal of Psychology*, **89**, 203–213.

Doleys, D. M. (1977). Behavioral treatments for nocturnal enuresis in children: A review of the recent literature. *Psychological Bulletin*, **84**, 30–54.

Doleys, D. M., Ciminero, A. R. and Tollison, J. W. (1977). Dry-bed training and retention control training: A comparison. *Behavior Therapy*, **8**, 541–548.

Edelstein, B. A., Keaton-Brasted, C. and Burg, M. M. (1984). Effects of caffeïne withdrawal on nocturnal enuresis, insomnia and behavior restraints. *Journal of Consulting and Clinical Psychology*, **52**, 857–862.

Fielding, D. (1985). Factors associated with drop-out, relapse and failure in the conditioning treatment of nocturnal enuresis. *Behavioural Psychotherapy*, **13**, 174–185.

Fincham, F. D. and Spettell, C. (1984). The acceptability of dry-bed training as treatment of nocturnal enuresis. *Behavior Therapy*, **15**, 388–394.

Geffken, G., Johnson, S. B. and Walker, D. (1986). Behavioral interventions for childhood nocturnal enuresis: The differential effect of bladder capacity on treatment progress and outcome. *Health Psychology*, **5**, 261–272.

Haan, E. de and Hoogduin, K. (1981). Over enuresis nocturna bij adolescenten en volwassenen (About nocturnal enuresis with adults and young adults). *Directieve Therapie*, **4**, 349–359.

Harris, L. S. and Purohit, A. P. (1977). Bladder training and enuresis: A controlled trial. *Behaviour Research and Therapy*, **15**, 485–490.

Keating, J. C. Jr, Butz, R. A., Burke, E. and Heimberg, R. G. (1983). Dry-bed training without a urine alarm: Lack of effect of setting and therapist contact with child. *Journal of Behavior Therapy and Experimental Psychiatry*, **14**, 109–115.

Kimmel, H. D. and Kimmel, E. (1970). An instrumental conditioning method for the treatment of enuresis. *Journal of Behavior Therapy and Experimental Psychiatry*, **1**, 121–123.

Kolko, D. J. (1987). Simplified inpatient treatment of nocturnal enuresis in psychiatrically disturbed children. *Behavior Therapy*, **2**, 199–212.

Londen, A. van (1986). Enuresis: Definities, begrippen, oorzaken en gevolgen. In: van Londen, A. (Ed.) *Enuresis*. Lisse: Swets & Zeitlinger, pp. 3–8.

Londen, A. van (1989). *Wektraining*. Utrecht: dissertation.

Lovibond, S. H. (1964). *Conditioning and enuresis*. Oxford: Pergamon Press.

Mountjoy, P. T., Ruben, D. H. and Bradford, T. S. (1984). Recent technological advancements in the treatment of enuresis. *Behavior Modification*, **8**, 291–315.

Mowrer, O. H. and Mowrer, W. M. (1938). Enuresis: A method for its study and treatment. *The American Journal of Orthopsychiatry*, **8**, 436–459.

Muellner, S. R. (1960). Development of urinary control in children: A new concept in cause, prevention and treatment. *Journal of Urology*, **84**, 714–716.

Mulder, G. A. L. A., Hedeman Joosten, A. P. S., Londen, A. van and Son, M. J. M. van (1988). The effectiveness of dry-bed training as a therapy for nocturnal enuresis in adults. Paper presented at the World Behaviour Therapy Congress, Edinburgh.

Paschalis, A. P., Kimmel, H. O. and Kimmel, E. C. (1972). Further study of diurnal instrumental conditioning in the treatment of enuresis nocturna. *Journal of Behavior Therapy and Experimental Psychiatry*, **3**, 253–256.

Resnick, M. I. and King, L. R. (1976). Urinary incontinence. In: Kelalis, P. and King, L. (Eds) *Clinical Pediatric Urology (I)*. Philadelphia: W. B. Saunders.

Sacks, S. and DeLeon, G. (1983). Conditioning functional enuresis: Follow-up after retraining. *Behaviour Research and Therapy*, **21**, 693–694.

Son, M. J. M. van, Beunderman, R., Duyvis, D. and Rientsma, M. (1984). Enuresis nocturna bij volwassenen en gedragstherapie. *Tijdschrift voor Psychotherapie*, **10**, 404–408.

Sorotzkin, B. (1984). Nocturnal enuresis: Current perspectives. *Clinical Psychology Review*, **4**, 293–316.

Tanagho, E. A. (1979). The neurophysiology of micturition. In: Miranda, S. and Voogt, H. J. (Eds) *Current and Future trends in Urology*. Utrecht: Bunge.

Timmreck, Th. C. (1983). Behavioral therapy for night bedwetting in children with parents as therapists. *JPN-MHS*, **21**, 31–37.

Turner, R. K. and Taylor, P. D. (1974). Conditioning treatment of nocturnal enuresis in adults: Preliminary findings. *Behaviour Research and Therapy*, **12**, 41–52.

Index